Tuberculosis

Guest Editors

ALIMUDDIN ZUMLA, FRCP, PhD(Lond), FRCPath
H. SIMON SCHAAF, MMed Paed, DCM, MD Paed

CLINICS IN
CHEST MEDICINE

www.chestmed.theclinics.com

December 2009 • Volume 30 • Number 4

SAUNDERS an imprint of ELSEVIER, Inc.

W.B. SAUNDERS COMPANY
A Division of Elsevier Inc.

1600 John F. Kennedy Boulevard ● Suite 1800 ● Philadelphia, Pennsylvania 19103

http://www.theclinics.com

CLINICS IN CHEST MEDICINE Volume 30, Number 4
December 2009 ISSN 0272-5231, ISBN-13: 978-1-4377-1804-1

Editor: Sarah E. Barth
Developmental Editor: Theresa Collier

Clinics in Chest Medicine (ISSN 0272-5231) is published quarterly by Elsevier Inc., 360 Park Avenue South, New York, NY 10010-1710. Months of issue are March, June, September, and December. Periodicals postage paid at New York, NY and additional mailing offices. Subscription prices are $274.00 per year (domestic individuals), $432.00 per year (domestic institutions), $133.00 per year (domestic students/residents), $300.00 per year (Canadian individuals), $530.00 per year (Canadian institutions), $373.00 per year (international individuals), $530.00 per year (international institutions), and $186.00 per year (international and Canadian students/residents). International air speed delivery is included in all Clinics subscription prices. All prices are subject to change without notice. **POSTMASTER:** Send address changes to Clinics in Chest Medicine, Elsevier Health Sciences Division, Subscription Customer Service, 3251 Riverport Lane, Maryland Heights, MO 63043. **Customer Service: Telephone: 1-800-654-2452** (U.S. and Canada); **1-314-447-8871** (outside U.S. and Canada). **Fax: 1-314-447-8029. E-mail: journalscustomerservice-usa@elsevier.com** (for print support); **journalsonlinesupport-usa@elsevier.com** (for online support).

Reprints. For copies of 100 or more of articles in this publication, please contact the Commercial Reprints Department, Elsevier Inc., 360 Park Avenue South, New York, NY 10010-1710. Tel.: 212-633-3812; Fax: 212-462-1935; E-mail: reprints@elsevier.com.

Clinics in Chest Medicine is covered in *MEDLINE/PubMed (Index Medicus), Current Contents/Clinical Medicine, EMBASE/ Excerpta Medica, Science Citation Index,* and *ISI/BIOMED.*

Printed and bound in the United Kingdom

Transferred to Digital Print 2011

Contributors

GUEST EDITORS

ALIMUDDIN ZUMLA, FRCP, PhD(Lond), FRCPath
Professor, University College London
Medical School, London,
United Kingdom

H. SIMON SCHAAF, MMed Paed, DCM, MD Paed
Professor, Desmond Tutu TB Centre,
Department of Paediatrics and Child Health,
Faculty of Health Sciences, Stellenbosch
University, and Tygerberg Children's Hospital,
South Africa

AUTHORS

SAVVAS ANDRONIKOU, MBBCh, FCRad, FRCR, PhD
Diagnostic Imaging Working Group, Medecins
Sans Frontiers, Plantage middenlaan,
Amsterdam, The Netherlands; Department of
Radiology, University of Cape Town, Anzio
Road, Observatory, Cape Town, South Africa

HELEN AYLES, MD, PhD
Clinical Research Unit, Department of
Infectious and Tropical Disease, London
School of Hygiene and Tropical Medicine,
London, United Kingdom;
ZAMBART project, University of Zambia,
Lusaka, Zambia

GAVIN J. CHURCHYARD, MD
Aurum Institute for Health Research,
Houghton, Johannesburg;
Nelson R Mandela School of Medicine,
University of Kwa-Zulu Natal, Durban;
and University of Cape Town, Cape Town,
South Africa

MARK F. COTTON, MBChB, MMed(Paed), FCPaed(SA), DCH(SA), DTM&H, PhD
Children's Infectious Diseases Clinical
Research Unit, Department of Paediatrics
and Child Health, Faculty of Health Science,
University of Stellenbosch, Tygerberg
Academic Hospital, Tygerberg,
South Africa

ADELARD I. DE BACKER, MD, PhD
Department of Radiology,
Sint-Lucas Hospital, Groenebriel, Ghent,
Belgium

KEERTAN DHEDA, MBBCh, FCP (SA), FCCP, PhD (Lond)
Associate Professor and Consultant Physician
in Respiratory Medicine, Division of
Pulmonology and UCT Lung Institute,
Department of Medicine, Lung Infection and
Immunity Unit, University of Cape Town;
Associate Professor and Consultant Physician
in Respiratory Medicine, Institute of Infectious
Diseases and Molecular Medicine, University
of Cape Town, South Africa; and Senior
Lecturer and Honorary Consultant,
Department of Infection, Centre for Infectious
Diseases and International Health, UCL,
London, United Kingdom

T. MARK DOHERTY, PhD
Professor, Department of Infectious Disease
Immunology, Statens Serum Institute,
København, Denmark

DOROTHY FALLOWS, PhD
The Public Health Research Institute,
University of Medicine and Dentistry
of New Jersey, Newark, New Jersey

KATHERINE FLOYD, MA, MSc, PhD
HIV/AIDS, Tuberculosis & Malaria, World
Health Organization, Geneva, Switzerland

PHILIPPE GLAZIOU, MD, MSc
HIV/AIDS, Tuberculosis & Malaria,
World Health Organization, Geneva,
Switzerland

PETER GODFREY-FAUSSETT, MD, PhD
Clinical Research Unit, Department of
Infectious and Tropical Disease, London
School of Hygiene and Tropical Medicine,
London, United Kingdom; ZAMBART project,
University of Zambia, Lusaka, Zambia

STEPHEN M. GRAHAM, MD, PhD
Department of Paediatrics, Centre
for International Child Health,
Murdoch Children's Research
Institute, Royal Children's Hospital,
University of Melbourne, Victoria,
Australia; International Union Against
Tuberculosis and Lung Disease,
Paris, France

WILLEM A. HANEKOM, MBChB, DCH, FCP
Associate Professor and Co-Director
South African TB Vaccine Initiative,
University of Cape Town, Cape Town,
South Africa

TONY HAWKRIDGE, MBChB
Aeras Global TB Vaccine Foundation, Africa
Office, South Africa

GILLA KAPLAN, PhD
The Public Health Research Institute,
University of Medicine and Dentistry of
New Jersey, Newark, New Jersey

KATHARINA KRANZER, MD
The Desmond Tutu HIV Centre, Institute of
Infectious Disease and Molecular Medicine,
Faculty of Health Sciences, University
of Cape Town, Cape Town, South Africa;
and Department of Infectious and Tropical
Diseases, Clinical Research Unit, London
School of Hygiene and Tropical Medicine,
London, United Kingdom

PAUL-HENRI LAMBERT, MD
Centre of Vaccinology, University of Geneva;
Chairman SC TB Vaccine Initiative, Geneva,
Switzerland

CHRISTOPH LANGE, MD, PhD
Division of Clinical Infectious Diseases,
Medical Clinic, Research Centre Borstel,
Borstel, Germany

STEPHEN D. LAWN, MD
The Desmond Tutu HIV Centre, Institute
of Infectious Disease and Molecular
Medicine, Faculty of Health Sciences,
University of Cape Town, Cape Town,
South Africa; and Department of Infectious
and Tropical Diseases, Clinical
Research Unit, London School
of Hygiene and Tropical Medicine,
London, United Kingdom

CHRISTIAN LIENHARDT, MD, PhD
Stop TB Partnership and Stop
TB Department, World Health Organization,
Geneva, Switzerland

ZHENKUN MA, PhD
Global Alliance for TB Drug Development,
New York, New York

**BEN J. MARAIS, MMed Paed,
FCPaed(SA), PhD**
Department of Paediatrics and Child Health,
Faculty of Health Sciences, Stellenbosch
University, Tygerberg, South Africa

**GRAEME MEINTJES, MBChB, MRCP(UK),
FCP(SA), Dip HIV Man(SA)**
Institute of Infectious Diseases and
Molecular Medicine, Faculty of Health
Sciences, University of Cape Town,
Observatory; Division of Infectious
Diseases and HIV Medicine, Department
of Medicine, University of Cape Town,
Observatory; and Infectious Diseases Unit,
GF Jooste Hospital, Manenberg, South Africa

GIOVANNI BATTISTA MIGLIORI, MD
WHO Collaborating Centre for TB and Lung
Diseases, Fondazione S. Maugeri, Care and
Research Institute/TBNET Secretariat
(TuBerculosis Network European
Trialsgroup)/Stop TB Italy, Tradate, Italy

JESSICA MINION, MD
Medical Resident & Graduate Scholar,
Department of Epidemiology, Biostatistics
& Occupational Health, McGill University,
Montreal, Quebec, Canada

ANTHONY P. MOLL, MBChB, BSc
Chief Medical Officer, Church of Scotland,
Hospital, Tugela Ferry, South Africa

PHILIP ONYEBUJOH, MD
Tropical Disease Research, World Health
Organization, Geneva, Switzerland

MADHUKAR PAI, MD, PhD
Assistant Professor, Department of
Epidemiology, Biostatistics & Occupational
Health, McGill University, Montreal, Quebec,
Canada

MARK D. PERKINS, MD
Chief Scientific Officer, Foundation for
Innovative New Diagnostics, Geneva,
Switzerland

**HELENA RABIE, MBChB, FCPaed(SA),
MMed Paed**
Children's Infectious Diseases Clinical
Research Unit, Department of Paediatrics
and Child Health, University of Stellenbosch
and Tygerberg Children's Hospital,
Tygerberg Hospital, Parow, South Africa

MARIO RAVIGLIONE, MD, FRCP (UK)
HIV/AIDS, Tuberculosis & Malaria, World
Health Organization, Geneva, Switzerland

MORGAN D'ARCY RICHARDSON, RN, MS
HIV/TB Global Program, PATH, Seattle,
Washington

GRAHAM A. ROOK, MD
Centre for Infectious Diseases &
International Health, Windeyer Institute
of Medical Sciences, Royal Free and
University College Medical School,
London, United Kingdom

**H. SIMON SCHAAF, MMed Paed,
DCM, MD Paed**
Professor, Desmond Tutu TB Centre,
Department of Paediatrics and Child Health,
Faculty of Health Sciences, Stellenbosch
University, and Tygerberg Children's Hospital,
South Africa

**JOHAN F. SCHOEMAN, MMed Paed,
FCPaed(SA), MD**
Professor, Department of Paediatrics and Child
Health, Faculty of Health Sciences, University
of Stellenbosch, Tygerberg, South Africa

HOJOON SOHN, MPH
Doctoral Candidate, Department
of Epidemiology, Biostatistics &
Occupational Health, McGill University,
Montreal, Quebec, Canada; Foundation
for Innovative New Diagnostics,
Geneva, Switzerland

GIOVANNI SOTGIU, MD, PhD
Hygiene and Preventive Medicine Institute,
University of Sassari, Sassari, Italy

**GUY E. THWAITES, MA, MBBS, MRCP,
FRCPath, PhD**
Department of Microcrobiology, Imperial
College, South Kensington, London,
United Kingdom

FILIP M. VANHOENACKER, MD, PhD
Department of Radiology, Sint-Maarten
Hospital, Duffel-Mechelen, Belgium;
University Hospital Antwerp, UZA,
University of Antwerp, Wilrijkstraat,
Edegem, Belgium

ROBERT S. WALLIS, MD, FIDSA,
Senior Medical Director, Clinical Group Lead,
Anti-Infectives, Pfizer Global Research &
Development, New London, Connecticut

**ROBERT J. WILKINSON, MA, BM,
BCh, PhD, DTM&H, FRCP**
Institute of Infectious Diseases
and Molecular Medicine, Faculty
of Health Sciences, University
of Cape Town, Observatory;
Division of Infectious Diseases and HIV
Medicine, Department of Medicine,
University of Cape Town, Observatory;
Infectious Diseases Unit, GF Jooste
Hospital, Manenberg, South Africa; and
Division of Medicine, Imperial College
London, London; National
Institute for Medical Research,
Mill Hill, United Kingdom

ROBIN WOOD, FCP MMed
Professor, The Desmond Tutu HIV Centre,
Institute of Infectious Disease and Molecular
Medicine, Faculty of Health Sciences,
University of Cape Town, Cape Town,
South Africa

ALIMUDDIN ZUMLA, FRCP, PhD(Lond), FRCPath
Professor, University College
London Medical School, London,
United Kingdom

ALICE ZWERLING, MSc
Doctoral Candidate, Department of
Epidemiology, Biostatistics & Occupational
Health, McGill University, Montreal, Quebec,
Canada

Contents

Tuberculosis (TB) ranks second only to human immunodeficiency virus as a cause of death from an infectious agent (1.77 million deaths from TB in 2007). Global targets for reductions in the epidemiologic burden of TB have been set for 2015 and 2050 within the context of the Millennium Development Goals and the Stop TB Partnership. Achieving these targets is the focus of national and international efforts in TB control, and demonstrating whether or not they are achieved is of major importance. This article discusses: the methods used by the World Health Organization to estimate the global burden of TB; estimates of incidence, prevalence, and mortality for 2007, combined with assessment of progress toward the 2015 targets for reductions in these indicators based on trends since 1990 and projections up to 2015; trends in TB notifications and case detection rates; and prospects for elimination of TB by 2050.

The emergence of multidrug-resistant (MDR) and, more recently, of extensively drug resistant (XDR) strains of *Mycobacterium tuberculosis* is a real threat to achieve tuberculosis (TB) control and elimination globally. More than 510,000 new cases of MDR-TB occur each year and XDR-TB cases are recognized in every setting where there has been the capacity to detect them, particularly in Eastern Europe. MDR- and XDR-TB control in Europe and the United States are heavily affected by what happens globally, as the majority of cases occurring in these countries originate in high TB-burden areas of the world. Scaling-up of culture- and drug susceptibility testing capacities and the expanded use of high-technology assays for rapid determination of resistance represent the prerequisites to achieve better control of MDR- and XDR-TB. Most cases with MDR- and XDR-TB in Europe and the United States can be treated successfully if well-designed regimens based on available second- and third-line anti-TB drugs are used and surgical options are carefully considered. Nevertheless, the development of new (more effective and less toxic) drugs to treat patients infected by MDR- and XDR-TB strains with or without active disease are urgently needed. Adherence to internationally agreed standards of care and control practices is imperative to achieve TB control.

Available data show that Africa, together with the Americas and western and central Europe, reported the lowest prevalence of multidrug-resistant tuberculosis

(MDR-TB). However, sub-Saharan Africa has a high TB incidence and the highest human immunodeficiency virus (HIV) prevalence in the world, and because of the high number of TB cases, Africa still presents 14% of the global burden of new MDR-TB cases. Until recently, Africa and South America were deprived of second-line antituberculosis drugs, preventing the development of extensively drug-resistant TB (XDR-TB). Current efforts, introducing improved laboratory infrastructure and second-line TB treatment in resource-limited countries, need to be carried out with care to minimize the development of MDR/XDR-TB in these countries. Recent diagnostic developments now need evaluation and implementation in resource-limited areas, and delays in diagnosis also need to be addressed. Outcomes for MDR/XDR-TB have improved, but prevention of MDR/XDR-TB by early diagnosis and treatment, improvement of adherence, and proper infection control remains the mainstay for the future.

Great progress has been made over the past few years in HIV testing in patients who have tuberculosis (TB) and in the scale-up of antiretroviral therapy. More than 3 million people in resource-limited settings were estimated to have started antiretroviral therapy by the end of 2007 and 2 million of these were in sub-Saharan Africa. However, little is known about what impact this massive public health intervention will have on the HIV-associated TB epidemic or how antiretroviral therapy might be used to best effect TB control. This article provides an in-depth review of these issues.

Despite a decade of success in improving cure rates for tuberculosis (TB), diagnosis and case detection remain a major obstacle to TB control. This article reviews the existing evidence base on TB diagnostics, describes the progress of new technologies, and ends with a review of cost-effectiveness and modeling studies on the potential effect of new diagnostics in TB control.

This article reviews the ongoing role of imaging in the diagnosis of tuberculosis (TB) and its complications. A modern imaging classification of TB, taking into account both adults and children and the blurring of differences in the presentation patterns, must be absorbed into daily practice. Clinicians must not only be familiar with imaging features of TB but also become expert at detecting these when radiologists are unavailable. Communication between radiologists and clinicians with regard to local constraints, patterns of disease, human immunodeficiency virus (HIV) coinfection rates, and imaging parameters relevant for management (especially in drug resistance programs) is paramount for making an impact with imaging, and preserving clinician confidence. Recognition of special imaging, anatomic and vulnerability differences between children and adults is more important than trying to define patterns of disease exclusive to children.

Update on Tuberculosis of the Central Nervous System: Pathogenesis, Diagnosis, and Treatment 745

Guy E. Thwaites and Johan F. Schoeman

Tuberculous meningitis is the most dangerous form of tuberculosis, yet our understanding of disease pathogenesis is based upon studies performed in the 1920s, our diagnostic methods are dependent upon those developed in the 1880s, and our treatment has advanced little since the introduction of isoniazid in the 1950s. The authors focus this review on three important questions. First, how does *Mycobacterium tuberculosis* reach the brain? Second, what is the best way of identifying patients who require early empiric antituberculosis therapy? Third, what is the best way of managing tuberculous hydrocephalus?

Toward an Optimized Therapy for Tuberculosis? Drugs in Clinical Trials and in Preclinical Development 755

Zhenkun Ma and Christian Lienhardt

Tuberculosis (TB) continues to be one of the greatest challenges in the global public health arena. Current therapeutic agents against TB are old and inadequate, particularly in the face of many new challenges. Multidrug-resistant TB (MDR-TB) has become prevalent in many parts of the world and extensively drug-resistant TB (XDR-TB) is rapidly emerging. There are few or essentially no effective drugs available to treat these drug-resistant forms of TB. TB and human immunodeficiency virus (HIV) coinfection has become another major problem in areas with high prevalence of HIV infection. Simultaneous treatment of TB and HIV is difficult due to the severe drug-drug interactions between the first-line rifamycin-containing TB therapy and antiretroviral agents. However, there have been some encouraging developments in TB drug research and development within the past decade. At present there are 6 compounds, including 3 novel agents, in late stages of clinical development. There are even larger numbers of compounds and projects in the TB drug pipeline at the discovery stage and in early stages of clinical development, mainly targeting treatment shortening and drug resistance. Despite these encouraging developments, the current TB drug pipeline is not sufficient to address the multitude of challenges inherent in the current standard of TB therapy. A stronger TB drug pipeline and a new paradigm for the development of novel TB drug combinations are needed.

Advances in Immunotherapy for Tuberculosis Treatment 769

Gavin J. Churchyard, Gilla Kaplan, Dorothy Fallows, Robert S. Wallis, Philip Onyebujoh, and Graham Rook

Immunotherapies have the potential to improve the outcome in all patients with tuberculosis (TB) including those with multidrug-resistant (MDR)-TB and extensively drug-resistant (XDR)-TB. Immunotherapy for TB may shorten duration of treatment and reduce pathology in individuals cured by chemotherapy, potentially preventing recurrence. Currently none of the available candidate agents have proof of efficacy for use in MDR-TB or XDR-TB. Further development and evaluation of existing immunotherapeutic agents is required to identify an effective agent that can be used adjunctively with chemotherapy to improve treatment outcomes for drug-susceptible TB, MDR-TB, and XDR-TB. With a range of potential immunotherapeutics, some of which have been produced to good manufacturing practice (GMP) standards and are registered for other indications in humans, the immunotherapy option should no longer be ignored.

Clinics in Chest Medicine

RELATED INTEREST

Primary Care: Clinics in Office Practice June 2009 (Vol. 36, No. 2)
Obesity Management
Ann Rodden and Vanessa Diaz, *Guest Editors*

Endocrinology and Metabolism Clinics of North America September and
December 2008 (Vol. 37, Nos. 3 and 4)
Obesity: Brain—Gut and Inflammation Connection: Parts I and II
Eddy Karnieli, MD, *Guest Editor*

THE CLINICS ARE NOW AVAILABLE ONLINE!

Access your subscription at:
www.theclinics.com

Preface

Clinics in Chest Medicine

THE CLINICS ARE NOW AVAILABLE ONLINE!

Access your subscription at:
www.theclinics.com

Preface

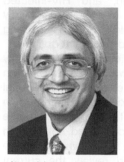
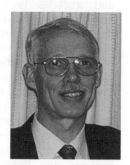

Alimuddin Zumla, FRCP, PhD(Lond), FRCPath   H. Simon Schaaf, MMed Paed, DCM, MD Paed
Guest Editors

To support World TB Day, Elsevier has kindly commissioned this special December 2009 issue of the *Clinics in Chest Medicine* series, which focuses on tuberculosis (TB). World TB Day is commemorated globally every year on March 24 and is meant to build public awareness that TB today remains, alongside HIV/AIDS, one of the top two leading causes of death from any infectious diseases worldwide. It was on March 24, 1882, that Professor Robert Koch, a German scientist, astounded the scientific community by announcing that he had discovered a microbial cause for TB; the bacillus *Mycobacterium tuberculosis*. At the time of Koch's announcement in Berlin, TB was rampaging through all of Europe and the Americas, causing the death of one out of every seven people. Koch's amazing discovery opened the way toward diagnosing and curing TB. In 1982, on the 100th anniversary of Koch's discovery of *M tuberculosis*, the International Union Against Tuberculosis and Lung Disease (IUATLD) proposed that March 24 be proclaimed as official World TB Day. In 1996, the World Health Organization (WHO) joined with the IUATLD and other concerned organizations to increase the impact of World TB Day for generating worldwide advocacy in efforts to effectively reduce the number of TB cases and work towards eradication of TB.

WHO declared TB a "global emergency" over a decade ago. Yet, despite the availability of effective treatment for TB, it continues to kill more than 1.7 million people every year. This is equal to nearly 4700 deaths a day, which is 1 person every 20 seconds! TB appears to be a disease of poverty and of the disadvantaged, affecting mostly young adults in their most productive years. TB is also a leading killer of people infected with HIV. HIV-infected people co-infected with TB are up to 50 times more likely to develop active TB in their lifetime than people who are HIV-negative. The vast majority of TB deaths are in the developing world, particularly in Asia and Africa. One third of the world's population is currently infected with the *M tuberculosis* bacillus. One in 10 people infected with TB bacilli will become sick with active TB in their lifetime. TB is a contagious disease that normally spreads through the airborne route. If not treated appropriately, each person with active TB infects on average 10 to 15 people every year. Globally, nearly 4 out of 10 TB cases are still not being properly detected and treated. The emergence of multidrug-resistant TB (MDR-TB) and extensively drug-resistant TB (XDR-TB) in recent years is an ominous sign and threatens global TB control.

This unique issue of *Clinics in Chest Medicine* on TB consists of 13 comprehensive articles on selected TB topics. These were written by internationally renowned TB experts from all over the globe and cover a broad range of important subject areas. The first article, written by Philipe Glaziou, Katherine Floyd, and Mario Raviglione, gives an update of the huge global burden and epidemiology of TB (incidence and prevalence) in various regions of the world. They remind us that TB ranks second only to HIV as a cause of death from an infectious agent. Global targets for reductions in the epidemiologic burden of TB have been set for 2015 and 2050 within the context of the Millennium Development Goals and by the Stop TB Partnership. National and international efforts in TB control focus on achieving these targets.

Clin Chest Med 30 (2009) xiii–xviii
doi:10.1016/j.ccm.2009.08.020

chestmed.theclinics.com

The authors discuss the methods WHO uses to estimate the global burden of TB. The article also presents estimates of incidence, prevalence, and mortality for 2007, and uses trends since 1990 to assess progress and formulate projections towards the 2015 targets for reductions in key indicators. Furthermore, the article notes trends in TB notifications and case-detection rates, and assesses prospects for elimination of TB by 2050.

In the next article, Giovanni B. Migliori, Morgan D. Richardson, Giovanni Sotgiu, and Christoph Lange review the emergence of MDR-TB and, more recently, of XDR-TB strains of *M tuberculosis*. In emphasizing that these are real threats to achieving TB control and elimination globally, the authors note that over 510,000 new cases of MDR-TB occur each year, and XDR-TB cases are recognized in every setting where there has been the capacity to detect them, particularly in Eastern Europe. Global trends significantly affect MDR- and XDR-TB control in Europe and the United States because the majority of cases occurring in these regions originate in high TB-burden areas of the world. The scaling up of culture- and drug-susceptibility testing capacities and the expanded use of high-technology assays for rapid determination of resistance represent the prerequisites to achieve better control of MDR- and XDR-TB. The majority of cases with MDR- and XDR-TB in Europe and the United States can be treated successfully if well-designed regimens based on available second- and third-line anti-TB drugs are used and surgical options are carefully considered. The authors conclude that the development of new, more effective, and less toxic drugs to treat patients infected by MDR- and XDR-TB strains with or without active disease are urgently needed.

Simon Schaaf, Anthony P. Moll, and Keertan Dheda illustrate in their article that sub-Saharan Africa bears the burden of both very high TB incidence and the highest HIV prevalence in the world. Because of the high number of TB cases, Africa presents 14% of the global burden of new MDR-TB cases. Until recently, Africa and South America as continents were relatively deprived of second-line anti-TB drugs, which prevented the development of XDR-TB. Current efforts to introduce improved laboratory infrastructure and second-line TB treatment in resource-limited countries need to be done with great care to minimize the development of MDR- and XDR-TB in these countries. Recent diagnostic developments have improved our ability to rapidly diagnose MDR- and XDR-TB. These developments now need evaluation and implementation in resource-limited areas. Patient and health care worker delays in diagnosis also need to be addressed to start early

and effective treatment. Transmission of MDR- and XDR-TB is common, and HIV-infected patients and children are at special risk. New drugs in development and old drugs revisited bring new hope for current limited-treatment options.

The HIV-associated TB epidemic is currently undermining progress towards the Millennium Development Goals for TB control, and additional interventions must be used in combination with the Directly Observed Therapy, Short-course (DOTS) strategy in resource limited settings. In the next article, Stephen D. Lawn, Katharina Kranzer, and Robin Wood review the current thinking on the HIV-TB problem. They state that

> ...the HIV-associated TB epidemic is one of the greatest stumbling blocks to progress towards the Millennium Development Goals for TB control. Conversely, scale-up of antiretroviral therapy (ART) is one of the largest public health interventions of our time.

Observational cohort studies in a wide range of settings have demonstrated that the use of ART is associated with a 54% to 92% reduction in TB incidence rates and a halving of the risk of TB recurrence. ART is also a potent means of reducing mortality rates among those with HIV-associated TB, causing reductions of 64% to 95%. Thus, ART confers huge benefits to the individual patient, yet limited data are available concerning the effects of ART on TB rates at a population level. Mathematical modeling and a range of empiric observations suggest that the effect of ART may be limited, largely because of the high burden of TB that occurs prior to ART initiation and the persistence of TB rates several-fold higher than background rates during long-term ART. Thus, they conclude that ART is likely to have limited impact on lifetime cumulative risk of TB.

Despite a decade of success in improving TB cure rates, techniques for rapid and accurate diagnosis and case detection are lacking, posing as a major obstacle to TB control. TB diagnosis, even today, continues to rely heavily on such tools as direct smear microscopy, solid media culture, chest radiography, and tuberculin skin testing—tools that often perform poorly and require infrastructure frequently unavailable in the periphery of the health system where patients first seek care. The limitations of the existing diagnostics toolbox have been exposed by the HIV epidemic and by the emergence of MDR- and XDR-TB. Diagnostic delays and failures of health systems often result in missed or late diagnoses with serious consequences for TB patients. Madhukar Pai, Jessica Minion, Hojoon Sohn, Alice Zwerling, and

Mark D. Perkins present a formidable review of the existing evidence base on TB diagnostics, describe the progress in development of new technologies, and conclude with a review of cost-effectiveness and modeling studies on potential impact of new diagnostics in TB control.

Savvas Andronikou, Filip M. Vanhoenacker, and Adelard I. De Backer demonstrate vividly the ongoing role of imaging in the diagnosis of TB and its complications. They describe a modern imaging classification of TB that takes into account both adults and children and the blurring of differences in the presentation patterns. They emphasize that clinicians must not only be familiar with imaging features of TB, but also must become expert at detecting these when radiologists are unavailable. To preserve clinician confidence and gain the full benefits of imaging, communication between radiologists and clinicians with regard to local constraints, patterns of disease, HIV co-infection rates, and imaging parameters relevant for management (especially in drug-resistance programs) is paramount. The authors conclude that the ability to recognize special imaging, anatomic, and vulnerability differences between children and adults is more important than trying to define patterns of disease exclusive to children.

Central nervous system (CNS) TB accounts for approximately 1% of all of disease caused by *M tuberculosis*, but kills and disables more sufferers than any other form of TB. TB meningitis is the most common form of CNS TB and is characterized by a slowly progressive granulomatous inflammation of the basal meninges that, if left untreated, results in hydrocephalus, brain infarction, and death. Guy E. Thwaites and Johan F. Schoeman reiterate, in their article, that TB meningitis is the most dangerous form of TB, yet our understanding of disease pathogenesis is based upon studies performed in the 1920s, our diagnostic methods depend on those developed in the 1880s, and our treatment has advanced little since the introduction of isoniazid in the 1950s. The authors pose three important questions: (1) How does *M tuberculosis* reach the brain? (2) What is the best way of identifying patients who require early empirical anti-TB therapy? and (3) What is the best way of managing TB hydrocephalus? These questions represent challenges for future research on TB of the CNS.

Zhenkun Ma and Christian Lienhardt remind us that current drugs against TB are old and inadequate, particularly in the face of many new challenges. They lament the failure to develop anti-TB drugs over the past 4 decades. MDR-TB has become prevalent in many parts of the world, and XDR-TB is emerging rapidly.

There are few safe and effective drugs available to treat these drug-resistant forms of TB. TB-HIV co-infection has become another major problem in areas with a high HIV infection prevalence. Simultaneous treatment of TB and HIV is difficult because of the drug-drug interactions between the first-line rifamycin-containing TB therapy and ART. In summarizing some encouraging developments in the field of TB drug research and development during the past decade, the authors list six compounds—two fluoroquinolones, a diarylquinoline, two nitroimidazoles, and a rifamycin—in late stages of clinical development. The fluoroquinolones (gatifloxacin and moxifloxacin) and the rifamycin (rifapentine) belong to known classes of antibiotics and are currently being studied for their potential to shorten the duration of therapy against drug-susceptible TB. The diarylquinoline TMC-207 and the nitroimidazoles PA-824 and OPC-67683 are new molecular entities that have a novel mechanism of action. These three novel agents are currently being studied for their potential in the treatment of both drug-susceptible and drug-resistant disease. The authors mention several other potentially promising new drugs in the TB drug pipeline, which are in the early phases of development. Despite these encouraging advances, they suggest that too few TB drugs are in the development pipeline to produce enough new drugs to accommodate the rational selection of novel TB drug combinations.

Drug-resistant TB is difficult and expensive to treat in HIV-infected patients, and the compromised immune system adds to poor treatment outcomes. Gavin Churchyard, Gilla Kaplan, Dorothy Fallows, Robert Wallis, Philip Onyebujoh, and Graham Rook, in their article, review current immunotherapies developed for improving treatment outcomes of TB. They point out that immunotherapies have the potential to improve the outcome in all TB patients, including those with MDR-TB and XDR-TB. Currently, none of the available candidate immunotherapeutic agents has proven effective against MDR-TB and XDR-TB. Further development and evaluation of these agents are required to find an effective agent that can be used adjunctively with chemotherapy to shorten the duration of treatment for drug-susceptible TB and improve the treatment outcomes for MDR-TB and XDR-TB. The authors list a range of currently available potential immunotherapeutics, some of which have been produced to Good Manufacturing Practice standards. The immunotherapy option can no longer be ignored, they implore. Further development and evaluation of existing immunotherapy agents are required to find an effective agent that can be used adjunctively with chemotherapy. The authors argue that it is ethically unacceptable to neglect the immunotherapy option for TB.

The changing face of TB, with epidemics fuelled by HIV and urbanization in much of the world, and a relative increase in the importance of latent TB as a source of cases in richer countries, has led to a demand for more robust, clinically applicable tools to measure disease activity, cure, and relapse. As a result, research aiming to identify biomarkers of *M tuberculosis* infection and disease has flourished. Mark Doherty, Robert S. Wallis, and Alimuddin Zumla (who chaired the recent WHO Special Programme for Research and Training in Tropical Diseases and European Commission joint expert meeting on biomarkers for TB) discuss the current views on biomarker development for TB. Biomarkers are needed not only to improve the process of making diagnoses, but also for assessing disease status and risk of progression to disease or of relapse. Such assessments are needed to open critical bottlenecks in the development of new vaccines and drugs. While the technologies listed above present a wide array of potential targets, only two of them—the venerable TB skin test and the interferon-gamma release assays—can be considered clinically useful, and they operate at the simplest level, merely detecting infection. One of the major hindrances so far in progress against TB has been the difference between clinical definitions and end points used by research groups.

The TB-associated immune reconstitution inflammatory syndrome (TB-IRIS) is a frequent early complication of ART used to treat HIV-1 infection, especially in countries where TB is prevalent. Graeme Meintjes, Helena Rabie, Robert J. Wilkinson, and Mark F. Cotton present their sentinel observations of TB-IRIS in clinical practice in South Africa. TB-IRIS is characterized by an exaggerated inflammatory response towards the antigens of *M tuberculosis* that results in clinical deterioration in patients experiencing immune recovery during early ART. Two forms of TB-IRIS are recognized: paradoxical and unmasking. Paradoxical TB-IRIS manifests with new or recurrent TB symptoms or signs in patients being treated for TB during early ART, and unmasking TB-IRIS is characterized by an exaggerated, unusually inflammatory initial presentation of TB during early ART. The authors review and highlight the incidence, clinical features, risk factors, treatment, and prevention of TB-IRIS in both adult and pediatric patients.

Effective vaccines against infectious diseases have led to the control of several viral and bacterial infections. Decades after the discovery of *M tuberculosis*, the development of a test for TB infection, and initial production of drugs to treat the disease, TB remains a major cause of morbidity and mortality in many developing countries. An effective vaccine against *M tuberculosis* has eluded the scientific community. Paul-Henri Lambert, Tony Hawkridge, and Willem A. Hanekom review the current efforts at developing a TB vaccine. They feel that unless a safer and more effective vaccine and regimen are found, TB rates are unlikely to decline in high-burden countries. Significant challenges in the TB vaccine field include the lack of good animal models of disease, the absence of immune correlates of protection, the chronic nature of the disease itself, and the difficulties in making an accurate and reliable diagnosis of TB disease in vaccine target groups. Despite these challenges, the authors note that significant progress has been made in recent years. A number of TB candidate vaccines have shown promise in preclinical studies and are now entering Phase I through IIB clinical trials. The authors speculate that there is a reasonable prospect for a safer, more effective vaccination schedule to become standard of care within a decade.

Finally, the article by Ben J. Marais, Helen Ayles, Stephen M. Graham, and Peter Godfrey-Faussett gives a critical assessment of the approach to TB preventive therapy in children and adults, and discusses the underlying treatment rationale and issues of concern. TB control remains poor in many developing countries, especially those worst affected by poverty and the HIV epidemic. The authors recommend that preventive therapy for all high-risk individuals following documented TB exposure should be regarded as standard of care. However, they caution that there is limited evidence of effectiveness because implementation and adherence are often poor. The tasks of excluding active disease in HIV-infected individuals and of handling the additional burden on health care services are particular challenges in resource-limited settings. There is a need to implement and evaluate preventive therapy strategies in a variety of settings to better inform policy and practice. A failure has been the exclusion of national policy makers in discussion of preventive therapy studies right from the start of development of the interventions. There is a need to implement and evaluate preventive therapy strategies in a variety of settings to better inform policy and practice.

This issue will be enormously valuable to all those respiratory and chest physicians, infectious diseases specialists, general physicians, scientists, and epidemiologists who want to get updated with current thinking on TB.

ACKNOWLEDGEMENTS

We would like to thank the publisher, Elsevier, and its editorial staff member Sarah Barth for rapidly agreeing to do an issue of *Clinics in Chest Medicine* for World TB Day. This brave and laudable decision by a medical journal publisher, which greatly enhances the combined global effort against TB, has led to the production of one of the most comprehensive and up-to-date treatises on several important areas of TB. All contributing authors have produced excellent, high-quality, up-to-date articles that reflect the time and effort they put into developing this exceptional issue for World TB Day. Our sincere thanks go to all of them for their invaluable contribution. Master Adam Zumla kindly provided word processing assistance to Professor Zumla in the development of the issue. In achieving this complicated task, we were supported unflinchingly at all stages by Ms. Sarah Barth, Elsevier editor, to whom we are very grateful. We also thank our families—particularly our wives, Mrs. Farzana Zumla and Mrs. Françoise Schaaf—for their forbearance and patience during the development of this issue.

Alimuddin Zumla, FRCP, PhD(Lond), FRCPath
Department of Infection
University College London Medical School
Windeyer Institute of Medical Sciences
46 Cleveland Street
London W1T 4JF, UK

H. Simon Schaaf, MMed Paed, DCM, MD Paed
Department of Pediatrics and Child Health
Desmond Tutu Tuberculosis Centre
Stellenbosch University
Tygerberg Children's Hospital
PO Box 19063
Tygerberg 7505, South Africa

E-mail addresses:
a.zumla@ucl.ac.uk (A. Zumla)
hss@sun.ac.za (H.S. Schaaf)

DEDICATION

To all those dedicated scientists, doctors, health personnel, and policy makers who have committed their lives to the control of TB worldwide, and to all patients who suffer from TB and those who have succumbed to TB.

Global Burden and Epidemiology of Tuberculosis

Philippe Glaziou, MD, MSc*, Katherine Floyd, MA, MSc, PhD,
Mario Raviglione, MD, FRCP (UK)

KEYWORDS

- Tuberculosis • Epidemiology • Burden
- Incidence • Prevalence • Mortality

Drugs that can cure most cases of tuberculosis (TB) have been available since the late 1940s. However, with 1.77 million deaths from TB in 2007, the disease ranks second only to the human immunodeficiency virus (HIV) as a cause of death from an infectious agent.[1] The number of new cases that occur each year also continues to grow, reaching 9.3 million in 2007.[2] Following neglect of the disease during the 1980s,[3,4] TB control has been high on the international public health agenda since the early 1990s. The dramatic effect of the HIV epidemic on the number of TB cases and deaths in Africa, show that short-course chemotherapy is one of the most cost-effective health care interventions,[5,6] and most recently global concern about the emergence of multi- and extensively drug-resistant TB (MDR and XDR-TB),[7] have further emphasized the urgent need to address tuberculosis effectively on a global scale.

Global targets for reductions in the epidemiologic burden of TB have been set for 2015 and 2050 within the context of the Millennium Development Goals (MDGs) and by the Stop TB Partnership (**Box 1**). The principal targets (so-called impact targets) are that the incidence rate should be falling by 2015 (MDG 6 Target 6.c), that prevalence and death rates should be halved by 2015 compared with their level in 1990, and that TB should be eliminated as a public health problem by 2050. Reaching these impact targets is the focus of national and international efforts in TB control, and the World Health Organization (WHO) has established a Global Task Force on TB Impact Measurement[8] to ensure the best possible evaluation of whether or not they are achieved. Besides the impact targets, 2 further global targets focusing on program performance are: to detect at least 70% of incident cases; and to successfully treat 85% of those cases that are detected. The WHO's recommended approach for achieving these targets is the Stop TB Strategy (**Box 2**). The strategy comprises best practices in the diagnosis and treatment of patients with active TB, approaches to address major epidemiologic and system challenges of today, and the promotion of research for innovations. It was launched in 2006 and underpins the Global Plan 2006–2015, a comprehensive and budgeted plan to reach the global targets.[9–11]

Each year, the WHO publishes estimates of TB incidence, prevalence, and mortality at global, regional, and country levels, along with an analysis of progress toward achievement of global targets.[2] Drawing on that work, this paper covers 4 major topics: the methods used by the WHO to estimate the global burden of TB; the estimates of incidence, prevalence, and mortality for 2007, combined with assessment of progress toward the 2015 targets for reductions in these indicators based on trends since 1990 and projections up to 2015; trends in TB notifications and case detection rates; and prospects for elimination of TB by 2050. Specific attention is given to estimates of the global burden of MDR-TB and TB/HIV, and to differences in notification rates between men and women.

Stop TB Department, World Health Organization, 1211 Geneva 27, Switzerland
* Corresponding author.
E-mail address: glazioup@who.int (P. Glaziou).

Clin Chest Med 30 (2009) 621–636
doi:10.1016/j.ccm.2009.08.017

chestmed.theclinics.com

Box 1
Goals, target and indicators for TB control

Health in the MDGs

Goal 6: Combat HIV/AIDS, malaria, and other diseases

 Target 6c: halt and begin to reverse the incidence of malaria and other major diseases

 Indicator 6.9: incidence, prevalence, and death rates associated with TB

 Indicator 6.10: proportion of TB cases detected and cured under DOTS

Stop TB Partnership targets

 By 2005: at least 70% of people with sputum smear-positive TB will be diagnosed (ie, under the DOTS strategy), and at least 85% successfully treated. The targets of a case detection rate of at least 70% and a treatment success rate of at least 85% were first set by the World Health Assembly of WHO in 1991.

 By 2015: the global burden of TB (per capita prevalence and death rates) will be reduced by 50% relative to 1990 levels.

 By 2050: the global incidence of active TB will be less than 1 case per million population per year.

METHODS USED TO ESTIMATE TUBERCULOSIS INCIDENCE, PREVALENCE AND MORTALITY
Incidence

The number of new TB cases per capita each year (incidence) is the central measure of progress toward the ultimate goal of eliminating TB as a public health problem (see **Box 1**).[13] It is not feasible to measure incidence by counting cases arising in cohorts under continuous observation because such studies would require cohorts of hundreds of thousands of people. Surveys of infection using tuberculin skin testing have been used in the past to derive estimates of incidence of TB disease, but the interpretation of such surveys is often difficult[8] and their performance unpredictable. The best alternative is to estimate incidence from routine surveillance systems in which case reports are more or less complete, such that notifications are a close proxy of incidence. This is possible in countries such as the Netherlands, the United Kingdom and the United States, where there is a long tradition of reporting TB morbidity and mortality[2,8] and where operational research has been used to quantify the

(small) fraction of cases that are treated but not notified to surveillance systems.

However, surveillance systems in most countries are not yet comprehensive enough to provide a direct measure of TB incidence. Many cases are either treated but not notified (eg, when cases are treated in the private sector) or go undiagnosed (eg, when people with TB do not access health care). In these countries, estimating incidence (its absolute value and trend) requires an evaluation of the quality and coverage of available TB notification data. The WHO framework for such evaluation, which has 3 major components, is shown in **Fig. 1**. The first component covers evaluation of data quality: analysis of the completeness of reporting, whether there are duplicate or misclassified records,[14] and the internal and external consistency of national and subnational data (internal consistency means data are consistent over time and space, or that variation can be explained; external consistency means that data are consistent with existing evidence about the epidemiology of TB).[15] The second component involves analysis of the extent to which trends in notifications reflect trends in incidence rates and/or the extent to which they reflect changes in other factors (such as programmatic efforts to find and treat more cases). A recent example from Kenya illustrates how the effect of the HIV epidemic and case-finding efforts on trends in TB notifications can be separated, and used to improve estimates of trends in TB incidence rates.[16] The third component of the framework recognizes that, even when available, notification data are complete (reports are available from all reporting units) and of high quality, and when they seem to be a good proxy of trends in TB incidence, they are not sufficient to estimate TB incidence in absolute terms. To do this, an analysis of the fraction of TB cases that are being captured in official notification systems is required.[17] The major reasons why cases are missed from official notification data include laboratory errors,[18] lack of notification of cases by public[17] and private providers,[19] failure of cases accessing health services to be identified as TB suspects,[20] and lack of access to health services.[21] Operational research (such as capture-recapture studies) and supporting evidence (such as whether prescriptions for TB drugs are available in the private sector, and the knowledge, attitudes, and practices of staff managing TB suspects in primary health care facilities) can be used to assess the fraction of cases that are missing from official notification data.[22–26] Incidence can then be estimated as notifications divided by the fraction of cases being recorded in official notification systems. The WHO is working

Box 2
StopTB Strategy

The Stop TB Strategy[10,12]

Vision, goal, objectives, and targets

Vision

A WORLD FREE OF TB

Goal

To dramatically reduce the global burden of TB by 2015 in line with the MDGs and the Stop TB Partnership targets

Objectives

- Achieve universal access to high-quality diagnosis and patient-centered treatment
- Reduce the human suffering and socioeconomic burden associated with TB
- Protect poor and vulnerable populations from TB, TB/HIV, and multidrug-resistant TB (MDR-TB)
- Support development of new tools and enable their timely and effective use

Targets

- MDG 6, Target 8: ... halted by 2015 and begun to reverse the incidence ...
- Targets linked to the MDGs and endorsed by the Stop TB Partnership:
  - By 2005: detect at least 70% of new sputum smear-positive TB cases and cure at least 85% of these cases
  - By 2015: reduce prevalence of and death due to TB by 50% relative to 1990
  - By 2050: eliminate TB as a public health problem (<1 case per million population)

Components of the Stop TB Strategy

1. Pursue high-quality DOTS expansion and enhancement

   - Secure political commitment, with adequate and sustained financing
   - Ensure early case detection and diagnosis through quality-assured bacteriology
   - Provide standardized treatment with supervision and patient support
   - Ensure effective drug supply and management
   - Monitor and evaluate performance and impact

2. Address TB-HIV, MDR-TB, and the needs of poor and vulnerable populations

   - Scale-up collaborative TB/HIV activities
   - Scale-up prevention and management of MDR-TB
   - Address the needs of TB contacts, and of poor and vulnerable populations

3. Contribute to health system strengthening based on primary health care

   - Help improve health policies, human resource development, financing, supplies, service delivery, and information
   - Strengthen infection control in health services, other congregate settings, and households
   - Upgrade laboratory networks and implement the Practical Approach to Lung Health (PAL)
   - Adapt successful approaches from other fields and sectors, and foster action on the social determinants of health

4. Engage all care providers

   - Involve all public, voluntary, corporate, and private providers through Public-Private Mix (PPM) approaches
   - Promote use of the International Standards for Tuberculosis Care (ISTC)

5. Empower people with TB and communities through partnership

   - Pursue advocacy, communication, and social mobilization
   - Foster community participation in TB care
   - Promote use of the Patients' Charter for Tuberculosis Care

6. Enable and promote research

   - Conduct program-based operational research and introduce new tools into practice
   - Advocate for and participate in research to develop new diagnostics, drugs, and vaccines

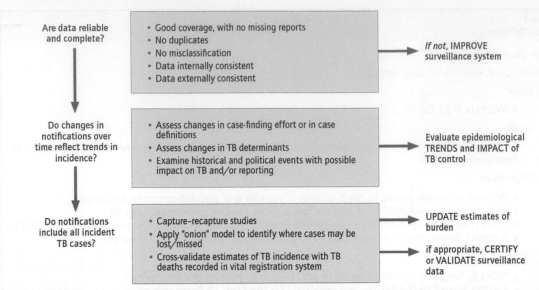

Fig. 1. Framework for estimation and measurement of TB incidence using surveillance data. (*Adapted from* WHO. Global tuberculosis control 2009: surveillance, planning, financing. Geneva: World Health Organization; 2009; with permission.)

closely with countries to use this framework to review and update estimates of TB incidence on a regular basis.

Prevalence

There are 2 methods for estimating the prevalence of TB disease. The first is direct measurement using a cross-sectional population-based survey.[27,28] In recent years, several countries have successfully measured the prevalence of TB disease through such surveys,[29–32] despite logistic challenges and high operational costs. With an estimated prevalence of 100 cases per 100,000 population, a sample size of around 200,000 and a budget of US$ 1–2 million are usually required.[27] Because prevalence typically falls more quickly than TB incidence in response to control efforts, a series of surveys conducted at wide intervals (eg, 10 years) can be useful for capturing large changes in the epidemiologic burden of TB in high-burden countries.[8] In countries where the burden of TB is lower, prevalence is best estimated indirectly as TB incidence multiplied by the average duration of disease. In the most recent series of WHO estimates, prevalence was estimated directly from survey data for 12 countries, and indirectly for 200 countries. To improve measurement of TB prevalence, the WHO Task Force on TB Impact Measurement has recommended that at least 1 nationwide survey should be undertaken in 21 global focus

countries (of which 12 are in Africa) between 2008 and 2015.

Mortality

The best way to measure the number of deaths from TB is via a national vital registration system in which deaths are coded according to the International Statistical Classification of Diseases (ICD-10), and data are of proven completeness and accuracy.[33] Few countries with a high burden of TB have vital registration systems, and where systems do exist there are often concerns about their completeness and accuracy. A recent review found that only 10% of the estimated 1.5 million TB-attributable deaths (in people negative for HIV) that occurred in 2005 were recorded in vital registration systems and reported to the WHO by August 2008.[33] The figures for the South-East Asia and Western Pacific regions, which account for 55% of the world's TB cases, were less than 0.1% and 2.6%, respectively. Sample vital registration combined with verbal autopsy may provide an alternative (albeit interim) solution when nationwide vital registration is not available, but this is not yet widely used. If neither national nor sample vital registration systems exist, mortality can be estimated as incidence multiplied by the case fatality rate[8]; the quality of such estimates depends on the accuracy of estimates of TB incidence and the case fatality rate. Case fatality rates in notified cases are measured directly in routine analysis of treatment outcomes.

THE GLOBAL EPIDEMIOLOGIC BURDEN OF TB: ESTIMATES FOR 2007, TRENDS SINCE 1990 AND PROJECTIONS UP TO 2015
Incidence

The WHO estimates that 9.27 million new cases of TB occurred in 2007 (139/100,000 population), compared with 9.24 million new cases (140/100,000 population) in 2006.[2] Of these 9.27 million new cases, an estimated 44% or 4.1 million (61/100,000 population) were new smear-positive cases. India, China, Indonesia, Nigeria, and South Africa rank first to fifth in the total number of incident cases (**Fig. 2**). Among the 15 countries with the highest estimated TB incidence rates, 13 are in Africa, a phenomenon linked to the effect of high rates of HIV coinfection[34] on the natural history of tuberculosis.

From series of notification data and surveys, the global incidence of TB per capita seems to have peaked in 2004 and is now in decline (**Fig. 3**). This peak and subsequent decline follow a similar pattern to the trend in HIV prevalence in the general population in Africa (**Fig. 4**).[35] Trends in incidence rates vary among regions (**Fig. 5**). Rates are falling in 7 of 9 epidemiologic subregions,[2] stable in Eastern Europe, and increasing only in African countries with a low prevalence of HIV. The resurgence of TB in Eastern European countries (mainly the former Soviet republics) can be explained by the major political, economic, and social disruption associated with the breakup of the Soviet Union at the beginning of the 1990s,

and related failures in TB control and provision of health care.[36]

Among the 9.27 million incident cases of TB in 2007, an estimated 1.37 million (14.8%) were HIV-positive.[2] In 2007, the African Region accounted for most (79%) HIV-positive TB cases, followed by the South-East Asia Region (mainly India) with 11% of total cases (**Fig. 6**). South Africa accounted for 31% of cases in the African Region. The global number of incident HIV-positive TB cases is estimated to have peaked in 2005 at 1.39 million. Direct measurements from provider-initiated HIV testing and counseling[37,38] in 2007 suggest that the relative risk of developing TB in HIV-positive people compared with HIV-negative people (the incidence rate ratio [IRR]) is 20.6 (95% confidence interval [CI] 15.4–27.5) in countries where the prevalence of HIV is more than 1% in the general population, 26.7 (95% CI 20.4–34.9) in countries where the prevalence of HIV in the general population is between 0.1% and 1%, and 36.7 (95% CI 11.6–116) in countries where the prevalence of HIV in the general population is less than 0.1%.[2]

Most of the current information about the proportion of TB cases with MDR-TB comes from drug susceptibility testing (DST) of samples from patients in whom MDR-TB is diagnosed in public health facilities under conditions defined by the WHO/IUATLD Global Project on Drug Resistance Surveillance (DRS).[39] These conditions include documented satisfactory performance of laboratories based on external quality assurance (EQA) and an adequate record of every patient's treatment history. Such data are available for new and retreatment cases for 113 and 102

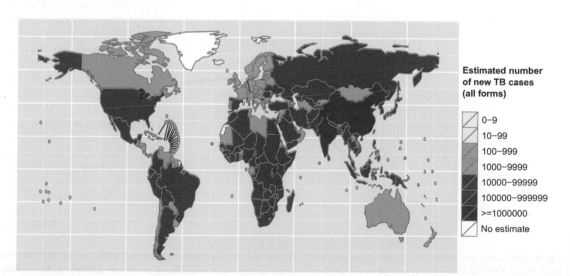

Estimated number of new TB cases (all forms)

- 0–9
- 10–99
- 100–999
- 1000–9999
- 10000–99999
- 100000–999999
- >=1000000
- No estimate

Fig. 2. Estimated number of new TB cases, by country, 2007.

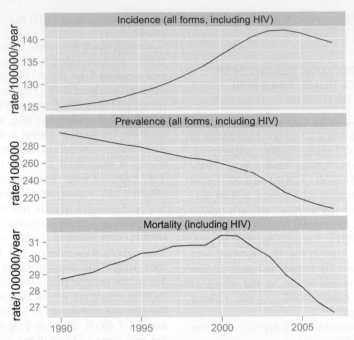

Fig. 3. Global rates of TB incidence, prevalence and mortality, including people with HIV, 1990 to 2007. (*Adapted from* WHO. Global tuberculosis control 2009: surveillance, planning, financing. Geneva: World Health Organization; 2009; with permission.)

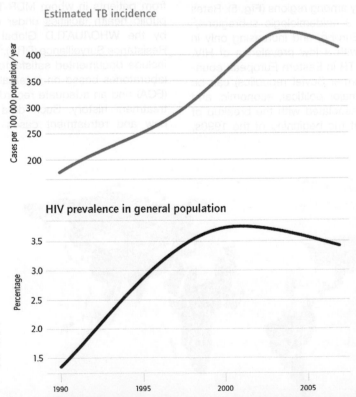

Fig. 4. Estimated incidence of TB and prevalence of HIV for the African subregion most affected by HIV (Africa high-HIV), 1990 to 2007. (*Adapted from* WHO. Global tuberculosis control 2009: surveillance, planning, financing. Geneva: World Health Organization; 2009; with permission.)

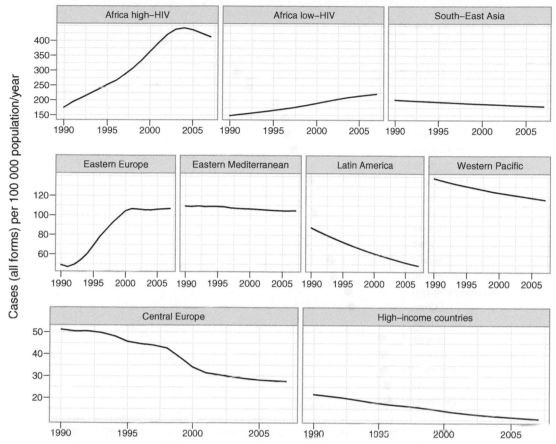

Fig. 5. Trends in incidence in 9 epidemiologic subregions, 1990 to 2007. The composition of each subregion is described in WHO Global TB Report.[2]

countries, respectively. Using a set of widely measurable independent variables that are predictive of the frequency of MDR-TB (such as gross national income (GNI) per capita, the ratio of retreatment to new patients, and the failure rate associated with first-line treatments), it is possible to estimate the frequency of MDR-TB in countries where it has not been measured directly.[40]

Among the estimated 9.27 million first episodes of TB that occurred in 2007 and an additional 1.16 million subsequent episodes of TB (episodes occurring in patients who had already experienced at least 1 previous episode of TB in the past and who had received at least 1 month of anti-TB treatment), an estimated 4.9% or 511,000 were cases of MDR-TB.[2] Of these, 289,000 were new cases (3.1% of all new cases, **Fig. 7**) and 221,000 were cases that had been previously treated for TB (19% of all previously treated cases). Of the 511,000 incident cases of MDR-TB in 2007, 349,000 (68%) were smear-positive. The highest estimated numbers of MDR-TB cases are in India

and China. The emergence of XDR-TB[41,42] has reinforced the need for updated plans to improve the performance of TB control, including prevention of resistance amplification, transmission of resistant strains, and the capacity to diagnose and treat adequately TB drug resistance.[43–45]

Prevalence

There were an estimated 13.7 million prevalent cases in 2007 (206/100,000 population), a slight decrease from 13.9 million in 2006. Of these 13.7 million prevalent cases, an estimated 687,000 (5%) were HIV-positive. From trends in TB incidence and assumptions about the duration of disease in different categories of cases, the global prevalence of TB is estimated to have been in decline since 1990 (**Fig. 8**). This decline is in marked contrast to the increase in TB incidence in the 1990s, which can be explained by a decrease in the average duration of disease as the fraction of cases treated in the DOTS programs

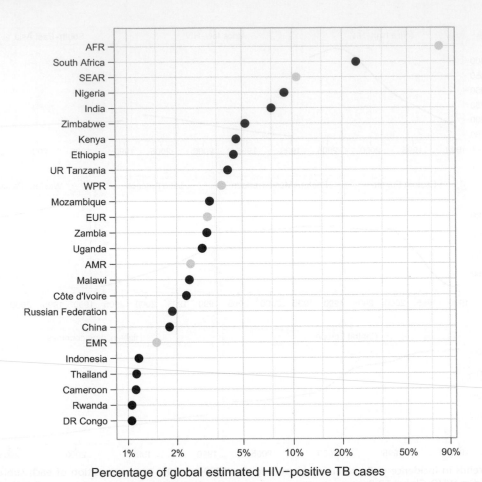

Fig. 6. Geographic distribution of the estimated number of HIV-positive TB cases in 2007. For each country (*dark circles*) and WHO region (*light gray circles*), the number of incident TB cases arising in people with HIV is shown as a percentage of the global total of such cases (note the scale on the horizontal axis). (*Adapted from* WHO. Global tuberculosis control 2009: surveillance, planning, financing. Geneva: World Health Organization; 2009; with permission.)

increased and a comparatively short duration of disease among HIV-positive cases specifically (which has partly compensated for an increase in the incidence of HIV-positive TB cases).

In the African and European regions, prevalence rates increased substantially during the 1990s, and by 2007 were still far above the 1990 level in the African Region and just back to the 1990 level in the European Region (see **Fig. 8**). With limited access to antiretroviral therapy (ART), HIV has probably had a smaller effect on TB prevalence than on incidence because the duration of TB among HIV-positive patients is relatively short: for people with advanced HIV infection, the progression to severe tuberculosis is rapid, with a marked reduction in life expectancy.[46] The gap between the 2015 targets and current prevalence rates in these 2 regions means that the world as a whole is unlikely to meet the target of halving

the 1990 prevalence rate by 2015 (see **Box 1** and **Fig. 8**).

Mortality

An estimated 1.32 million HIV-negative people (19.7/100,000 population) died of TB in 2007, and there were an additional 456,000 TB deaths among HIV-positive people; thus, the total number of deaths caused by tuberculosis was 1.77 million. Deaths from TB among HIV-positive people account for 23% of the estimated 2 million HIV deaths that occurred in 2007. The global TB mortality rate (including TB deaths in HIV-positive people) is estimated to have increased during the 1990s; this trend was reversed around the year 2000, and mortality rates are now in decline (see **Fig. 3**; **Fig. 9**). Mortality rates have been declining in the Eastern Mediterranean Region, the Region

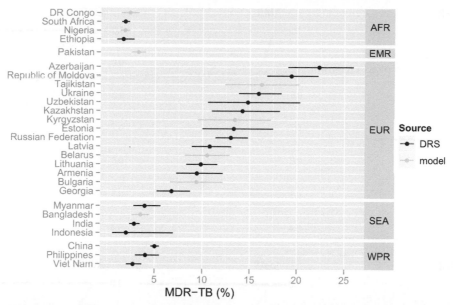

Fig. 7. Levels of MDR-TB in 27 priority countries for MDR-TB control, expressed as a percentage of new TB cases with no history of previous antituberculosis treatment (or <4 weeks of previous treatment). Estimates were measured directly from DRS (*black dots*) or indirectly using statistical modeling (*light gray dots*).

of the Americas, the South-East Asia Region, and the Western Pacific Region since 1990. In the African and European regions, mortality rates increased substantially during the 1990s. Although this trend has been reversed (around 2000 in the European Region and around 2005 in the African Region), mortality rates in 2007 were still far above the 1990 level in the African Region and just back to the 1990 level in the European Region. Projections indicate that neither region will reduce mortality rates back to even 1990 levels by 2015, and will certainly not halve mortality rates compared with 1990 (see **Fig. 9**). The gulf between the 2015 targets and current mortality rates in these 2 regions mean that the world as a whole is unlikely to meet the Stop TB Partnership target of halving the 1990 mortality rate by 2015.

TRENDS IN TB CASE NOTIFICATIONS AND RATES OF CASE DETECTION AND TREATMENT SUCCESS

The 196 countries reporting to the WHO in 2008 notified 5.6 million new and relapse cases in 2007, of which 2.6 million (46%) were new smear-positive cases. Notifications disaggregated by sex were reported for new pulmonary smear-positive TB cases by 170 countries. Of 2.55 million notifications, 1.65 million were male and 0.9 million were female, giving a male/female ratio of 1.8 for those aged 14 years and older. One of the factors associated with the male/female ratio in smear-positive TB patients is the prevalence of HIV in

the general population. More women than men are detected with TB in countries where the prevalence of HIV in the general population exceeds 1% (**Fig. 10**). The reasons for higher TB notification rates in men are poorly understood.[47] Possible explanations include biologic differences between men and women in certain age groups that affect the risk of being infected and the risk of infection progressing to active disease,[48] and differences in the societal roles of men and women that influence their risk of exposure to TB and access to care (gender differences).[49–51] The observation that TB notification rates tend to be more equal between men and women in countries with a high prevalence of HIV supports the hypothesis of biologic differences (which can be lessened by immunologic suppression caused by HIV), but other nonbiologic factors may play an important role.

The 2.6 million new smear-positive cases notified in 2007 represent 63% of the 4.1 million estimated cases. This is a small increase from a figure of 62% in 2006, following a slow increase from 35% to 43% between 1995 and 2001 and a more rapid increase from 43% to 60% between 2001 and 2005. The improvement that occurred between 2001 and 2007 was attributable mostly to increases in the numbers of new smear-positive cases reported in the Eastern Mediterranean, South-East Asia and Western Pacific regions. The case detection rate (defined as the ratio of newly notified cases over estimated incident

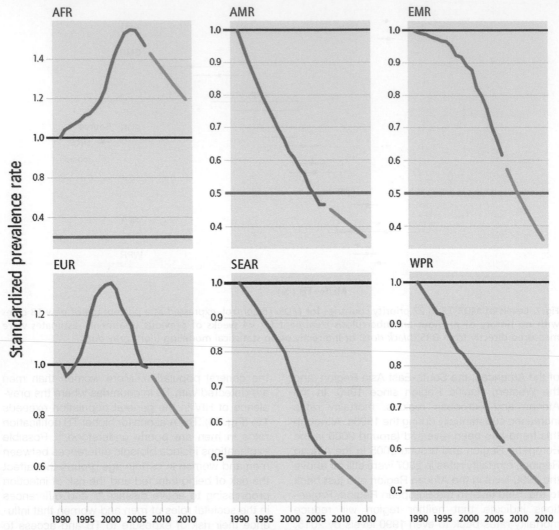

Fig. 8. Progress toward achieving the target of halving the prevalence of TB by 2015 compared with the 1990 level, by WHO region. The y-axis displays standardized prevalence rates, with the baseline set at the 1990 level in each region (*upper horizontal line*) and regional targets set at 50% of the 1990 level (*lower horizontal line*). Trends for 2008 to 2015 are forecast using an exponential regression of estimated prevalence rates over the period 2005 to 2007. (*Adapted from* WHO. Global tuberculosis control 2009: surveillance, planning, financing. Geneva: World Health Organization; 2009; with permission.)

cases) of smear-positive cases in 2007 was equal to or greater than 70% in the Western Pacific Region (78%) and the Region of the Americas (76%), followed by the South-East Asia Region (69%, **Fig. 11**). The African Region had the lowest case detection rate (47%).

Globally, the rate of treatment success was 85% in 2006. This means that 52% of the smear-positive cases estimated to have occurred in 2006 were detected and successfully treated. The target for treatment success was reached at global level in 2006 because of the high treatment success rates reported from the South-East Asia and Western Pacific Regions (87% and 92%,

respectively; the latter figure is high enough to warrant further validation of the data). Treatment success rates in other regions in 2006 were 75% in the African Region, 86% in the Eastern Mediterranean Region (where the target was reached for the first time in 2006), 70% in the European Region (the lowest recorded since 1996) and 75% in the Region of the Americas (**Fig. 12**).

CAN TB BE ELIMINATED BY 2050?

TB can be controlled by preventing infection, stopping progression from infection to active disease, and rapid detection and treatment of active

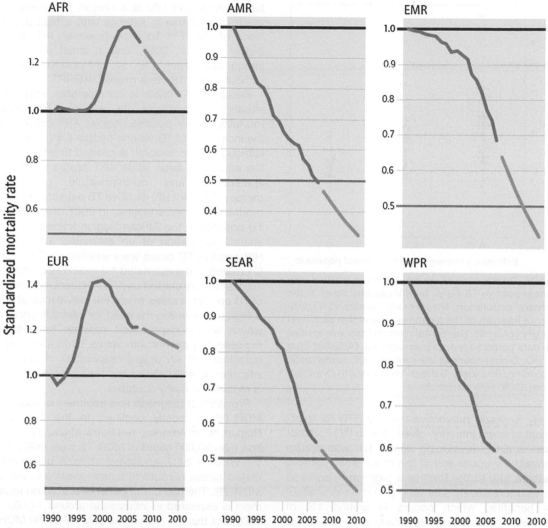

Fig. 9. Progress toward achieving the target of halving mortality from TB by 2015 compared with the 1990 level, by WHO region. The y-axis displays standardized mortality rates, with the baseline set at the 1990 level in each region (*upper horizontal line*) and regional targets set at 50% of the 1990 level (*lower horizontal line*). Trends for 2008 to 2015 are forecast using an exponential regression of estimated mortality rates over the period 2005 to 2007. The mortality rates represented in these graphs exclude deaths from TB in HIV-positive people. (*Adapted from* WHO. Global tuberculosis control 2009: surveillance, planning, financing. Geneva: World Health Organization; 2009; with permission.)

disease.[52,53] To date, only bacille Calmette-Guérin (BCG) vaccination (provided to more than 80% of the annual birth cohort) and treatment of active TB using first-line drugs have been implemented on a large scale.[54] With these interventions, global targets set for 2015 will be met in some regions, but on current trends, elimination (defined as an annual incidence of new cases of less than 1 per million population) will not be achieved by 2050.[55] In that year, even with full implementation of the Global Plan 2006–2015, the incidence rate will be about 100 times higher than the elimination target. To accelerate progress, wider application of existing interventions combined with development and implementation of new drugs, vaccines, and diagnostic tools is required, as set out in the Stop TB Strategy and the Global Plan to Stop TB.[9,11]

Mathematical modeling suggests that the 2050 target of TB elimination is most likely to be achieved if latent infection and active disease are treated.[56] This would be the result of an intervention on 2 separate pathways: preventing transmission from averting cases and minimizing transmission from active cases with their rapid detection and treatment. Randomized controlled trials (RCTs) have shown that up to 12 months of

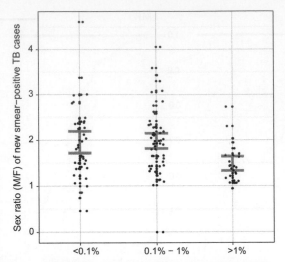

Fig. 10. Distribution of sex ratio (M/F) in notified new smear-positive TB cases, by HIV epidemic level in the general population. The error bars denote 95% confidence intervals of the mean sex ratio within each level of HIV epidemic. Horizontal random jitter was applied to data points to reduce over-plotting. (*Adapted from* WHO. Global tuberculosis control 2009: surveillance, planning, financing. Geneva: World Health Organization; 2009; with permission.)

daily isoniazid preventive therapy (IPT) for treatment of latent infection gives 25% to 92% protection against developing active TB, with results toward the upper end of this range when patients adhere fully to the treatment regimen.[57] Isoniazid is also a relatively safe drug (the main side effect is hepatitis, which occurs in around 1% of patients), and the exceptionally high risk of TB among people coinfected with *Mycobacterium*

tuberculosis and HIV is a reason for promoting much greater use in settings with a high prevalence of HIV.[58,59] To date, however, IPT is not widely used. In 2007, only a small proportion (much less than 1%) of HIV-positive people without active TB were treated with IPT.

Besides IPT, there is considerable scope to expand interventions to reduce TB-related mortality in HIV-positive people. ART decreases the incidence of TB among people living with HIV (although more research is needed to understand the impact of large scale ART programs on TB epidemics), and co-trimoxazole preventive therapy (CPT) for HIV-positive TB patients reduces mortality.[38,60] Nevertheless, in 2007 only 37% of TB patients in the African Region knew their HIV status, 0.2 million of an estimated 1.4 million HIV-positive TB cases were enrolled on CPT, and 0.1 million of the estimated 1.4 million HIV-positive TB cases were started on ART.[2] Recent expansion of TB control in areas where the prevalence of HIV is high has unveiled the need for infection control, where immunosuppressed patients have been exposed to patients with active TB in clinics and hospitals.[61,62] An urgent reappraisal of airborne infection control policies and their implementation is required in many countries.

Provision of diagnosis and treatment of cases of MDR-TB is mostly confined to the European Region, North America, and South Africa.[2] Globally, less than 30,000 cases of MDR-TB were notified to the WHO in 2007, equivalent to 8.5% of the estimated global number of smear-positive cases of MDR-TB. The number of patients started on treatment is expected to increase to around 14,000 in 2009, but this still represents only 4% of the MDR-TB cases estimated to exist globally. Urgent

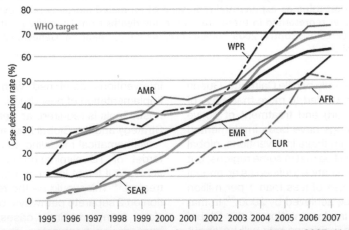

Fig. 11. Smear-positive case detection rate under DOTS, by WHO region, 1995 to 2007. Heavy line shows global DOTS case detection rate. (*Adapted from* WHO. Global tuberculosis control 2009: surveillance, planning, financing. Geneva: World Health Organization; 2009; with permission.)

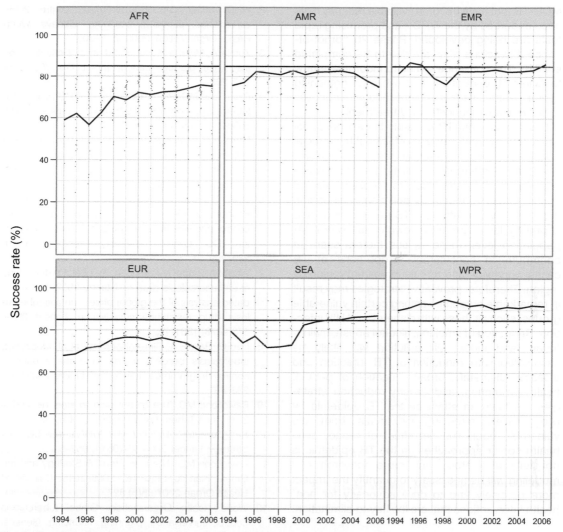

Fig. 12. Trends in TB treatment success rates by WHO region from 1994 to 2006. Each dot represents 1 country's success rate in the corresponding year. Horizontal jitter was applied randomly to avoid over-plotting. Black curves represent weighted averages of treatment success rates over time. The horizontal line represents the global target of 85% success rate.

improvements in the provision of services for laboratory culture, DST, and treatment are needed in many countries, with special urgency in the 27 high-burden countries for MDR-TB (see **Fig. 7**).

In addition to scaling up interventions related to treatment of latent infection, TB/HIV and MDR-TB, the Stop TB Strategy also emphasizes the importance of engaging all care providers in the public and the nonstate sectors to shorten delays to diagnosis, and ensure that treatment of all patients (in the public and nonstate sectors) meets international standards.[63] This means engaging medical services in prisons and the armed forces, private clinicians, nongovernmental organizations, faith-based organizations and mission services and

hospitals, and clinics in the corporate sector.[64–68] With less than two-thirds of estimated cases detected and notified to national TB control programs in 2007, there is considerable scope for earlier detection and better treatment of people with TB.

Beyond wider use of existing tools, research and development related to new drugs, new diagnostics, and new vaccines has accelerated in recent years.[55,69,70] For example, several pharmaceutical companies have embarked on the development of new anti-TB drugs, which may shorten treatment duration to 4 months or less; several drugs targeting MDR-TB are now in phase 1, 2, and 3 clinical trials.[71,72] New diagnostics for rapid detection of

MDR-TB that have become available recently have been endorsed by the WHO[73] and promising rapid tests are being developed. Phase 2b "proof-of-concept" vaccine trials are due to be completed in 2010. The challenge will be to incorporate new tools into TB control practices while strengthening overall health systems and ensuring wider access to prevention, diagnostic, and treatment.

Recognition that TB depends largely on social and economic determinants of ill health is crucial to achieve full control and elimination. Recent articles[74] have attempted to estimate the relative importance of factors such as smoking, alcohol abuse, diabetes, indoor air pollution, malnutrition that, like HIV, are affecting TB epidemiology and impeding faster progress toward its control. At population level, these various factors seem to contribute to considerable proportions of TB cases worldwide and to differing extent region by region. Therefore, preventive strategies may result in remarkable outcomes among certain vulnerable groups, such as those with diabetes and HIV infection. Reduction of smoking, alcohol abuse, malnutrition, and indoor air pollution will likely be associated with reduction of TB infection and disease. Ultimately, broad education of people, health promotion, and poverty-reduction strategies will have an effect on the TB epidemic by progressively removing individuals from the vulnerable pool. The net effect of broad, non–health sector approaches on the TB epidemic is not fully understood and more research and modeling will be necessary to quantify the impact more precisely and to drive advocacy for non-health interventions that are the key to elimination.

SUMMARY

Despite progress in our understanding of TB epidemiology and the availability of effective treatments, the number of new TB cases that occur each year is still rising, particularly in poor and otherwise disadvantaged populations.[75] To reverse this trend and achieve global targets set for 2015 and 2050, major and urgent scaling up of the interventions and approaches included in the Stop TB Strategy is needed in most countries, combined with the successful development and application of new drugs, diagnostics, and vaccines, and with a clearer understanding of the impact of social and economic determinants of ill health.

REFERENCES

1. WHO, editor. The global burden of disease: 2004 update. Geneva: World Health Organization; 2008. p. 11–2.

2. WHO, editor. Global tuberculosis control 2009: surveillance, planning, financing. Geneva: World Health Organization; 2009. p. 1–303.

3. Zumla A, Mwaba P, Huggett J, et al. Reflections on the white plague. Lancet Infect Dis 2009;9(3): 197–202.

4. Raviglione MC, Pio A. Evolution of WHO policies for tuberculosis control, 1948–2001. Lancet 2002; 359(9308):775–80.

5. Murray CJ, DeJonghe E, Chum HJ, et al. Cost effectiveness of chemotherapy for pulmonary tuberculosis in three sub-Saharan African countries. Lancet 1991;338(8778):1305–8.

6. Dye C, Floyd K. Tuberculosis. In: Jamison DT, Breman JG, Measham AR, et al, editors. Disease control priorities in developing countries. Washington, DC: Oxford University Press; 2006. p. 289–309.

7. Wright A, Zignol M, Van Deun A, et al. Epidemiology of antituberculosis drug resistance 2002–07: an updated analysis of the global project on anti-tuberculosis drug resistance surveillance. Lancet 2009; 373(9678):1861–73.

8. Dye C, Bassili A, Bierrenbach AL, et al. Measuring tuberculosis burden, trends, and the impact of control programmes. Lancet Infect Dis 2008;8(4): 233–43.

9. Raviglione MC. The global plan to stop TB, 2006–2015. Int J Tuberc Lung Dis 2006;10(3):238–9.

10. Raviglione MC, Uplekar MW. WHO's new Stop TB Strategy. Lancet 2006;367(9514):952–5.

11. Raviglione MC. The new Stop TB Strategy and the Global Plan to Stop TB, 2006–2015. Bull World Health Organ 2007;85(5):327.

12. World Health Organization. Global tuberculosis control: surveillance, planning, financing. Geneva: World Health Organization; 2007.

13. Dye C, Maher D, Weil D, et al. Targets for global tuberculosis control. Int J Tuberc Lung Dis 2006; 10(4):460–2.

14. Bierrenbach AL, Stevens AP, Gomes AB, et al. [Impact on tuberculosis incidence rates of removal of repeat notification records]. Rev Saude Publica 2007;41(Suppl 1):67–76 [Portuguese].

15. Dye C, Ottmani S, Laasri L, et al. The decline of tuberculosis epidemics under chemotherapy: a case study in Morocco. Int J Tuberc Lung Dis 2007;11(11):1225–31.

16. Mansoer J, Floyd K, Dye C, et al. New methods for estimating the tuberculosis case detection rate in high-HIV prevalence countries: the example of Kenya. Bull World Health Organ 2009;87:186–92.

17. Dye C, Scheele S, Dolin P, et al. Consensus statement. Global burden of tuberculosis: estimated incidence, prevalence, and mortality by country. WHO Global Surveillance and Monitoring Project. JAMA 1999;282(7):677–86.

18. Botha E, den Boon S, Lawrence KA, et al. From suspect to patient: tuberculosis diagnosis and treatment initiation in health facilities in South Africa. Int J Tuberc Lung Dis 2008;12(8):936–41.

19. Uplekar M, Pathania V, Raviglione M. Private practitioners and public health: weak links in tuberculosis control. Lancet 2001;358(9285):912–6.

20. Meintjes G, Schoeman H, Morroni C, et al. Patient and provider delay in tuberculosis suspects from communities with a high HIV prevalence in South Africa: a cross-sectional study. BMC Infect Dis 2008;8:72.

21. Veron LJ, Blanc LJ, Suchi M, et al. DOTS Expansion: will we reach the 2005 targets? Int J Tuberc Lung Dis 2004;8(1):139–46.

22. Baussano I, Bugiani M, Gregori D, et al. Undetected burden of tuberculosis in a low-prevalence area. Int J Tuberc Lung Dis 2006;10(4):415–21.

23. Borgdorff MW, Glynn JR, Vynnycky E. Using capture-recapture methods to study recent transmission of tuberculosis. Int J Epidemiol 2004;33(4):905–6 [author reply 7].

24. Cailhol J, Che D, Jarlier V, et al. Incidence of tuberculous meningitis in France, 2000: a capture-recapture analysis. Int J Tuberc Lung Dis 2005;9(7):803–8.

25. Crofts JP, Pebody R, Grant A, et al. Estimating tuberculosis case mortality in England and Wales, 2001–2002. Int J Tuberc Lung Dis 2008;12(3):308–13.

26. Na Vanh, Story A, Grant AD, et al. Record-linkage and capture-recapture analysis to estimate the incidence and completeness of reporting of tuberculosis in England 1999–2002. Epidemiol Infect 2008; 136(12):1606–16.

27. Glaziou P, van der Werf MJ, Onozaki I, et al. Tuberculosis prevalence surveys: rationale and cost. Int J Tuberc Lung Dis 2008;12(9):1003–8.

28. WHO, editor. Assessing tuberculosis prevalence through population-based surveys. Manila: World Health Organization; 2007. p. 1–235.

29. Soemantri S, Senewe FP, Tjandrarini DH, et al. Three-fold reduction in the prevalence of tuberculosis over 25 years in Indonesia. Int J Tuberc Lung Dis 2007;11(4):398–404.

30. Dye C, Fengzeng Z, Scheele S, et al. Evaluating the impact of tuberculosis control: number of deaths prevented by short-course chemotherapy in China. Int J Epidemiol 2000;29(3):558–64.

31. Tupasi TE, Radhakrishna S, Rivera AB, et al. The 1997 nationwide tuberculosis prevalence survey in the Philippines. Int J Tuberc Lung Dis 1999;3(6):471–7.

32. Hong YP, Kim SJ, Lew WJ, et al. The seventh nationwide tuberculosis prevalence survey in Korea, 1995. Int J Tuberc Lung Dis 1998;2:27–36.

33. Korenromp EL, Bierrenbach AL, Williams BG, et al. The measurement and estimation of tuberculosis mortality. Int J Tuberc Lung Dis 2009;13(3):283–303.

34. Corbett EL, Watt CJ, Walker N, et al. The growing burden of tuberculosis: global trends and interactions with the HIV epidemic. Arch Intern Med 2003; 163(9):1009–21.

35. UNAIDS. HIV epidemiology. Available at: http://www.unaids.org/en/KnowledgeCentre/HIVData/Epidemiology/latestEpiData.asp. 2009. Accessed March 7, 2009.

36. Shilova MV, Dye C. The resurgence of tuberculosis in Russia. Philos Trans R Soc Lond A 2001; 356(1411):1069–75.

37. WHO. WHO and UNAIDS issue new guidance on HIV testing and counseling in health facilities. Available at: http://www.who.int/mediacentre/news/releases/2007/pr24/en/index.html. 2007. Accessed April 7, 2009.

38. Harries AD, Zachariah R, Lawn SD. Providing HIV care for co-infected tuberculosis patients: a perspective from sub-Saharan Africa. Int J Tuberc Lung Dis 2009;13(1):6–16.

39. WHO, editor. Anti-tuberculosis drug resistance in the world, 4th report: the WHO/IUATLD Global Project on Anti-tuberculosis Drug Resistance Surveillance. 2008 edition. Geneva: World Health Organization; 2008. p. 1–142.

40. Zignol M, Hosseini MS, Wright A, et al. Global incidence of multidrug-resistant tuberculosis. J Infect Dis 2006;194(4):479–85.

41. Shah NS, Wright A, Bai GH, et al. Worldwide emergence of extensively drug-resistant tuberculosis. Emerg Infect Dis 2007;13(3):380–7.

42. Migliori GB, Loddenkemper R, Blasi F, et al. 125 years after Robert Koch's discovery of the tubercle bacillus: the new XDR-TB threat. Is "science" enough to tackle the epidemic? Eur Respir J 2007; 29(3):423–7.

43. Manissero D, Fernandez de la Hoz K. Surveillance methods and case definition for extensively drug resistant TB (XDR-TB) and relevance to Europe: summary update. Euro Surveill 2006;11(11):E061103.1.

44. Raviglione M. XDR-TB: entering the post-antibiotic era? Int J Tuberc Lung Dis 2006;10(11):1185–7.

45. Raviglione MC, Smith IM. XDR tuberculosis–implications for global public health. N Engl J Med 2007; 356(7):656–9.

46. Corbett EL, Charalambous S, Moloi VM, et al. Human immunodeficiency virus and the prevalence of undiagnosed tuberculosis in African gold miners. Am J Respir Crit Care Med 2004; 170(6):673–9.

47. Ottmani SE, Uplekar MW. Gender and TB: pointers from routine records and reports. Int J Tuberc Lung Dis 2008;12(7):827–8.

48. Thorson A, Long NH, Larsson LO. Chest X-ray findings in relation to gender and symptoms:

a study of patients with smear positive tuberculosis in Vietnam. Scand J Infect Dis 2007;39(1): 33–7.

49. Borgdorff MW, Nagelkerke NJ, Dye C, et al. Gender and tuberculosis: a comparison of prevalence surveys with notification data to explore sex differences in case detection. Int J Tuberc Lung Dis 2000;4(2):123–32.

50. Connolly M, Nunn P. Women and tuberculosis. World Health Stat Q 1996;49(2):115–9.

51. Somma D, Thomas BE, Karim F, et al. Gender and socio-cultural determinants of TB-related stigma in Bangladesh, India, Malawi and Colombia. Int J Tuberc Lung Dis 2008;12(7):856–66.

52. Dye C, Garnett GP, Sleeman K, et al. Prospects for worldwide tuberculosis control under the WHO DOTS strategy. Directly observed short-course therapy. Lancet 1998;352(9144):1886–91.

53. Dye C, Watt CJ, Bleed DM, et al. Evolution of tuberculosis control and prospects for reducing tuberculosis incidence, prevalence, and deaths globally. JAMA 2005;293(22):2767–75.

54. Enarson DA, Seita A, Fujiwara P. Global elimination of tuberculosis: implementation, innovation, investigation. Int J Tuberc Lung Dis 2003;7(12 Suppl 3): S328–32.

55. Lonnroth K, Raviglione M. Global epidemiology of tuberculosis: prospects for control. Semin Respir Crit Care Med 2008;29(5):481–91.

56. Dye C, Williams BG. Eliminating human tuberculosis in the twenty-first century. J R Soc Interface 2008; 5(23):653–62.

57. Sterling TR. New approaches to the treatment of latent tuberculosis. Semin Respir Crit Care Med 2008;29(5):532–41.

58. Woldehanna S, Volmink J. Treatment of latent tuberculosis infection in HIV infected persons. Cochrane Database Syst Rev 2004;(1):CD000171.

59. Churchyard GJ, Scano F, Grant AD, et al. Tuberculosis preventive therapy in the era of HIV infection: overview and research priorities. J Infect Dis 2007; 196(Suppl 1):S52–62.

60. Grimwade K, Sturm AW, Nunn AJ, et al. Effectiveness of cotrimoxazole prophylaxis on mortality in adults with tuberculosis in rural South Africa. AIDS 2005;19(2):163–8.

61. Bock NN, Jensen PA, Miller B, et al. Tuberculosis infection control in resource-limited settings in the era of expanding HIV care and treatment. J Infect Dis 2007;196(Suppl 1):S108–13.

62. Wells CD, Cegielski JP, Nelson LJ, et al. HIV infection and multidrug-resistant tuberculosis: the perfect storm. J Infect Dis 2007;196(Suppl 1): S86–107.

63. Hopewell PC, Pai M, Maher D, et al. International standards for tuberculosis care. Lancet Infect Dis 2006;6(11):710–25.

64. Lonnroth K, Uplekar M, Arora VK, et al. Public-private mix for DOTS implementation: what makes it work? Bull World Health Organ 2004;82(8):580–6.

65. Ambe G, Lonnroth K, Dholakia Y, et al. Every provider counts: effect of a comprehensive public-private mix approach for TB control in a large metropolitan area in India. Int J Tuberc Lung Dis 2005;9(5):562–8.

66. Lonnroth K, Uplekar M. Invest in breaking the barriers of public-private collaboration for improved tuberculosis care. Bull World Health Organ 2005; 83(7):558–9.

67. Floyd K, Arora VK, Murthy KJ, et al. Cost and cost-effectiveness of PPM-DOTS for tuberculosis control: evidence from India. Bull World Health Organ 2006; 84(6):437–45.

68. Pantoja A, Floyd K, Unnikrishnan KP, et al. Economic evaluation of public-private mix for tuberculosis care and control, India. Part I. Socio-economic profile and costs among tuberculosis patients. Int J Tuberc Lung Dis 2009;13(6):698–704.

69. Pai M, O'Brien R. New diagnostics for latent and active tuberculosis: state of the art and future prospects. Semin Respir Crit Care Med 2008;29(5):560–8.

70. Ly LH, McMurray DN. Tuberculosis: vaccines in the pipeline. Expert Rev Vaccines 2008;7(5): 635–50.

71. Diacon AH, Pym A, Grobusch M, et al. The diarylquinoline TMC207 for multidrug-resistant tuberculosis. N Engl J Med 2009;360(23):2397–405.

72. Nuermberger E, Mitchison DA. Once-weekly treatment of tuberculosis with the diarylquinoline R207910: a real possibility. Am J Respir Crit Care Med 2009;179(1):2–3.

73. World Health Organization. Molecular line probe assays for rapid screening of patients at risk of multi-drug-resistant tuberculosis (MDR-TB). Policy statement. WHO. 2008. Available at: www.who.int/tb/features_archive/policy_statement.pdf. Accessed June 28, 2009.

74. Lonnroth K, Jaramillo E, Williams BG, et al. Drivers of tuberculosis epidemics: the role of risk factors and social determinants. Soc Sci Med 2009;68(12): 2240–6.

75. Squire SB, Obasi A, Nhlema-Simwaka B. The global plan to stop TB: a unique opportunity to address poverty and the Millennium Development Goals. Lancet 2006;367(9514):955–7.

Multidrug-Resistant and Extensively Drug-Resistant Tuberculosis in the West. Europe and United States: Epidemiology, Surveillance, and Control

Giovanni Battista Migliori, MD[a],*,
Morgan D' Arcy Richardson, RN, MS[b],
Giovanni Sotgiu, MD, PhD[c], Christoph Lange, MD, PhD[d]

KEYWORDS
- MDR-TB • XDR-TB • Tuberculosis control
- Europe • United States • Epidemiology • Surveillance

The global tuberculosis (TB) epidemic has been complicated by the emergence of strains of *Mycobacterium tuberculosis* resistant to anti-TB drugs. Misuse of drugs to treat TB, for reasons related to prescribers, patients, and producers has given rise to various forms of drug-resistant TB.[1] The spread of multidrug-resistant TB (MDR-TB),[2–6] and more recently of extensively drug-resistant TB (XDR-TB)[7–9] is considered a real threat to achieving the global goal of TB control and elimination by 2050. The aims of this article are (1) to review the available information on epidemiology of MDR- and XDR-TB, (2) to discuss the role and organization of surveillance of MDR- and XDR-TB, (3) to discuss consensus strategies to control and care for MDR- and XDR-TB, and (4) to describe the priorities for research, focusing on Western countries (Europe and the United States).

DEFINITIONS AND METHODS

TB is generally treated with a standardized regimen of 4 first-line anti-TB drugs, including isoniazid, rifampicin, pyrazinamide, and ethambutol. Pan-susceptible TB is defined as TB susceptible to all first-line agents. MDR-TB is caused by *Mycobacteria* that are resistant to at least isoniazid and rifampicin, the 2 most potent first-line anti-TB drugs.[2–5,10] Whereas MDR-TB has been documented for many years, the term XDR-TB appeared in the literature for the first time in March 2006, in a report jointly published by the US Centers for Disease Control and Prevention (CDC) and the World Health Organization (WHO) to describe a severe form of disease, now defined as TB caused by strains of *M tuberculosis*, which are resistant to at least isoniazid and rifampicin (ie, MDR-TB), plus to any fluoroquinolone, and to at least 1 of 3 injectable drugs used in anti-TB treatment: capreomycin, kanamycin, or amikacin.[7,9,11,12] A European study has demonstrated recently that the occurrence of XDR-TB, as currently defined, has both a clinical value (predicting poor outcome) and an operational significance (confirming the loss of first-line drugs coupled with key second-line ones).[13]

[a] WHO Collaborating Centre for TB and Lung Diseases, Fondazione S. Maugeri, Care and Research Institute/TBNET Secretariat (TuBerculosis Network European Trialsgroup)/Stop TB Italy, Via Roncaccio 16, 21049, Tradate, Italy
[b] HIV/TB Global Program, PATH, 1800 K Street, NW, Suite 800, Washington, DC 20006, USA
[c] Hygiene and Preventive Medicine Institute, University of Sassari, Via Padre Manzella, 4 07100 Sassari, Italy
[d] Division of Clinical Infectious Diseases, Medical Clinic, Research Centre Borstel, Parkallee 35, 23845 Borstel, Germany
* Corresponding author.
E-mail address: giovannibattista.migliori@fsm.it (G.B. Migliori).

Clin Chest Med 30 (2009) 637–665
doi:10.1016/j.ccm.2009.08.015

For the purposes of this review, Europe is defined as the 53 countries that comprise the WHO European Region. In the context of MDR-TB control in Europe, it is important to consider TB epidemiology in Central and Eastern Europe as well, because a large proportion of cases originate in other countries of the region and the world.

The United States is defined as the 50 states and the territories over which the United States has jurisdiction, with a total of 68 units (including separate reporting by some large cities) reporting TB data to the CDC.

This review is based on a Medline search performed using the key words TB, MDR, XDR, Europe, and United States, covering the period 2004 to 2009. In addition, the CDC *Morbidity and Mortality Weekly Report* (MMWR) was searched from 1989 to the present for reports on MDR-TB and XDR-TB investigations in the United States. The articles identified were divided into 5 groups (epidemiology and risk factors, surveillance, clinical presentation and outcomes, control, research) and quoted in the review based on priority criteria.

The majority of the data from Europe reported here are derived from the WHO)/International Union Against TB and Lung Disease (IUATLD) Global Project on Drug Resistance Surveillance launched in 2004. The surveys are done at national level based on 3 main principles: representativeness, distinction between new (eg, treated for less than 1 month) and retreatment cases, and quality assurance of laboratory results by a TB Supranational Reference Laboratory (SRL).[4,6] The latest drug susceptibility testing (DST) data available were gathered from 90,726 patients in 83 countries and territories between 2002 and 2007.[6]

Additional data from Europe reported in this review are derived from the TBNET (TuBerculosis Network European Trials group) studies reporting epidemiologic and clinical data for all culture-confirmed TB cases (n = 4583) diagnosed consecutively by the TB clinical reference centers in Estonia (Tallin, Tartu), Germany (Borstel, Munich-Gauting, Grosshansdorf, Bad-Lippspringe), Italy (Sondalo, Milan, Rome), and Russian Federation (Archangels Oblast) between 1999 and 2006 (Italy and Germany: 2003–2006; Estonia: 2001–2004; Archangels Oblast: 1999–2001). Standard WHO definitions for MDR-TB, XDR-TB, and treatment outcome (treatment success, died, failure, default, and transferred out) were used in all the TBNET studies.[13–19]

Data from the United States are derived from the CDC's Division of TB Elimination annual surveillance reports, MMWR data, and queries performed using the CDC's Online TB Information System (OTIS).

EPIDEMIOLOGY

MDR-TB and XDR-TB are strong indicators of TB control program failures. Their epidemiology points to key global challenges for TB control and elimination. MDR-TB and XDR-TB occur for several reasons. First, providers may prescribe insufficient drug regimens for patients (eg, inadequate doses, inadequate numbers of drugs or incorrect drugs, or inadequate durations of treatment). Second, patients may not adhere to an appropriate regimen (ie, interrupting or discontinuing treatment). Third, drugs used may be of poor quality. All of these factors may contribute to development of *acquired* drug resistance in patients being treated for pan-sensitive TB. In addition, when MDR-TB and XDR-TB are left undetected or untreated, they may be transmitted directly from one individual to another, resulting in *primary* drug resistance in a previously untreated individual.

Only estimates are available regarding the total number of MDR-TB and XDR-TB cases globally, surveillance being hampered by a lack of adequate laboratory capacity for DST in many high-burden countries and even in the West, as discussed later in this article. Zignol and colleagues[5] estimated that 458,000 (95% confidence interval [CI] 321,000–689,000) incident MDR-TB cases occurred globally in 2003 (including new and retreatment cases). Because MDR-TB patients usually require treatment for 2 or more years, the prevalence of MDR-TB may be 3 times greater than its incidence,[20] suggesting that the true number of prevalent MDR-TB cases in the world today may approach or exceed 1 million.

The fourth report on global anti-TB drug resistance[4] informed the production of latest (2007) global estimates of the burden of MDR-TB (511,000 incident cases, 150,000 deaths) and XDR-TB cases (50,000 cases, 30,000 deaths). The median prevalence of MDR-TB in new TB cases was 1.6% (interquartile range [IQR] 0.6–3.9), ranging from 0% in 8 countries with low TB prevalence to 19.4% in Moldova and 22.3% in Baku, Azerbaijan. The prevalence of MDR-TB in new TB cases was greater than 6% in 15 settings, 12 of them being located (or corresponding to) countries of the former Soviet Union (FSU: Azerbaijan, Moldova, Ukraine, Russian Federation, Uzbekistan, Estonia, Latvia, Lithuania, Armenia, and Georgia). Considering the surveys performed in earlier stages of the project (Kazakhstan, Ivanovo Oblast in the Russian

Federation, and Dominican Republic), 14 out of 19 high MDR-TB burden territories were located in FSU countries (**Fig. 1**).[4,6]

The median prevalence of MDR-TB in previously treated TB cases was 11.7% (IQR 4.9–20.9). A reported 55.8% of retreatment cases in Baku (Azerbaijan) and 60% in Tashkent (Uzbekistan) had MDR-TB. Among the 17 settings reporting a prevalence of MDR-TB of more than 25% in retreatment cases, 9 were in FSU countries.[4,9]

Epidemiology of MDR- and XDR-TB in Europe

The distribution of MDR-TB and XDR-TB in the countries of Europe is highly variable, influenced by overall TB incidence, human movement, health program strengths and weaknesses, and economic and social factors. Population-based data on drug resistance are not available for many countries and laboratory capacity is weak in some areas, which further limit one's ability to draw conclusions on the epidemiology of drug resistance throughout the region.

In the European Union (EU) and EEA/EFTA (European Economic Area/European Free Trade Association) countries data on anti-TB drug resistance surveillance in 2007 were made available by 28 countries. Overall, the proportion of cases with MDR-TB among those tested was 4.0%. Cases resistant to one or more first-line anti-TB drugs were reported by all countries. The Baltic States,

Bulgaria, Germany, Spain, Romania, and the United Kingdom each reported 50 or more MDR-TB cases. The proportion of new cases with MDR-TB ranged from 0% to 17%, but was higher in the Baltic States (7%–17%). Drug resistance was commonly higher in cases of foreign origin compared with the native population. The proportion of combined MDR-TB cases (new and retreatment) is high and stable in the Baltic States; it decreased in Latvia (2004–2007), but these trends remained insignificant for primary MDR-TB cases. These results suggest that retreated cases are decreasing faster than incident ones in these countries. Despite variable quality, data in general showed a high prevalence of drug resistance in most non-EU Eastern European countries. Levels of MDR-TB in cases with no history of treatment for more than 1 month varied from 6.4% in Georgia to 30.9% in Uzbekistan.

Prevalence in retreated cases was much higher (32.7%–78.8%). The most recent figures indicate that XDR-TB cases comprise up to 15% of MDR-TB cases in some areas of Europe. (The data reported here are derived from the European Centre for Disease Prevention and Control [ECDC] surveillance and do not necessarily correspond precisely to the data reported later.)

According to the fourth global report on drug resistance, in the Established Market Economies region (both Western Europe and United States belong to this group of countries as defined by

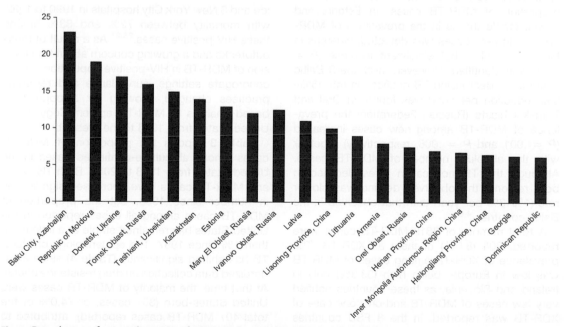

Fig. 1. Prevalence of more than 5% of MDR-TB in new TB cases in 19 countries.

WHO), out of 85,729 new TB cases, 724 (95% CI 573–942) were estimated to be MDR-TB (0.8%; 0.7%–1.1%). In Central Europe, out of 42,464 new TB cases, 416 (95% CI 166–2,170) were estimated to be MDR-TB (1%; 0.4%–5%), and in Eastern Europe both absolute number and proportion were much higher (out of 336,842 new TB cases, approximately 43,878 [95% CI 35,881–54,877] were estimated to be MDR-TB, ie, 13%; 11.8%–15.3%).

In Europe as a whole, the proportion of retreatment cases was consistently higher in XDR- than in MDR-TB cases (MDR-TB cases: 49.3%–58.7%; XDR-TB cases 75%–100%). The mean or median number of previous treatment regimens longer than 1 month (MDR-TB cases: 2–2.1; XDR-TB cases 2.4–3) and the number of drugs to which the strains of *M tuberculosis* were resistant (MDR-TB cases: 4–5.3; XDR-TB cases 5–6) similarly was higher in XDR- than in MDR-TB cases.[21]

Also among retreatment cases, the number and proportion of MDR-TB cases is higher in Eastern Europe, the figures being the following: Established Market Economies 413 (330–528), 8.2% (6.8%–10.2%); Central Europe 785 (303–2625), 9.8% (39%–31.3%); Eastern Europe 36,179 (29,216–43,769), 45.5% (41.8%–49.4%).[4,9]

Whereas the United States reported substantial reductions in both the prevalence of MDR-TB (among all TB cases, P = .005) and TB notification rates between 1994 and 2007, in most high-resource countries with low prevalence of TB (United Kingdom, France, and Germany) trends in MDR-TB were stable with a low number and proportion of MDR-TB cases. In Estonia and Latvia, stable trends in the prevalence of MDR-TB among new cases was detected, whereas in Lithuania a slow but significant increase (P = .012) was identified. However, in all the 3 Baltic countries a decreasing TB notification rate (5%–8% reduction per year) was found. In Orel and Tomsk Oblasts (Russian Federation) the prevalence of MDR-TB among new cases increased (P = .001 and P = .006, respectively) together with the absolute number of MDR-TB cases. Although the TB notification rates declined in both regions, the observed decline was slower rate (1%–3% per year) than that observed in the Baltic countries.[4,6]

A total number of 3818 MDR-TB cases were reported, 304 (8.0%) of them as XDR-TB. The prevalence of XDR-TB among cases of MDR-TB was low in Europe, being high (33.3%) only in Ireland and Slovenia, as these countries notified very few cases of MDR-TB and only one case of XDR-TB was reported. In the 8 FSU countries providing data, about 10% of all MDR-TB cases

were XDR-TB, ranging from 4% in Armenia to 23.7% in Estonia. Five of these countries reported 25 cases or more of XDR-TB. In Europe, only Russia (Tomsk Oblast) and Spain reported data for drug resistance stratified by human immunodeficiency virus (HIV) status: no significant association between MDR-TB and HIV infection was found. However, MDR-TB was significantly associated with HIV in Latvia (odds ratio [OR] 2.1, 95% CI 1.4–3.0) and Donetsk Oblast, Ukraine (OR 1.5, 1.1–2). In both countries, resistance to any TB drug was also significantly higher in HIV-positive than in HIV-negative patients (Latvia OR 1.5, 1.1–2.1; Donetsk Oblast OR 1.4, 1.1–1.8).[4,6]

Detailed information on the prevalence of MDR-TB in European countries is summarized in **Table 1**. The core information derived from the European TBNET studies is summarized in **Table 2**.

Epidemiology of MDR and XDR-TB in the United States

Before 1993 when collection of standardized data on drug resistance began in the United States and during the initial years of drug resistance surveillance, MDR-TB was noted most frequently in reports of TB outbreaks. A series of MDR-TB outbreaks in the late 1980s and early 1990s was reported in the MMWR, involving largely HIV-positive populations in congregate settings (hospitals, drug treatment programs, and prisons) and with very high mortality rates.[25] The most well-publicized of these was a cluster of outbreaks in 1 Florida and 3 New York City hospitals in 1990 to 1992, with mortality between 72% and 83% among these HIV-positive cases.[26,27] As a result of these outbreaks and a growing concern about transmission of MDR-TB in HIV-positive populations and in congregate settings, surveillance and reporting practices changed, allowing for a population-based analysis of MDR-TB epidemiology in the United States from 1993 to the present.

Table 3 reports the proportion of MDR-TB cases among all culture-confirmed cases in the United States from 1993 to 2007. Both TB cases and MDR-TB cases have decreased significantly in number since 1993, but the proportion of MDR-TB cases among all cases reported in the United States has remained stable at a little more than 1% since 1997. The epidemiology of MDR-TB has shifted significantly (**Table 4**) since standardized data collection on drug resistance began. At that time, the majority of MDR-TB cases were United States-born (301 cases, or 74.0% of the total 407 MDR-TB cases reported), attributed to a weakened public health infrastructure and poor

TB management practices that failed to prevent acquired drug resistance among TB patients.[26] Strengthening of TB control at the state and local levels received increased attention and financial support, resulting in a dramatic decrease in the number of TB cases overall and a concomitant decrease in MDR-TB cases in the United States-born population. Foreign-born cases now account for more than 80% of MDR-TB cases in the United States. However, this proportion may decrease as overseas screening guidelines for persons applying for immigration have changed. Screening of TB suspects identified by chest radiograph now includes smear, culture, and DST for all positive cultures.[2,3,10] Completion of treatment is required before immigration, so that these cases would no longer be reported as United States cases, and a significant decrease in both numbers and the proportion of foreign-born cases might be expected.

In 2007, the United States reported a total of 13,288 new cases of TB. Of these, 10,421 cases were confirmed by culture and 97.8% (10,190) had DST reported for at least isoniazid and rifampicin. A total of 125 MDR-TB cases (1.2% of those tested) and 2 XDR-TB cases were reported.

At least one XDR-TB case has been reported annually in the United States since reporting of drug resistance began. Between 1993 and 2007, a total of 83 XDR-TB cases were reported, with 18 cases reported in 1993, decreasing to 2 cases in 2007. **Table 2** reports the characteristics of the most significant United States studies on XDR-TB cases. Between the first half and the last half of the reporting period, some notable changes in the demographics of XDR-TB cases have occurred. First, there has been a marked shift from United States- to foreign-born populations. United States-born cases comprised 59% of XDR-TB cases diagnosed between 1993 and 1999, decreasing to 24% of total XDR-TB cases in the 2000 to 2007 cohort, whereas foreign-born cases increased from 38% to 76% during that period. At the same time, there has been a dramatic decrease in the proportion of XDR-TB patients who are also infected with HIV, from 44% in the first period to 12% in the last. However, the proportion of cases with unknown HIV status has remained relatively stable at around 40%, indicating a need for intensified HIV counseling and testing in this population of patients. As would be expected, age and ethnic/racial distributions have changed, tracking with the changes in place of birth and HIV status. Deaths during treatment have decreased from 31% to 12%, with a subsequent increase in those still on treatment (from 9% to 29%), reflecting the availability of additional

drugs and the evolution of treatment regimens. Out of 26 deaths that occurred among XDR-TB cases between 1993 and 2007, there were 21 confirmed HIV-positive patients, underlining the consistently poor treatment outcomes among HIV coinfected XDR-TB cases.

Available data have several limitations. The number of XDR-TB cases is a minimum estimate because of incomplete DST data. Although 57% of MDR-TB cases had DST results reported for at least 1 fluoroquinolone and at least 1 of the 3 second-line injectable drugs, only 22% had DST results reported for all drugs in the definition of XDR TB. In addition, aggregate reporting of drug resistance traditionally has been based only on initial DST results, not on drug resistance that develops during treatment. Another potential factor leading to underestimation of XDR-TB is related to negative culture results in approximately 20% of reported TB cases that are clinically diagnosed, on which DST could not be performed.

The geographic distribution of MDR- and XDR-TB across the United States is uneven, as is the TB burden in general. States that account for the majority of XDR-TB cases notified between 1993 and 2006 include New York (27 cases, of which 18 in New York City), California (11), New Jersey (3), Texas and Nevada (2), and 1 case each in Virginia, Ohio, Michigan, and Illinois. These states are characterized by a larger proportion of foreign-born or vulnerable and HIV-positive populations. Nine of 50 states have reported cases of XDR-TB.

Risk Factors for MDR- and XDR-TB in Europe and in the United States

Drug resistance is strongly associated with previous treatment. In previously treated patients, the probability of any resistance is more than 4-fold higher, and of MDR-TB more than 10-fold higher, than for untreated patients.[28] The findings of a recently published article indicate that MDR-TB and XDR-TB share common predictor variables; previous treatment of active TB disease is the covariate showing the strongest association.[29] Several studies confirmed the relationship between MDR-TB and prior exposure to anti-TB drugs, but the aforementioned was the first study to report that XDR-TB is associated with previous TB treatment even more strongly than MDR-TB.[29-33] In fact, the duration of previous treatment plays a key role in the generation of extremely resistant strains, clearly demonstrated by the higher proportion of retreated cases among MDR-TB and XDR-TB patients (44.5% and 66.7%, respectively) versus the percentage among non-MDR-TB patients (12.6 %). Previous anti-TB treatment

Table 1
Prevalence of MDR-TB in European Countries

Country	Year	Survey Method	No. of New Cases Tested	Prevalence of MDR-TB	No. of Retreatment Cases Tested	Prevalence of MDR-TB
Andorra	2005	Surveillance	9	0 (0%, 0–28.3)	NA	NA
Armenia	2007	Survey	552	52 (9.4%, 7–12.4)	340	147 (43.2%, 37.9–48.7)
Austria	2005	Surveillance	570	11 (1.9%, 1–3.5)	16	2 (12.5%, 1.6–38.3)
Azerbaijan, Baku City	2007	Survey	551	123 (22.3%, 18.5–26.6)	552	308 (55.8%, 49.7–62.4)
Belgium	2005	Surveillance	588	7 (1.2%, 0.5–2.5)	41	3 (7.3%, 1.5–19.9)
Bosnia and Herzegovina	2005	Surveillance	1035	4 (0.4%, 0.1–1)	106	7 (6.6%, 2.7–13.1)
Croatia	2005	Surveillance	586	3 (0.5%, 0.1–1.5)	61	3 (4.9%, 1–13.7)
Czech Republic	2005	Surveillance	562	7 (1.2%, 0.5–2.6)	20	6 (30%, 11.9–54.3)
Denmark	2005	Surveillance	307	5 (1.6%, 0.5–3.8)	18	0 (0%, 0–15.3)
Estonia	2005	Surveillance	316	42 (13.3%, 9.7–17.5)	71	37 (52.1%, 39.9–64.1)
Finland	2005	Surveillance	198	2 (1%, 0.1–3.6)	22	1 (4.5%, 0.1–22.8)
France	2005	Sentinel	1291	14 (1.1%, 0.6–1.8)	112	8 (7.1%, 3.1–13.6)
Georgia	2006	Survey	799	54 (6.8%, 5.1–8.8)	515	141 (27.4%, 23–32.3)
Germany	2005	Surveillance	3094	57 (1.8%, 1.4–2.4)	251	31 (12.4%, 8.5–17.1)
Iceland	2005	Surveillance	7	0 (0%, 0–34.8)	1	0 (0%, 0–95)
Ireland	2005	Surveillance	200	1 (0.5%, 0–2.8)	10	1 (10%, 0.3–44.5)
Israel	2005	Surveillance	211	12 (5.7%, 3–9.7)	3	0 (0%, 0–63.2)
Italy, 8 regions	2005	Surveillance	485	8 (1.6%, 0.7–3.2)	79	14 (17.7%, 10–27.9)
Latvia	2005	Surveillance	873	94 (10.8%, 8.7–13.2)	182	66 (36.3%, 29.3–43.7)

Lithuania	2005	Surveillance	1293	127 (9.8%, 8.2–11.7)	440	209 (47.5%, 42.8–52.3)
Luxembourg	2005	Surveillance	36	0 (0%, 0–8)	NA	NA
Malta	2005	Surveillance	11	0 (0.0%, 0.0–23.8)	NA	NA
Moldova	2006	Surveillance	825	160 (19.4%, 16.5–22.6)	2054	1044 (50.8%, 47.8–54)
Netherlands	2005	Surveillance	709	5 (0.7%, 0.2–1.6)	30	1 (3.3%, 0.1–17.2)
Norway	2005	Surveillance	193	3 (1.6%, 0.3–4.5)	8	0 (0%, 0–31.2)
Poland	2004	Surveillance	2716	8 (0.3%, 0.1–0.6)	522	43 (8.2%, 6–11.1)
Portugal	2005	Surveillance	1407	12 (0.9%, 0.4–1.5)	172	16 (9.3%, 5.4–14.7)
Romania	2004	Surveillance	849	24 (2.8%, 1.8–4.2)	382	42 (11%, 8–14.6)
Russia, Tomsk Oblast	2005	Surveillance	515	77 (15%, 11.8–18.7)	NA	NA
Russia, Orel Oblast	2006	Surveillance	317	28 (8.8%, 5.9–12.5)	30	5 (16.7%, 5.6–34.7)
Russia, Maryel Oblast	2006	Surveillance	304	38 (12.5%, 9–16.8)	NA	NA
Serbia	2005	Surveillance	1112	4 (0.4%, 0.1–0.9)	121	5 (4.1%, 1.4–9.4)
Slovakia	2005	Surveillance	248	4 (1.6%, 0.4–4.1)	56	4 (7.1%, 2–17.3)
Slovenia	2005	Surveillance	217	0 (0%, 0–1.4)	28	1 (3.6%, 0.1–18.3)
Spain, Galicia	2005	Surveillance	566	1 (0.2%, 0–1)	68	1 (1.5%, 0–7.9)
Spain, Aragon	2005	Surveillance	200	0 (0%, 0–1.5)	26	4 (15.4%, 4.4–34.9)
Spain, Barcelona	2005	Surveillance	NA	NA	NA	NA
Sweden	2005	Surveillance	425	2 (0.5%, 0.1–1.7)	17	2 (11.8%, 1.5–36.4)
Switzerland	2005	Surveillance	326	2 (0.6%, 0.1–2.2)	30	2 (6.7%, 0.8–22.1)
Ukraine, Donetsk Oblast	2006	Survey	1003	160 (16%, 13.6–18.6)	494	219 (44.3%, 39.9–48.8)
UK	2005	Surveillance	3428	23 (0.7%, 0.4–1)	271	7 (2.6%, 1–5.2)
Uzbekistan Tashkent	2005	Survey	203	30 (14.8%, 10.2–20.4)	85	51 (60%, 48.8–70.5)

Abbreviation: NA: not available.

Table 2
Clinical and epidemiologic features of drug-resistant cases enrolled in European and United States studies

Setting	Study	Total MDR Cohort Size (Country, Year)	MDR-TB/XDR-TB (n/n)	Representative Sample (MDR Coverage >65%)	Cohort Prevalence of HIV + (%) MDR vs XDR	No. of Drug Strains Resistant to: MDR vs XDR
Europe	Migliori, EID 2007[14]	137 (Italy, Germany, 2003–2006)	126/11	Yes (Italy 69%; Germany 12.6%)	MDR: 10 (9.2%) XDR: 0 (0%)	5 vs 8 (median)
	Migliori, ERJ 2007[13]	425 (Estonia, Italy, Germany, Russia, 1999–2006)	361/64	Yes (Estonia 100%; Italy 69%; Germany 12.6%; Russia (Archangelsk) 100%)	MDR: 17 (5%) XDR: 2 (3.2%)	5 vs 7 (median)
	Eker, EID 2008[22]	184 (Germany, 2004–2006)	177/7	Yes (65%)	MDR: 7 (4.9%) XDR: 0 (0%)	5 vs 9 (median)
United States	Chan, NEJM 2008[23]	174 (Denver, USA)	164/10	No	NA	NA
	Banerjee, CID 2008[24]	424 (California, USA, 1993–2006)	406/18	Yes (100% in California)	NA	NA

Abbreviations: CID, Clinical Infectious Diseases; EID, Emerging Infectious Diseases; ERJ, European Respiratory Journal; NA, not available; NEJM, New England Journal of Medicine.

Table 3
Incidence of MDR-TB in the United States among culture-positive cases, evaluated on 202,611 TB cases (1993–2007)

Year	No (%)	Yes (%)	Not Reported (%)	Total TB Cases/Year (%)[a]
		MDR		
1993	17218 (96.4)	484 (2.7)	159 (0.9)	17861 (100)
1994	17191 (97.1)	431 (2.4)	77 (0.4)	17699 (100)
1995	16765 (97.7)	327 (1.9)	62 (0.4)	17154 (100)
1996	16077 (98.1)	250 (1.5)	62 (0.4)	16389 (100)
1997	15065 (98.3)	201 (1.3)	60 (0.4)	15326 (100)
1998	14116 (98.4)	155 (1.1)	77 (0.5)	14348 (100)
1999	13319 (98)	157 (1.2)	109 (0.8)	13585 (100)
2000	12407 (98.1)	144 (1.1)	95 (0.8)	12646 (100)
2001	12113 (98.3)	152 (1.2)	59 (0.5)	12324 (100)
2002	11322 (98.3)	155 (1.3)	39 (0.3)	11516 (100)
2003	11159 (98.6)	116 (1)	48 (0.4)	11323 (100)
2004	10966 (98.4)	128 (1.1)	55 (0.5)	11149 (100)
2005	10508 (98.1)	123 (1.1)	80 (0.7)	10711 (100)
2006	10203 (97.3)	117 (1.1)	166 (1.6)	10486 (100)
2007	9739 (96.5)	119 (1.2)	236 (2.3)	10094 (100)
Total	198168	3059 ($R^2 = 0.851$)	1384	202611

[a] Multidrug-resistant is not available if the value of "Verification Criteria" is other than "Positive Culture". This affects totals and percentages.
Data from Online Tuberculosis Information System (OTIS). National Tuberculosis Surveillance System, United States, 1993–2007. Accessed at http://wonder.cdc.gov/tb-v2007.html on June 7, 2009.

increased the chance of multidrug resistance fivefold (OR 5.41) and MDR-TB occurred significantly more in people aged 25 to 44 (OR 2.5) and 45 to 64 years (OR 1.89). Alcohol abuse (OR 1.56) was also an independent risk factor for MDR-TB due to its impact on TB treatment adherence. Among the patients younger than 25 years, female gender (OR 7.81) and place of birth outside the host country (in data from Estonia), mainly in individuals coming from the FSU (OR 79.7), were strongly associated with MDR-TB.

Immigration, mainly from high MDR-TB prevalence countries, could increase the risk of being infected by a resistant strain not only among foreign-born people but also native individuals.[29,34] MDR-TB may affect young adults, which may result in increased rates of TB transmission to their children. Moreover, HIV-infected children are at increased risk of TB, and there is strong evidence that TB is more common in children living in households affected by TB. On the other hand, living in an urban area resulted in significantly less likelihood of having MDR-TB (OR 0.21).

The independent variables associated with XDR-TB were previous anti-TB treatment (OR 4.01) and

homelessness (OR 3.35); homeless people, living in poor conditions and malnourished, usually have reduced access to health care assistance, prolonging the period of infectiousness and, consequently, increasing the risk of mycobacterial transmission among their close contacts.

Another important issue, frequently described by several investigators, is the high rate of defaulting from treatment and treatment failure among socially disadvantaged patients, including alcohol abusers and homeless people.[29,35,36]

Previous reports have described the association between MDR-TB and HIV-infection, and a European meta-analysis well described the higher risk (OR 3.52) of developing active MDR-TB disease.[30,32] High TB prevalence in prisons and transmission of resistant strains related to overcrowding and inability to isolate resistant cases is internationally well documented (relative risk for MDR-TB is 1.9).[36,37]

SURVEILLANCE

TB (and MDR-TB) surveillance is an epidemiologic tool designed to monitor the spread of the disease

Table 4
Incidence of MDR-TB in the United States among new cases according to place of birth, 1993–2007

	New MDR-TB Cases		
Year	Total	United States-born (%)	Foreign-born (%)
1993	407	301 (74)	103 (26)
1994	353	238 (67)	110 (33)
1995	254	169 (67)	85 (33)
1996	207	105 (51)	101 (49)
1997	155	76 (49)	79 (51)
1998	132	55 (42)	76 (58)
1999	127	39 (31)	88 (69)
2000	120	38 (32)	82 (68)
2001	118	34 (29)	84 (71)
2002	130	36 (28)	94 (72)
2003	92	24 (26)	68 (74)
2004	102	26 (25)	76 (75)
2005	98	19 (19)	78 (81)
2006	94	17 (18)	77 (82)
2007	98	20 (20)	78 (80)

to establish patterns of progression. The main role of TB and MDR-TB surveillance is to observe, predict, and minimize the harm caused by outbreaks and epidemics/pandemics, as well as to decipher the key risk factors involved. A core component of TB and MDR-TB surveillance is represented by case reporting.[6,38] As TB/MDR-TB surveillance benefits from collecting the key information required to achieve TB control (and eventually, elimination), the organization of surveillance in Europe and in the United States is described here in terms of variables and flow.[39–41] Accurate identification and timely reporting of both active TB disease and latent TB infection have been considered essential to achieve TB elimination: both Europe and the United States have committed to reaching elimination, defined as less than 1 case per million population annually.[41–43]

Surveillance of MDR- and XDR-TB in Europe

Following the recommendations of the Wolfheze Conference convening representatives of all European (Western and Eastern) countries,[39–44] TB surveillance was launched in Europe in 1996 as a European Commission-funded project under the name of "EuroTB." Individual information on TB notification for the previous calendar year has been collected annually. The project was based at the Institut de Veille Sanitaire (InVS) in France. Since January 2008, the ECDC and the WHO

Regional Office for Europe jointly coordinate European TB surveillance. The aim of the new TB and MDR-TB surveillance system is to ensure collection of high-quality standardized TB data from all the 53 countries in the WHO European Region. Designated surveillance institutions are in charge of collecting national data, reported to a common database. Data from the EU and EEA/EFTA countries are validated and processed in the platform of The European Surveillance System (TESSy), whereas data from the other countries are validated and processed in the Centralized Information System for Infectious Diseases (CISID) platform. The procedures and methods guiding European TB Surveillance activities are those strongly recommended by European advisors nominated by ECDC, WHO, and International Union Against Tuberculosis and Lung Disease. Several variables are analyzed: number of TB notifications, pulmonary or extrapulmonary diseases, concomitant HIV infection, resistance to anti-TB drugs, treatment outcomes, cases among immigrants.

Drug resistance is low in most EU countries other than FSU states. Drug resistance surveillance (DRS) methodology varies across countries, and data on the result of DST for isoniazid, rifampicin, ethambutol, and streptomycin at the start of anti-TB treatment are reported as "susceptible" or "resistant." Proportions of drug-resistant cases are calculated using as a denominator those cases with DST results available for at least isoniazid and rifampicin. DST results may be collected routinely for all culture-positive TB cases notified, or for cases included in specific surveys or diagnosed in/referred to selected laboratories. Geographic coverage of DRS is partial in some countries. The representativeness of diagnostic DST data depends on the routine use of culture and DST at TB diagnosis.[44–46] Of the 21 countries that had more than one laboratory performing DST, national external quality assurance schemes existed in 13; national reference laboratories (NRL) had participated in international quality assurance for DST. Concordance with SRL was 100% for both isoniazid and rifampicin in 18 countries, and 89% to 99% for one or both drugs in another 5 countries.

In summary, TB surveillance has to be improved even in industrialized countries of Europe, where case notification to the central level occurs within a median period of 7 days, independent of mandatory notification requirements. The mean completeness of TB case-reporting was estimated to be 93.5% (range 65%–100%). Integration between HIV and TB registries is performed in a few countries, and in others, both databases are cross-matched periodically.

Surveillance of MDR- and XDR-TB in the United States

MDR-TB has had a significant impact on surveillance practices in the United States. Following the well-publicized outbreaks of MDR-TB in the late 1980s and early 1990s described earlier, the CDC convened an MDR-TB Task Force to develop a plan for addressing MDR-TB in the United States.[47] The Task Force identified 4 problem areas related to United States surveillance and epidemiology: (1) inadequate surveillance systems, (2) lack of data on the extent of MDR-TB transmission in congregate settings and the community, (3) lack of data on risk factors for MDR-TB infection and disease among populations at high risk such as health workers, and (4) lack of information specific to HIV-infected populations and MDR-TB.

Key surveillance recommendations included promoting DST for all culture-positive cases; modifying the standardized national Report of a Verified Case of Tuberculosis (RVCT) form to include DST results as data elements; upgrading the national TB reporting system to an electronic format; and providing financial and technical support to state-level programs to accomplish increased surveillance. Routine testing for drug resistance to first-line agents (at least isoniazid and rifampicin, and often ethambutol and streptomycin) and data collection on DST patterns of all

culture-positive TB cases began in 1993. DST results for second-line agents are also reported on the RVCT as appropriate for MDR-TB cases. As a result, the United States is one of the few countries (aside from South Korea and Latvia) where population-based data on drug resistance are presently available.

In addition, the CDC formed an outbreak investigation team at the national level to provide support to states for complex MDR-TB outbreak investigation and containment (as well as TB outbreaks in general). Sentinel surveillance activities were recommended for tracking infection in health care workers and others at risk for infection, and measures were taken to enhance surveillance related to TB/HIV coinfection.

Since 2004, the CDC have offered genotyping services (for all isolates) to detect potential outbreaks or clusters of TB and MDR-TB to all 68 reporting regions that have a cooperative agreement with the CDC. States must apply to participate in the genotyping service, which is performed by laboratories in California and Michigan. The CDC also support the TB Epidemiologic Studies Consortium (TBESC), with task orders that include molecular epidemiology of MDR-TB to further characterize dynamics of MDR-TB transmission, identify risk factors, and propose interventions.[48] The results of this work are not yet available.

The electronic national TB surveillance system (NTSS) collects data on the following through the RVCT: demographic variables, including country of birth; clinical data on diagnosis and treatment; laboratory data on diagnosis, monitoring, and drug resistance; risk factor variables, including occupation (eg, health care worker, institutional staff), substance abuse, homelessness, congregate setting residence, HIV status, and similar factors; and treatment outcome variables. All variables are well defined in a data dictionary, and staff at the state level is trained and responsible for data quality checks and aggregate reporting to the national level through the electronic NTSS.

Why Surveillance is Still Unable to Provide Reliable Figures and Why Special Studies are Needed

Whereas most European countries and the United States have equipped their surveillance to monitor MDR-TB, the situation remains challenging for XDR-TB. In Europe, the first evidence that surveillance systems were unable to provide timely information on the occurrence of XDR-TB cases was represented by the media storm following publication[49] of the first study reporting poor outcomes for

XDR-TB cases (XDR-TB cases having a relative risk of death 5.45 times higher than MDR-TB cases).[14]

The surveillance system was unable to detect these cases simply because the entire set of XDR-TB defining drugs was not systematically tested. This problem has been underlined in the majority of studies investigating or commenting on XDR-TB[21,50] and by official documents.[51]

To provide timely detection of incident XDR-TB cases, the following conditions need to be met in low TB incidence countries as well: (1) adequate technical capacity to test all isolated MDR-TB strains for all XDR-TB defining drugs by quality-assured laboratories; (2) policy in force ensuring referral of all strains from culture/first-line DST laboratories to second-line DST referral laboratories; (3) links between the notification system and the reference laboratories established to ensure that second-line DST results are available; and (4) availability, within the surveillance system, of the appropriate fields necessary to record the information on the XDR-defining drugs on which DST is performed in reference laboratories.

Furthermore, surveillance systems should be equipped to report treatment outcomes for at least 24 months following treatment initiation to capture the outcomes of MDR- and XDR-TB cases.

Although the different countries of Europe are taking action to improve their surveillance systems, most of the information presently available on XDR-TB is based on "ad hoc" designed studies.[21,50]

CLINICAL PRESENTATION AND OUTCOMES

The initial clinical presentation of patients with drug-resistant TB in most cases does not differ from that of patients with TB due to drug-susceptible strains of M tuberculosis. In fact, clinical presentation of patients with MDR- and XDR-TB may be variable (**Fig. 2**). However, extrapulmonary involvement and progressive disease in patients with a previous history of anti-TB treatment may be more frequently expected.

Data from a large retrospective cohort (>5550 cases) recruited 10 years ago (including a European cohort from Italy and Ivanovo Oblast, Russian Federation) provided evidence that standard short-course chemotherapy, based on first-line drugs, was inadequate to treat patients with MDR-TB.[52] A study from Russia demonstrated a high relapse rate (27.8%) of MDR-TB cases declared "successfully" cured with standard short-course chemotherapy regimens (WHO Category 1 and 2) within a median time of 8 months (2.46 recurrences were observed in 100 person-months).[53]

As M tuberculosis drug resistance increases, it has become more obvious that the clinical outcome is mostly dependent on the degree of M tuberculosis drug resistance, availability of second- and third-line drugs, and adherence to the therapy.[19,22,53–58] Risk factors for adverse

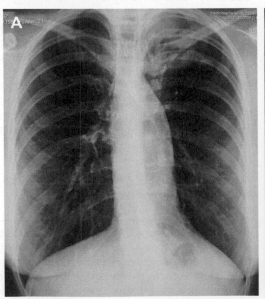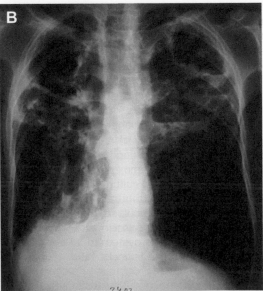

Fig. 2. *Mycobacterium tuberculosis* drug resistance cannot be identified by radiographic imaging. A 21-year-old woman with isolated left upper lobe infiltrate (*A*) and a 38-year-old man with extensive bilateral cavities (*B*), both presenting with pulmonary TB due to MDR strains of *M tuberculosis*.

treatment outcome in patients with MDR-TB and XDR-TB have recently been reviewed in detail.[21,59,60] These factors include delayed treatment initiation,[61] prior treatment with anti-TB drugs, resistance to fluoroquinolones or to capreomycin, HIV seropositivity, and other immunosuppressive conditions.[15,17,21,22,54–56,58,62–70]

The treatment of patients with MDR-TB and XDR-TB relies on drugs that are less potent, need to be administered for a much longer time, and are substantially more toxic than those used to treat TB caused by drug-susceptible strains (**Table 5**). In contrast, the costs of a second-line drug regimen are much higher: up to thousands of dollars compared with about US $20 cost per patient for the standard 6-month short-course, first-line chemotherapy regimen (WHO Category 1).

The optimal duration of any given combination of anti-TB drugs for treatment of MDR- and XDR-TB has not been defined in controlled clinical trials, although WHO has recently provided suggestions that are described here.[71] In addition, the role of single drugs or drug combinations in effective MDR-TB and XDR-TB treatment is difficult to investigate in double-blinded, placebo-controlled, prospective clinical trials due to ethical considerations and cost. Especially the effectiveness of treatment with third-line antituberculosis drugs (amoxicillin-clavulanate, clarithromycin, clofazimine, linezolid, called Group 5 drugs in the WHO guidelines, see **Table 5**) is difficult to ascertain. Long-term treatment of patients with MDR- and XDR-TB with linezolid at a regular daily dosage of 600 mg twice a day was shown recently to be related to severe toxicity with little additional benefit in clinical outcome in a large retrospective cohort study.[72] Promising treatment options, like meropenem-clavulanate, which were recently reported in the news will need to be investigated clinically before they can be recommended for clinical use.[73]

In Europe, treatment outcome data in patients with MDR-TB showing cure rates of 60% to 75% have been reported in Estonia, Latvia, and the Russian Federation since 2004.[10] The proportion of MDR-TB patients who were successfully treated ranged from 77% among new cases to 69% among previously treated patients.[74] A recent report confirmed that XDR-TB has higher probability of death, longer hospitalization, longer treatment duration, and delayed microbiological conversion compared with MDR-TB at TB reference centers in Italy and Germany.[15]

However, earlier observations from the Tugela Ferry outbreak in the Republic of South Africa that XDR-TB is untreatable have not been confirmed in other areas of the world.[75] A recent systematic review on MDR-TB and XDR-TB included 2 studies from North-America and 3 studies from Europe.[13,14,21–24] This review showed that XDR-TB can be successfully treated in more than 50% of patients (**Table 6**). However, treatment duration is significantly longer and outcomes are in general poorer than for non–XDR-TB patients.

Surgical resection of infected lung tissue has been proven to be a useful strategy in the treatment of MDR- and XDR-TB.[76–79] Indications for surgical interventions include (1) severe drug resistance with a high probability of treatment failure of medical therapy alone, (2) localized disease with good chances for complete or nearly complete resection and adequate expected postoperative lung function, and (3) sufficient activity of anti-TB drugs to ensure postsurgery stump healing.[79,80] Anti-TB treatment should be offered for at least 3 months before the surgical intervention.[80,81] Surgical interventions complementing individualized chemotherapy regimens guided by DST have led to treatment success rates in patients with MDR-TB of greater than 90% in several studies, but success rates in patients with XDR-TB are lower, as would be expected.[21,78,82–88]

Designing an Optimal Drug Regimen

Recommendations for the management of patients with MDR- and XDR-TB have recently been reviewed.[59,60,89–92]

A method of grouping anti-TB drugs based on potency, experience of use, and drug class can be used to design an empirical regimen for the treatment of suspected MDR-TB cases (see **Table 5**).[55,71] The general principles for designing a regimen are reported in **Table 7**. Treatment outcomes are optimized if patients with MDR- or XDR-TB receive timely and adequate empirical therapy including multiple drugs with which the patient has not been treated before.[57,65]

To achieve a regimen designed to treat the majority of patients with a minimum of 4 effective drugs as is recommended, it may be necessary to use 5, 6, or more drugs to cover all the possible patterns of resistance when DST results for second-line agents are not yet available. As summarized in **Table 7**, an injectable agent and a fluoroquinolone form the core of the preferred regimen.

The latest WHO guidelines propose different treatment strategies for individuals suspected to harbor MDR-TB strains.[71] Treatment regimens including second-line anti-TB drugs can considerably improve cure rates and reduce transmission.[56,64,66,93–96] Depending on specific country conditions, treatment protocols may recommend a standardized treatment regimen for all MDR-TB

Table 5
Antituberculosis drugs, dosages, adverse effects, and drug interactions

Antituberculous Drugs	Recommended Daily Dosage	Common Adverse Effects (Not Exclusive)	Drug Interactions	Comments
1. First-line oral agents (Group 1)				
Isoniazid	5 mg/kg OD should not exceed 300 mg/d, consider always to coadminister vitamin B6	Elevated transaminases; hepatitis; peripheral neuropathy; GI intolerance; CNS toxicity	May increase phenytoin and carbamazepine levels; INH drug levels may be decreased by corticosteroids	Avoid administration if preexisting liver damage; avoid alcohol; also available for IV or IM injection
Rifampicin	10 mg/kg OD >50 kg: 600 mg <50 kg: 450 mg	Elevation of liver enzymes; hepatitis; hypersensitivity; fever; GI disorders: anorexia, nausea, vomiting, abdominal pain; discoloration (orange or brown) of urine, tears and other body fluids; thrombopenia	Many drug interactions: induces cytochrome P450, reduces effectiveness of oral contraceptive pill	Monitor liver functions; inform the patient about discoloration of urine; also available for IV injection
Ethambutol	15–25 mg/kg OD maximum 2.0 g/d	Optic neuritis; hyperuricemia; peripheral neuropathy (rare)	Antacids may decrease absorption, ethionamide may increase adverse effects of EMB	Baseline screen for visual acuity and color perception, (repeated monthly); contraindicated in pts with preexisting lesions of optic nerve; also available for IV injection
Pyrazinamide	30 mg/kg OD maximum 2.0 g/d	Arthralgia, hyperuricemia, toxic hepatitis, GI discomfort	Ethionamid may increase the risk of hepatotoxicity	Asymptomatic hyperuricemia; monitor liver functions; not available for IV injection
2. Injectables (Group 2)				
Streptomycin IV/IM administration only	0.75–1 g OD <50 kg: 0.75 g/d >50 kg: 1 g/d maximum cumulative dose 50 g	Auditory and vestibular nerve damage (nonreversible); renal failure (usually reversible); allergies; Nausea; rash, neuromuscular blockade	Cave: other nephrotoxic or ototoxic drugs: do not coadminister together with penicillins in the same tubing system	Audiometry; cumulative dose should not be exceeded; monitor renal function closely

Amikacin IV administration only	0.75–1 g OD <50 kg: 0.75 g/d >50 kg: 1 g/d maximum cumulative dose 50 g	Auditory and vestibular nerve damage (nonreversible); renal failure (usually reversible); allergies; Nausea; rash, neuromuscular blockade	Cave: other nephrotoxic or ototoxic drugs; do not coadminister together with penicillins in the same tubing system; avoid nondepolarizing muscle relaxants	Audiometry; monitor renal function closely; consider IV port implantation to avoid long-term IM treatment
Capreomycin IV/IM administration only	0.75–1 g OD <50 kg: 0.75 g/d >50 kg: 1 g/d maximum cumulative dose 50 g	Auditory and vestibular nerve damage (nonreversible); renal failure (usually reversible); Bartter-like syndrome; allergies; neuromuscular blockade	Cave: other nephrotoxic or ototoxic drugs; do not coadminister together with penicillins in the same tubing system; avoid nondepolarizing muscle relaxants	Audiometry; monitor renal function and electrolytes in serum and urine closely; consider IV port implantation to avoid long-term IM treatment
Kanamycin IV administration only	375–500 mg BID <50 kg: 0.75 g/d >50 kg: 1 g/d maximum cumulative dose 50 g	Auditory and vestibular nerve damage (nonreversible); renal failure (usually reversible); allergies; Nausea; rash, neuromuscular blockade	Cave: other nephrotoxic or ototoxic drugs; do not coadminister together with penicillins in the same tubing system; avoid nondepolarizing muscle relaxants	Audiometry; monitor renal function and electrolytes in serum and urine closely; consider IV port implantation to avoid long-term IM treatment
3. Fluoroquinolones (Group 3)				
Levofloxacin Also available for IV injection	500–1000 mg OD	Gastrointestnal discomfort, CNS disorders, tendon rupture (rare); Hypersensitivity; C. diff. colitis	Antacids, calcium, zinc, iron and other cations (milk products) significantly decrease	Avoid other drugs know to prolong the QT interval; Likely very good antituberculosis activity, increasing drug resistance is expected because of widespread use of fluoroquinolones against LRTI

(continued on next page)

Table 5
(continued)

Antituberculous Drugs	Recommended Daily Dosage	Common Adverse Effects (Not Exclusive)	Drug Interactions	Comments
Ciprofloxacin Also available for IV injection	500–750 mg BID	Gastrointestinal discomfort, CNS disorders, tendon rupture (rare); Hypersensitivity; C. diff. colitis	Antacids, calcium, zinc, iron and other cations (milk products) significantly decrease ciprofloxacin levels	Avoid other drugs know to prolong the QT interval; Likely very good antituberculosis activity, increasing drug resistance is expected because of widespread use of fluoroquinolones against LRTI
Moxifloxacin Also available for IV injection	400 mg OD	Gastrointestinal discomfort; headache; dizziness, hallucinations; increased transaminases QT prolongation; C diff. colitis	Antacids, calcium, zinc, iron and other divalent or trivalent cations significantly decrease moxifloxacin levels	Avoid other drugs know to prolong the QT interval; Likely very good antituberculosis activity, increasing drug resistance is expected because of widespread use of fluoroquinolones against LRTI
4. Second-line oral agents (Group 4)				
Rifabutin	150–450 mg OD consider to monitor drug levels	Anemia; GI discomfort; discoloration (orange or brown) of urine and other body fluids; uveitis; elevated liver enzymes	Weaker inductor of cytochrome P450 than rifampicin	Monitor LFTs; In HIV-infected pts on ARTs generally preferred instead of rifampicin; inform the patient about discoloration of urine
Ethionamid	0,75–1 g OD	Severe GI intolerance; nausea; vomiting; hepatitis; CNS disorders	Aggravates risk of neurotoxicity of cycloserine (should be avoided in pts with a history of seizures); transient increase in INH levels	Severe GI side effects and orthostatic hypotension limit its use

Drug	Dosage	Adverse effects	Interactions	Remarks
Prothionamide	0,75–1 g OD	Severe GI intolerance; nausea; vomiting; hepatitis; CNS disorders	Aggravates risk of neurotoxicity of cycloserine (should be avoided in pts with a history of seizures); transient increase in INH levels	Severe GI side effects and orthostatic hypotension limit its use
Cycloserine	250 mg TID maximum 1000 mg/day	CNS disorders, anxiety, confusion, dizziness, psychosis, seizures, headache	Aggravates CNS side effects of INH and ethionamide/prothionamide	Contraindicated in pts with a history of epilepsy; CNS side effects occur usually within the first 2 weeks
Terizidone	250 mg TID maximum 1000 mg/day	CNS disorders, anxiety, confusion, dizziness, psychosis, seizures, headache	Aggravates CNS side effects of INH and prothionamide	Contraindicated in epileptics; CNS side effects occur usually within the first 2 weeks
Para-aminosalicylic acid	4 g TID	GI intolerance; nausea; diarrhea; vomiting; hypersensitivity	May increase drug levels of INH and may aggravate risk of ethionamide hepatotoxicity; decreases digoxin absorption	Delayed release granules should be taken with acidic food or drink; contraindicated in patients with severe renal impairment (risk of crystalluria); rare risk of fatal hepatitis
Thiacetazone	50 mg TID	Hypersensitivity; GI intolerance; vertigo; hepatitis	Possible aggravation of aminoglycoside-induced ototoxicity	Should be avoided in HIV+ individuals because of increased risk of Stevens-Johnson-syndrome
5. Oral reserve drugs with uncertain antituberculosis activity (Group 5)				
Linezolid	600 mg OD (recommended for 600 mg BID dosage for MRSA and VRE infections)	Thrombopenia, anemia, neuropathy	Avoid coadministration with buspirone, meperidone, fluoxetine, and serotonin 5HT1 receptor agonists	Frequent adverse effects. Once daily dosage with 600 mg likely as effective as twice daily dosage with fewer adverse effects
Clofazimine	100 mg OD	Ichthyosis; gastrointestinal discomfort nausea; vomiting; discoloration of the skin	Aluminum-magnesium antacid may decrease the absorption of clofazimine substantially	Licensed for the treatment of multibacillary leprosy

(continued on next page)

Table 5
(continued)

Antituberculous Drugs	Recommended Daily Dosage	Common Adverse Effects (Not Exclusive)	Drug Interactions	Comments
Amoxicillin-clavunate	875–125 mg BID or 500–250 mg TID	GI discomfort; diarrhea; rash	Allopurinol may increase the risk of rash; avoid concurrent administration of tetracyclines	Rash typically appears after the first week of treatment; avoid in the setting of infectious mononucleosis
Clarithromycin	500 mg BID	GI discomfort	Clarithromycin is a substrate and inhibitor of CYP 3A-4. Inhibitors of CYP 3A-4 may increase clarithromycin serum levels while inducers of CYP 3A-4 may decrease the serum levels	Azithromycin has a better tissue penetration than clarithromycin and is better tolerated, but clinical data are lacking on its efficacy in the treatment of TB

Abbreviations: ART, antiretroviral therapy; BID, twice per day; C diff, *Clostridium difficile*; CNS, central nervous system; EMB, ethambutol; GI, gastrointestinal; HIV, human immuno-deficiency virus; INH, isoniazid; IM, intramuscular; IV, intravenous; LFT, liver function test; LRTI, lower respiratory tract infection; MRSA, methicillin-resistant *Staphylococcus aureus*; OD, once per day; pts, patients; TID, 3 times per day; VRE, vancomycin-resistant enterococci.

Table 6
Treatment efficacy end-points in European and United States studies on MDR-TB and XDR-TB

Setting	Study	Times to Conversion	Treatment Success MDR vs XDR n (%)	Failure MDR vs XDR n (%)	Death MDR vs XDR n (%)	Follow-up (Months)
Europe	Migliori, EID 2007[14]	SS: 41 vs 110 days C: 58 vs 97.5 days (median)	45 (35.7%) vs 0	NA	8 (6.3%) vs 4 (36.4%) P: <0.001; RR: 5.45	42 (median)
	Migliori, ERJ 2007[13]	SS: 56 vs 110 days C: 60 vs 168 days (median)	165 (45.7%) vs 22 (34.4%)	32 (8.9%) vs 12 (18.7%) P: 0.016; RR: 2.12	43 (11.9%) vs 14 (21.9%) P: 0.03; RR: 1.84	42 (median)
	Eker, EID 2008[22]	SS: 53.5 vs 88 days C: 61.5 vs 117 days (median)	105 (59.3%) vs 4 (57.1%)	1 (0.6%) vs 0	14 (7.9%) vs 1 (14.3%) P: 0.5; RR: 1.81	48 (median)
United States	Chan, NEJM 2008[23]	NA	164/10	NA	Hazard ratio (XDR) 2.5 P: 0.07	NA
	Banerjee, CID 2008[24]	C: 98.5 vs 195 days (median)	345 (66%) vs 7 (41.2%)	NA	80 (15.3%) vs 5 (29.4%) P: 0.4; RR: 1.41	NA

Abbreviations: C, controls; CID, Clinical Infectious Diseases; EID, Emerging Infectious Diseases; ERJ, European Respiratory Journal; NA, not available; NEJM, New England Journal of Medicine; RR, relative risk; SS, study subjects.

cases (eg, in countries where DST is not widely available), or may alternatively recommend individualized treatment based on individual DST results. If standardized combinations of second-line drugs are chosen, representative national DRS data on predominant resistance patterns to specific treatment categories are needed. An alternative approach is to design a regimen based on the individual history of previous anti-TB therapy, and eventually redesign it guided by individual DST. Relevant laboratory capacity is necessary if this option is chosen, as DST on most second-line drugs must be performed.

Although the individual patient's treatment duration should be guided by sputum smear and culture conversion, in general an injectable agent should be continued for at least the first 6 months of treatment. The entire treatment should be no less than 18 months *after* culture conversion. Extension to 24 months may be indicated in patients defined as "chronic cases" with extensive pulmonary damage.[71,97] In clinical practice, the treatment with second- and third-line antituberculosis chemotherapy in MDR- and XDR-TB is frequently influenced by the occurrence of adverse drug events. A larger proportion of patients who are being treated with a fluoroquinolone-containing regimen will likely be cured after 12 months of therapy.[58,98] Unfortunately, reliable indicators to individually guide the duration of anti-TB drug treatment are not available.

MDR- AND XDR-TB CONTROL: CHALLENGES

Within the United States, MDR- and XDR-TB control and prevention is built on the following actions: (1) case management (primarily nurse-based) of TB patients through the public health system to ensure completion of treatment and prevent additional development of drug resistance; (2) DST for all culture-confirmed cases of TB and use of rapid DST methods for cases with a high suspicion of drug resistance and prompt initiation of appropriate treatment; (3) limiting access to first- and second-line anti-TB drugs to prescription only; (4) infection control to prevent transmission; (5) contact investigation to identify and treat contacts with active disease or latent TB infection; and (6) revised overseas screening guidelines for persons applying for immigration to the United States and requirements for complete, documented treatment of identified TB cases before immigration.[99,100]

Although the burden of drug-resistant TB is low in the United States, several challenges must be faced to reach the goal of TB elimination. First,

Table 7
General principles for designing an empirical regimen to treat MDR-TB

Basic Principles	Comments
1. Use at least 4 drugs of know effectiveness or highly likely to be effective	Effectiveness is supported by several factors (more of them are present more likely is the drug will be effective): A. Susceptibility is there at DST B. No previous history of treatment failure with the drug C. No known close contacts with resistance to the drug D. DRS indicates resistance is rare in similar patients E. No common use of the drug in the area If at least 4 drugs are not certain to be effective, use 5–7 drugs depending on the specific drugs and level of uncertainty
2. Do not use drugs for which resistance crosses over	A. Rifamycins (rifampicin, rifabutin, rifapentin, rifalazil): have high level of cross-resistance B. Fluoroquinolones: variable cross-resistance; in vitro data show some higher-generation agent remain susceptible when lower-generation are resistant (clinical significance of the phenomenon still unknown) C. Aminoglycosides and polypeptides: not all cross-resistant; in general only kanamycin and amikacin fully cross-resistant
3. Eliminate drugs likely to be not safe for the patient	A. Known severe allergy or difficult-to-manage intolerance B. High risk of severe adverse effects including: renal failure, deafness, hepatitis, depression and/or psychosis C. Unknown or questionable drug quality
4. Include drugs from groups 1–5 in a hierarchical order, based on potency	A. Use any group 1 (oral first-line) drugs that are likely to be effective (see section 1 of this table) B. Use an effective injectable aminoglycoside or polypeptide (group 2 drugs) C. Use a fluoroquinolone (group 3) D. Use the remaining group 4 drugs to make a regimen consisting of at least 4 effective drugs. For regimens with ≤4 effective drugs, add second-line drugs most likely to be effective, to give up to 5–7 drugs in total, with at least 4 of them highly likely to be effective. The number of drugs will depend on the degree of uncertainty E. Use group 5 drugs as needed so that at least 4 drugs are likely to be effective
5. Be prepared to prevent, monitor, and manage adverse effects for each of the drugs selected	A. Ensure laboratory services for hematology, biochemistry, serology, and audiometry are available B. Establish a clinical and laboratory baseline before starting the regimen C. Initiate treatment gradually for a difficult-to-tolerate drug, splitting daily doses of Eto/Pto, Cs, and PAS D. Ensure ancillary drugs are available to manage adverse effects E. Organize intake supervision for all doses

Abbreviations: Cs, cycloserine; DST, drug susceptibility testing; Eto, ethionamide; PAS, para-aminosalicylic acid; Pto, prothionamide.

expertise in TB diagnosis and treatment has dwindled as the burden of TB has decreased, leaving many jurisdictions without experienced TB providers. In addition, although laboratory capacity is far greater than in much of the world, the ability to do second-line DST is still concentrated within only a few laboratories in the United States. Third, the TB burden overseas plays a significant role in shaping TB epidemiology in the United States, particularly the epidemiology of MDR- and XDR-TB. This recognition has prompted the Federal Tuberculosis Task Force to recommend further United States engagement in technical assistance and support for TB control overseas, particularly in the countries from which it receives the majority of cases, as a key component of addressing domestic MDR- and XDR-TB control.[47]

Many of the issues discussed earlier are also applicable to Western Europe, the key difference being that the proximity of settings with high burden of MDR- and XDR-TB in the neighboring Eastern European countries makes the threat of drug-resistant TB ever more tangible. As a result, several EU-led initiatives have been launched under the auspices of the ECDC, the European Commission, Member States, and relevant stakeholders. An EU Framework Action Plan was launched in 2008, setting control of MDR- and XDR-TB as a priority area and recognizing the need for extending the benefits of TB control to the most vulnerable populations as a matter of equity and public health importance in preventing TB morbidity and mortality.[101] A TB surveillance system for the EU and extending to the entire WHO European Region is in place and provides a reliable monitoring tool for the MDR-TB epidemic. Progress made by the Baltic States, which are experiencing stabilization of overall MDR-TB rates and a decline in secondary MDR-TB, in dealing with this problem may provide an example that can be of use in similar settings and contexts.[45]

In 2007, to combat the emerging threat, WHO and partners formulated a policy to address the MDR- and XDR-TB epidemic globally.[102] The major recommendation of the panel was to improve general TB control globally to prevent the selection of MDR- and XDR-TB mutants, and then to better organize early diagnosis and effective treatment of the existing cases. The WHO developed a broader approach, having the DOTS (Directly Observed Treatment, Short-course) strategy as the element of continuity; the new Stop TB Strategy was prepared to achieve the TB-related Millennium Development Goal, eg, making TB incidence decline steadily.[103] As summarized in **Table 8**, the Strategy consists of 6 elements: (1) pursue high-quality DOTS expansion and enhancement; (2) address TB/HIV, MDR-TB, and other challenges; (3) contribute to health system strengthening; (4) engage all care providers; (5) empower people with TB and communities; and (6) enable and promote research.

To combat the MDR- and XDR-TB epidemic, a WHO-convened Task Force developed a Global MDR-TB and XDR-TB Response Plan (2007–2008), and in April 2009 a governmental conference was organized in China to develop the Beijing Call for Action,[51,104] committing the 27 high MDR-TB burden countries to a specific set of actions for MDR- and XDR-TB containment and prevention.

Seven additional recommendations[1] were developed to prevent and control XDR-TB, including:

1. Preventing XDR-TB through basic strengthening TB and HIV control. The new Stop TB strategy and the Global Plan to Stop TB are the key reference documents to guide these priority interventions.[103,105]
2. Improving management of individuals suspected to be affected by XDR-TB through accelerated access to laboratory facilities, with rapid DST test for rifampicin and isoniazid resistance, and DST for MDR-TB cases, as well as improved detection of cases suspected of harboring MDR strains both in high and low HIV prevalence settings.
3. Strengthening management of XDR-TB and treatment design in both HIV-negative and positive individuals, through adequate use of second-line drugs and patient-centered approaches to ensure support and supervision.
4. Standardizing the definition of XDR-TB.
5. Increasing health care worker infection control and protection mainly (but not exclusively) in high HIV prevalence settings.
6. Implementing immediate XDR-TB surveillance activities through the existing network of SRLs and NRLs.
7. Initiating advocacy, communication, and social mobilization activities to inform and raise awareness about TB and XDR-TB.

Within the framework of these recommendations, the United States Agency for International Development in collaboration with the WHO and other partners has developed a tool (the MDR/XDR-TB Assessment and Monitoring Tool) to be used for preparing national or subnational plans for MDR/XDR-TB prevention and control; providing baseline information and monitoring progress; providing data and analysis to prepare Green Light Committee (GLC) and Global Fund to Fight AIDS, TB and Malaria (GFATM) applications; providing information to guide requests for external technical assistance; and providing information to guide donor investment in MDR/XDR-TB interventions.[106]

PRIORITIES FOR RESEARCH

Research priorities to improve MDR and XDR-TB prevention and control can be identified at all levels, including basic, applied, and operational research. A summary of the relevant priorities for TB- and MDR-TB related research are summarized in **Table 9**.

As the main focus of this review is on MDR-TB control, the new diagnostics and new drugs issues are specifically addressed, leaving out the new vaccines. The rationale as to why these 2 areas

---

Table 8
WHO-recommended StopTB Strategy to reach the 2015 Millennium Development Goals

1.   Pursue high-quality DOTS expansion and enhancement

   - Secure political commitment, with adequate and sustained financing
   - Ensure early case detection, and diagnosis through quality-assured bacteriology
   - Provide standardized treatment with supervision, and patient support
   - Ensure effective drug supply and management
   - Monitor and evaluate performance and impact

2.   Address TB-HIV, MDR-TB, and the needs of poor and vulnerable populations

   - Scale up collaborative TB/HIV activities
   - Scale up prevention and management of multidrug-resistant TB (MDR-TB)
   - Address the needs of TB contacts, and of poor and vulnerable populations, including
     women, children, prisoners, refugees, migrants and ethnic minorities

3.   Contribute to health system strengthening based on primary health care

   - Help improve health policies, human resource development financing, supplies, service
     delivery and information
   - Strengthen infection control in health services, other congregate settings and households
   - Upgrade laboratory networks, and implement the Practical Approach to Lung Health (PAL)
   - Adapt successful approaches from other fields and sectors, and foster action on the social
     determinants of health

4.   Engage all care providers

   - Involve all public, voluntary, corporate and private providers through Public-Private Mix
     (PPM) approaches
   - Promote use of the International Standards for TB Care (ISTC)

5.   Empower people with TB, and communities through partnership

   - Pursue advocacy, communication and social mobilization
   - Foster community participation in TB care
   - Promote use of the Patients' Charter for TB Care

6.   Enable and promote research

   - Conduct program-based operational research, and introduce new tools into practice
   - Advocate for and participate in research to develop new diagnostics, drugs and vaccines

---

are so relevant for MDR-TB control is also discussed.

Rationale for MDR-TB Research Priorities: Prevention First of All

Drug resistance is largely a man-made phenomenon: under selective pressure caused by inadequate regimens or monotherapy, genetic mutants emerge to replace original strains, thus making an initially pan-susceptible strain a resistant one (**Table 10**). Subsequent cycles generate multiresistant strains, including MDR-TB, and when second-line drugs are wrongly used (often by including a single drug to a failing regimen) XDR-TB may result.[107,108] The risk of mutation for the majority of the first-line anti-TB antibiotics is 10^{-9}, whereas the risk for isoniazid resistance is 10^{-8}. Rifampicin resistance

has been proposed as molecular marker for MDR-TB.[107]

Prevention of selection of new MDR-TB resistance requires sound application of the WHO Stop TB Strategy, acting on the different components of the treatment delivery process chain: from uninterrupted supply of quality drugs to patient-centered support.[109]

Improved Diagnostic Tools

In contrast to the de novo development of drug resistance, the transmission of MDR- and XDR-strains of *M tuberculosis* is becoming an increasing problem in settings where the prevalence of TB and MDR-TB is high and that of HIV is increasing (for example, FSU countries). It is necessary to immediately interrupt the MDR- and XDR-TB ongoing transmission

Table 9
Overview of research priorities relevant for TB and MDR-TB control

Research Aarea	Specific Research Activities
Improving diagnosis for TB and MDR-TB	Improving program performance and human resource development
	Improving existing diagnostics
	Developing new diagnostics
	Incorporating new/improved diagnostics into diagnostic algorithms at program level
	Developing methods to monitor disease activity
	Improving diagnostics for latent infection
	Strengthening research capacity and operational research
	Establishing and maintaining research resources
Improving treatment of TB and MDR-TB	Facilitating drug research and development of new drugs and treatment regimens
	Enhancing clinical trial site capacity
	Building evidence base for adoption of new regimens
	Tailoring existing treatment strategies
	Developing and validating surrogate end points and biomarkers
	Assessing mathematical models for simulation of efficacy and costs
Improving prevention of TB and MDR-TB	Facilitating drug research and development of new vaccines
	Enhancing operational research to improve program performances (case-finding and treatment success)
	Improving infection control
Strengthening social research and the global agenda on TB and MDR-TB	Reducing risk and vulnerability to TB
	Addressing effect of poverty on health-seeking behavior
	Ascertaining effects of sex inequality
	Identifying effect of community factors on health services and DOTS programs
Scaling-up operational and implementation research on TB and MDR-TB	Building close collaboration between researchers, national control programs, Ministry of Health, and other partners
	Engaging all health care providers
	Empowering patients and communities
	Enabling and promoting research
	Assessing adherence-support strategies
Promoting immunopathogenesis studies on TB and MDR-TB	Assessing use of adjunctive immunotherapy
	Developing approaches to detect and manage immune reconstitution inflammatory response
	Investigating and using new information on immunopathogenesis
	Identifying immune correlates of protection
	Investigating geographic diversity of preexisting immune status of vaccine target population
Improving program performance and human resource development	Increasing human resource development at individual and institutional level in both low and high TB incidence countries
	Focusing on Western-Eastern and Northern-Southern partnership

through early diagnosis and effective treatment.[110] Novel diagnostic line probe assays, like the new GenoType *M tuberculosis* drug resistance second-line (MTBDRsl) assay (Hain Lifescience, Nehren, Germany) provide a reliable new tool for the detection of XDR strains of *M tuberculosis* within 1 to 2 days directly in clinical specimens.[111]

Diagnosis of latent TB infection specifically caused by drug-resistant strains is currently not possible. Yet, early diagnosis and exact identification of drug resistance during *M tuberculosis*

Table 10
Causes for the selection of drug-resistant strains of *M tuberculosis*

1.	Unknown multidrug resistance treated by standard therapy and lack of knowledge of previous therapy regimens	Dearth of proper diagnostic facilities and laboratories in poorer nations means health care workers are forced to engage in the kind of symptom-based guesswork leading to misdiagnosis; the consequence is the increased likelihood of prescribing the wrong medications. Sputum culture and DST are not performed and patients receive standard, empirical chemotherapy
2.	Use of nonstandardized drug regimens and/or use of drugs of low quality	Prescription of inadequate amounts of antimicrobials or ineffective drugs (poor pharmacokinetic and dynamic profiles) could increase mutation rate as a stress response. It is necessary to maintain treatment until the bacterial population is extinct (Ehrlich's advice: "hit hard and hit early")
3.	Dual infection with strains of different drug susceptibility	The antibiotic action acts as an environmental pressure; allowing mutant strains to survive; they will pass resistant trait to their offspring, resulting in a fully resistant bacterial population
4.	Addition of single drugs to a failing regimen	The occurrence of multiple drug resistance arising as a result of several sequences of mono-therapy is known as "sequential regimen" resistance mechanism
5.	Nonadherence	It is associated to sub-inhibitory concentrations of the drugs. This finding has led to the emphasis on the importance of full supervision of drug taking (Directly Observed Therapy; DOT) and support for patient adherence through a patient-centered approach to care
6.	Nonavailability of drugs	Poverty and inadequate access to drugs continue to be a major force in the development of resistance. In many developing countries drugs are freely available, but only to those who can afford them. Most patients are forced to resort to poor quality counterfeit, or truncated treatment courses that invariably lead to more rapid selection of resistant organisms

latency could have a substantial impact on TB control. The early diagnosis of drug resistance in *M tuberculosis* infection should be a priority target of future research activities.

Development of New Drugs

For more than 40 years, not a single new drug has been developed and licensed for the treatment against TB. Under these circumstances and under constant evolutionary pressure of the same anti-TB drugs, it was only a matter of time before drug resistance of *M tuberculosis* emerged as a serious problem. The emergence of MDR- and XDR-TB has spurred interest in the development of new drugs. The first report of a Phase 2 clinical trial of a promising new diarylquinoline compound to be used for the treatment of MDR- and XDR-TB cases has been published recently.[112] Other nitro-imidazole, diamine, and pyrrole compounds are being investigated in clinical Phase 1 or 2 drug

trials, yet none of the compounds will have passed Phase 3 to be available before the year 2011 (**Table 11**). Randomized clinical trials are now urgently needed to develop new regimens for improved treatment outcomes of patients with MDR- and XDR-TB.[113,114] The development of new potent drugs with a low toxicity profile, allowing for shorter and more effective treatment against TB, and the exploration of the role of possible adjunctive therapies, such as vitamin D supplementation, are a priority for the future.[115]

Operational Research for MDR-TB Control

Research on new diagnostics and drugs (and vaccines) involves both basic and applied research. In a way it involves also operational research, as new diagnostic and treatment approaches after clinical trials must be tested at the program level.

Furthermore, operational research is necessary to implement adequate infection control

Table 11
Examples of new antituberculosis drugs under clinical development[a]

Advanced Preclinical Evaluation	Phase 1	Phase 2
TB Oxazolidinone PNU-100480 Pfizer	Diamine SQ-109 Pfizer	Diarylquinoline TMC-207 Tibotec
TBK-613 - Quinolone TB Alliance, various clinical research organizations	Pyrolle-LL3858 Lupin Pharmaceuticals	Rifapentine TBTC-29 Sanofi Pasteur, TBTC, CDC
		Nitro-dihydro-imidazooxazole OPC-67683 Otsuka Pharmaceuticals Nitroimidazole-oxazine PA-824 TB Alliance

Drugs such as Moxifloxacin and Linezolid, which are already licensed for other indications and used in the treatment against MDR- and XDR-TB, are in clinical evaluation.

[a] http://www.stoptb.org/wg/new_drugs/projects.asp.

measures, particularly in setting at high prevalence of both MDR-TB and HIV infection, and to optimize support for patient adherence to a long and difficult treatment regimen.

SUMMARY

The global MDR-TB epidemic (511,000 new cases and 150,000 deaths estimated annually) has presently a case-fatality rate of 293.5 per 1000 affected individuals, whereas XDR-TB (50,000 cases and 30,000 deaths estimated) has a case-fatality rate of 600 per 1000 affected cases. These statistics mean that every day 410.9 deaths occur from MDR-TB and 82.2 from XDR-TB in every setting where there has been the capacity and the willingness to detect them. The main pitfalls to be faced are the following:

- The laboratory network is not fully equipped to identify resistance to second-line drugs and diagnose XDR-TB. Furthermore, the availability and affordability of high-technology assays is limited to rich countries.
- Although a high proportion of MDR-TB cases can be cured, treatment of MDR-TB is difficult and expensive. Despite some new light on the topic, the response to treatment of XDR-TB cases is still suboptimal, with higher probability of death and longer hospital and treatment duration compared with MDR-TB cases.
- The prevalence of MDR-TB correlates well with poor TB control practices, while the emergence and spread of XDR-TB is due to the improper regulation and use of second-line anti-TB drugs. Therefore, prevention of drug resistance through adherence to proper standards of care and control is imperative, and a top priority for all TB control efforts.[1,11]

ACKNOWLEDGMENTS

Special gratitude is extended to Dr Davide Manissero, ECDC TB program coordinator, Stockholm, Sweden, and Dr Rosella Centis and Dr Lia D'Ambrosio, WHO Collaborating Center for TB and Lung Diseases, Fondazione S. Maugeri, Care and Research Institute, Tradate, Italy, for their important contributions.

REFERENCES

1. Matteelli A, Migliori GB, Cirillo D, et al. Multidrug-resistant and extensively drug-resistant *Mycobacterium tuberculosis*: epidemiology and control. Expert Rev Anti Infect Ther 2007;5(5):857–71.
2. Pablos-Méndez A, Raviglione MC, Laszlo A, et al. Global surveillance for antituberculosis-drug resistance, 1994–1997. N Engl J Med 1998;338(23):1641–9.
3. Espinal MA, Laszlo A, Simonsen L, et al. Global trends in resistance to antituberculosis drugs. World Health Organization-International Union against Tuberculosis and Lung Disease Working Group on Anti-Tuberculosis Drug Resistance Surveillance. N Engl J Med 2001;344(17):1294–303.
4. WHO, IUATLD. Anti-tuberculosis drug resistance in the world: fourth global report. Geneva: World Health Organization; 2009.
5. Zignol M, Hosseini MS, Wright A, et al. Global incidence of multidrug-resistant tuberculosis. J Infect Dis 2006;194(4):479–85.
6. Wright A, Zignol M, Van Deun A, , et alGlobal Project on Anti-Tuberculosis Drug Resistance Surveillance. Epidemiology of antituberculosis drug resistance 2002-07: an updated analysis of the Global Project on Anti-Tuberculosis Drug Resistance Surveillance. Lancet 2009;373(9678):1861–73.

7. Shah NS, Wright A, Drobniewski F, et al. Extreme drug resistance in tuberculosis ("XDR-TB"): global survey of supranational reference laboratories for *Mycobacterium tuberculosis* with resistance to second-line drugs. Int J Tuberc Lung Dis 2005; 9(Suppl 1):S77.

8. Holtz TH, Riekstina V, Zarovska E, et al. XDR-TB: extreme drug-resistance and treatment outcome under DOTS-Plus, Latvia, 2000–2002. Int J Tuberc Lung Dis 2005;9(Suppl 1):S258.

9. Centers for Disease Control and Prevention. Emergence of *Mycobacterium tuberculosis* with extensive resistance to second-line drugs- worldwide. Morb Mortal Wkly Rep 2006;55:301–5.

10. Nathanson E, Lambregts-van Weezenbeek C, Rich ML, et al. Multidrug-resistant tuberculosis management in resource-limited settings. Emerg Infect Dis 2006;12(9):1389–97.

11. Migliori GB, Loddenkemper R, Blasi F, et al. 125 years after Robert Koch's discovery of the tubercle bacillus—the new XDR-TB threat. Is "science" enough to tackle the epidemic? Eur Respir J 2007;29:423–7.

12. Holtz TH, Cegielski JP. Origin of the term XDR-TB. Eur Respir J 2007;30:396.

13. Migliori GB, Besozzi G, Girardi E, et al. Clinical and operational value of the extensively drug-resistant tuberculosis definition. Eur Respir J 2007;30(4): 623–6.

14. Migliori GB, Ortmann J, Girardi E, et al. Extensively drug-resistant tuberculosis, Italy and Germany. Emerg Infect Dis 2007;13(5):780–2.

15. Migliori GB, Lange C, Centis R, et al. Resistance to second-line injectables and treatment outcomes in multidrug-resistant and extensively drug-resistant tuberculosis cases. Eur Respir J 2008;31(6): 1155–9.

16. Migliori GB, Lange C, Girardi E, et al. Extensively drug-resistant tuberculosis is worse than multidrug-resistant tuberculosis: different methodology and settings, same results. Clin Infect Dis 2008; 46(6):958–9.

17. Migliori GB, Lange C, Girardi E, et al. Fluoroquinolones: are they essential to treat multidrug-resistant tuberculosis? Eur Respir J 2008;31(4): 904–5.

18. Migliori GB, Sotgiu G, Richardson MD, et al. Consensus not yet reached on key drugs for XDR-TB treatment. Clin Infect Dis 2009;49:315–6.

19. Migliori GB, Sotgiu G, Richardson MD, et al. MDR-TB and XDR-TB: drug resistance and treatment outcomes. Eur Resp J 2009;34:778–9.

20. Blower SM, Chou T. Modeling the emergence of the "hot zones": tuberculosis and the amplification dynamics of drug resistance. Nat Med 2004; 10(10):1111–6.

21. Sotgiu G, Ferrara G, Matteelli A, et al. Epidemiology and clinical management of XDR-TB: a systematic review by TBNET. Eur Respir J 2009;33(4):871–81.

22. Eker B, Ortmann J, Migliori GB, et al. Multidrug- and extensively drug-resistant tuberculosis, Germany. Emerg Infect Dis 2008;14(11):1700–6.

23. Chan ED, Strand MJ, Iseman MD. Treatment outcomes in extensively resistant tuberculosis. N Engl J Med 2008;359:657–9.

24. Banerjee R, Allen J, Westenhouse J, et al. Extensively drug-resistant tuberculosis in California, 1993–2006. Clin Infect Dis 2008;47:450–7.

25. Extensively drug-resistant tuberculosis—United States, 1993-2006. MMWR Morb Mortal Wkly Rep 2007;56(11):250–3.

26. CDC. Reported tuberculosis in the United States, 2005: *Mycobacterium tuberculosis*. Atlanta (GA): US Department of Health and Human Services, CDC; 2006. Available at: http://www.cdc.gov/tb/statistics/reports/surv2005/PDF/TBSurvFULLReport.pdf. Accessed September 18, 2009.

27. Frieden TR, Sterling T, Pablos-Mendez A, et al. The emergence of drug-resistant tuberculosis in New York City. N Engl J Med 1993;328:521–6.

28. Espinal MA, Laserson K, Camacho M, et al. Determinants of drug-resistant tuberculosis: analysis of 11 countries. Int J Tuberc Lung Dis 2001;5(10):887–93.

29. Kliiman K, Altraja A. Predictors of extensively drug-resistant pulmonary tuberculosis. Ann Intern Med 2009;150(11):766–75.

30. Casal M, Vaquero M, Rinder H, et al. A case-control study for multidrug-resistant tuberculosis: risk factors in four European countries. Microb Drug Resist 2005;11(1):62–7.

31. Falzon D, Infuso A, Aït-Belghiti F. In the European Union, TB patients from former Soviet countries have a high risk of multidrug resistance. Int J Tuberc Lung Dis 2006;10(9):954–8.

32. Faustini A, Hall AJ, Perucci CA. Risk factors for multidrug resistant tuberculosis in Europe: a systematic review. Thorax 2006;61(2):158–63.

33. Granich RM, Oh P, Lewis B, et al. Multidrug resistance among persons with tuberculosis in California, 1994-2003. JAMA 2005;293(22):2732–9.

34. Clark CM, Li J, Driver CR, et al. Risk factors for drug-resistant tuberculosis among non-US-born persons in New York City. Int J Tuberc Lung Dis 2005;9(9):964–9.

35. Jakubowiak WM, Bogorodskaya EM, Borisov SE, et al. Risk factors associated with default among new pulmonary TB patients and social support in six Russian regions. Int J Tuberc Lung Dis 2007; 11(1):46–53.

36. Ruddy M, Balabanova Y, Graham C, et al. Rates of drug resistance and risk factor analysis in civilian

and prison patients with tuberculosis in Samara Region, Russia. Thorax 2005;60(2):130–5.

37. Coker R, McKee M, Atun R, et al. Risk factors for pulmonary tuberculosis in Russia: case-control study. BMJ 2006;332(7533):85–7.

38. M'ikanatha NM, Lynfield R, Van Beneden CA, et al. Infectious disease surveillance. London: Wiley-Blackwell; 2007.

39. Rieder HL, Watson JM, Raviglione MC, et al. Surveillance of tuberculosis in Europe. Recommendations of a Working Group of the World Health Organization (WHO) and the European Region of the International Union Against Tuberculosis and Lung Disease (IUATLD) for uniform reporting on tuberculosis cases. Eur Respir J 1996;9:1097–104.

40. Schwoebel V, Lambregts-van Weezenbeek CS, Moro ML, et al. Standardisation of antituberculosis drug resistance surveillance in Europe. Recommendations of a World Health Organization (WHO) and the European Region of the International Union Against Tuberculosis and Lung Disease (IUATLD) Working Group. Eur Respir J 2000;16:364–71.

41. Schwoebel V, Lambregts CS, Moro ML, et al. European recommendations on surveillance of antituberculosis drug resistance. Euro Surveill 2000; 5(10):104–6.

42. Clancy L, Rieder HL, Enarson DA, et al. Tuberculosis elimination in the countries of Europe and other industrialized countries. Eur Respir J 1991; 4(10):1288–95.

43. Broekmans JF, Migliori GB, Rieder HL, et al. European framework for tuberculosis control and elimination in countries with a low incidence. Recommendations of the World Health Organization (WHO), International Union Against Tuberculosis and Lung Disease (IUATLD) and Royal Netherlands Tuberculosis Association (KNCV) Working Group. Eur Respir J 2002;19(4):765–75.

44. Rieder HL, Zellweger JP, Raviglione MC, et al. Tuberculosis control in Europe and international migration. Eur Respir J 1994;7(8):1545–53.

45. Tuberculosis situation in the European Union in 2007. Available at: http://ecdc.europa.eu/en/Health_Topics/tuberculosis/special_report/Tuberculosis_surveillance_report_rev1.pdf. Accessed June 10, 2009.

46. Mor Z, Migliori GB, Althomsons SP, et al. Comparison of tuberculosis surveillance systems in low-incidence industrialised countries. Eur Respir J 2008;32(6):1616–24.

47. Centers for Disease Control and Prevention (CDC). Plan to combat extensively drug-resistant tuberculosis: recommendations of the Federal Tuberculosis Task Force. MMWR Recomm Rep 2009;58(RR-3): 1–43.

48. Available at: http://www.cdc.gov/tb/topic/research/TBESC/committee_members.htm. Accessed September 18, 2009.

49. Migliori GB, Cirillo DM, Spanevello A, et al. Ripped from the headlines: how can we harness communications to control TB? Eur Respir J 2007;30(2):194–8.

50. Migliori GB, Richardson MD, Lange C. Of blind men and elephants: making sense of extensively drug-resistant tuberculosis. Am J Respir Crit Care Med 2008;178(10):1000–1.

51. Available at: http://www.who.int/tb_beijingmeeting/media/en_call_for_action.pdf. Accessed September 18, 2009.

52. Espinal MA, Kim SJ, Suarez PG, et al. Standard short-course chemotherapy for drug-resistant tuberculosis: treatment outcomes in 6 countries. JAMA 2000;283(19):2537–45.

53. Migliori GB, Espinal M, Danilova ID, et al. Frequency of recurrence among MDR-TB cases 'successfully' treated with standardised short-course chemotherapy. Int J Tuberc Lung Dis 2002;6(10):858–64.

54. Park SK, Kim CT, Song SD. Outcome of chemotherapy in 107 patients with pulmonary tuberculosis resistant to isoniazid and rifampin. Int J Tuberc Lung Dis 1998;2(11):877–84.

55. Chan ED, Laurel V, Strand MJ, et al. Treatment and outcome analysis of 205 patients with multidrug-resistant tuberculosis. Am J Respir Crit Care Med 2004;169(10):1103–9.

56. Leimane V, Riekstina V, Holtz TH, et al. Clinical outcome of individualised treatment of multidrug-resistant tuberculosis in Latvia: a retrospective cohort study. Lancet 2005;365(9456):318–26.

57. Turett GS, Telzak EE, Torian LV, et al. Improved outcomes for patients with multidrug-resistant tuberculosis. Clin Infect Dis 1995;21(5):1238–44.

58. Yew WW, Chan CK, Chau CH, et al. Outcomes of patients with multidrug-resistant pulmonary tuberculosis treated with ofloxacin/levofloxacin-containing regimens. Chest 2000;117(3):744–51.

59. Chan ED, Iseman MD. Multidrug-resistant and extensively drug-resistant tuberculosis: a review. Curr Opin Infect Dis 2008;21(6):587–95.

60. Yew WW, Leung CC. Management of multidrug-resistant tuberculosis: Update 2007. Respirology 2008;13(1):21–46.

61. Telzak EE, Sepkowitz K, Alpert P, et al. Multidrug-resistant tuberculosis in patients without HIV infection. N Engl J Med 1995;333(14):907–11.

62. Goble M, Iseman MD, Madsen LA, et al. Treatment of 171 patients with pulmonary tuberculosis resistant to isoniazid and rifampin. N Engl J Med 1993;328(8):527–32.

63. Chiang CY, Enarson DA, Yu MC, et al. Outcome of pulmonary multidrug-resistant tuberculosis: a 6-yr follow-up study. Eur Respir J 2006;28(5):980–5.

64. Tahaoğlu K, Törün T, Sevim T, et al. The treatment of multidrug-resistant tuberculosis in Turkey. N Engl J Med 2001;345(3):170–4.

65. Park MM, Davis AL, Schluger NW, et al. Outcome of MDR-TB patients, 1983-1993. Prolonged survival with appropriate therapy. Am J Respir Crit Care Med 1996;153(1):317–24.

66. Flament-Saillour M, Robert J, Jarlier V, et al. Outcome of multi-drug-resistant tuberculosis in France: a nationwide case-control study. Am J Respir Crit Care Med 1999;160(2):587–93.

67. Pearson ML, Jereb JA, Frieden TR, et al. Nosocomial transmission of multidrug-resistant *Mycobacterium tuberculosis*. A risk to patients and health care workers. Ann Intern Med 1992; 117(3):191–6.

68. Fischl MA, Daikos GL, Uttamchandani RB, et al. Clinical presentation and outcome of patients with HIV infection and tuberculosis caused by multiple-drug-resistant bacilli. Ann Intern Med 1992;117(3):184–90.

69. Edlin BR, Tokars JI, Grieco MH, et al. An outbreak of multidrug-resistant tuberculosis among hospitalized patients with the acquired immunodeficiency syndrome. N Engl J Med 1992;326(23): 1514–21.

70. Drobniewski F, Eltringham I, Graham C, et al. A national study of clinical and laboratory factors affecting the survival of patients with multiple drug resistant tuberculosis in the UK. Thorax 2002;57(9):810–6.

71. Guidelines for the programmatic management of drug-resistant tuberculosis; Emergency update 2008. Available at: http://whqlibdoc.who.int/publications/2008/9789241547581_eng.pdf. Accessed September 18, 2009.

72. Migliori GB, Eker B, Richardson MD, et al. A retrospective TBNET assessment of linezolid safety, tolerability and efficacy in MDR-TB. Eur Respir J 2009;34:387–93.

73. Hugonnet JE, Tremblay LW, Boshoff HI, et al. Meropenem-clavulanate is effective against extensively drug-resistant *Mycobacterium tuberculosis*. Science 2009;323(5918):1215–8.

74. Spigelman MK. New tuberculosis therapeutics: a growing pipeline. J Infect Dis 2007;196(Suppl 1): S28–34.

75. Gandhi NR, Moll A, Sturm AW, et al. Extensively drug-resistant tuberculosis as a cause of death in patients co-infected with tuberculosis and HIV in a rural area of South Africa. Lancet 2006; 368(9547):1575–80.

76. Kwon YS, Kim YH, Suh GY, et al. Treatment outcomes for HIV-uninfected patients with multidrug-resistant and extensively drug-resistant tuberculosis. Clin Infect Dis 2008;47(4):496–502.

77. Mitnick CD, Shin SS, Seung KJ, et al. Comprehensive treatment of extensively drug-resistant tuberculosis. N Engl J Med 2008;359(6):563–74.

78. Kim DH, Kim HJ, Park SK, et al. Treatment outcomes and long-term survival in patients with extensively drug-resistant tuberculosis. Am J Respir Crit Care Med 2008;178(10):1075–82.

79. Wang H, Lin H, Jiang G. Pulmonary resection in the treatment of multidrug-resistant tuberculosis: a retrospective study of 56 cases. Ann Thorac Surg 2008;86(5):1640–5.

80. Iseman MD, Madsen L, Goble M, et al. Surgical intervention in the treatment of pulmonary disease caused by drug-resistant *Mycobacterium tuberculosis*. Am Rev Respir Dis 1990;141(3):623–5.

81. Pomerantz M, Brown JM. Surgery in the treatment of multidrug-resistant tuberculosis. Clin Chest Med 1997;18(1):123–30.

82. Chiang CY, Yu MC, Bai KJ, et al. Pulmonary resection in the treatment of patients with pulmonary multidrug-resistant tuberculosis in Taiwan. Int J Tuberc Lung Dis 2001;5(3):272–7.

83. Kir A, Inci I, Torun T, et al. Adjuvant resectional surgery improves cure rates in multidrug-resistant tuberculosis. J Thorac Cardiovasc Surg 2006; 131(3):693–6.

84. Naidoo R. Active pulmonary tuberculosis: experience with resection in 106 cases. Asian Cardiovasc Thorac Ann 2007;15(2):134–8.

85. Park SK, Lee CM, Heu JP, et al. A retrospective study for the outcome of pulmonary resection in 49 patients with multidrug-resistant tuberculosis. Int J Tuberc Lung Dis 2002;6(2):143–9.

86. Pomerantz BJ, Cleveland JC Jr, Olson HK, et al. Pulmonary resection for multi-drug resistant tuberculosis. J Thorac Cardiovasc Surg 2001;121(3):448–53.

87. Shiraishi Y, Nakajima Y, Katsuragi N, et al. Resectional surgery combined with chemotherapy remains the treatment of choice for multidrug-resistant tuberculosis. J Thorac Cardiovasc Surg 2004; 128(4):523–8.

88. Sung SW, Kang CH, Kim YT, et al. Surgery increased the chance of cure in multi-drug resistant pulmonary tuberculosis. Eur J Cardiothorac Surg 1999;16(2):187–93.

89. Grant A, Gothard P, Thwaites G. Managing drug resistant tuberculosis. BMJ 2008;28:337.

90. Mitnick CD, Appleton SC, Shin SS. Epidemiology and treatment of multidrug resistant tuberculosis. Semin Respir Crit Care Med 2008;29(5):499–524.

91. Jassal M, Bishai WR. Extensively drug-resistant tuberculosis. Lancet Infect Dis 2009;9(1):19–30.

92. LoBue P. Extensively drug-resistant tuberculosis. Curr Opin Infect Dis 2009;22(2):167–73.

93. Geerligs WA, Van Altena R, De Lange WCM, et al. Multidrug-resistant tuberculosis: long-term

treatment outcome in the Netherlands. Int J Tuberc Lung Dis 2000;4(8):758–64.

94. Narita M, Alonso P, Lauzardo M, et al. Treatment experience of multidrug-resistant tuberculosis in Florida, 1994–1997. Chest 2001;120(2):343–8.

95. Viskum K, Kok-Jensen A. Multidrug-resistant tuberculosis in Denmark 1993-1995. Int J Tuberc Lung Dis 1997;1(4):299–301.

96. Ferrara G, Richeldi L, Bugiani M, et al. Management of multidrug-resistant tuberculosis in Italy. Int J Tuberc Lung Dis 2005;9(5):507–13.

97. Treatment of tuberculosis: guidelines for national programmes. 3rd edition. Geneva: World Health Organization; 2003. (WHO/CDS/TB/2003.313). Available at: http://www.popline.org/docs/1528/278861.html. Accessed September 18, 2009.

98. Pérez-Guzmán C, Vargas MH, Martínez-Rossier LA, et al. Results of a 12-month regimen for drug-resistant pulmonary tuberculosis. Int J Tuberc Lung Dis 2002;6(12):1102–9.

99. Centers for Disease Control and Prevention (CDC). National action plan to combat multidrug-resistant tuberculosis. MMWR Morb Mortal Wkly Rep 1992; 41(RR-11):1–48.

100. US Centers for Disease Control and Prevention. CDC immigration requirements: technical instructions for tuberculosis screening and treatment. 2007.

101. Framework action plan to fight TB in the EU. Available at: http://ecdc.europa.eu/pdf/080317_TB_Action_plan.pdf. Accessed June 10, 2009.

102. Control of XDR-TB—update on progress since the Global XDR-TB Task Force Meeting, Geneva, Switzerland; October 9–10, 2006. Available at: http://www.who.int/tb/xdr/globaltaskforce_update_feb07.pdf. Accessed August 7, 2007.

103. World Health Organisation. The global plan to stop TB 2006-2015. Available at: http://www.stoptb.org/globalplan/plan_main.asp. Accessed August 7, 2007.

104. World Health Organisation. The global MDR-TB and XDR-TB response plan 2007-2008. Available at: http://www.who.int/tb/publications/2007/global_response_plan.pdf. Accessed September 18, 2009.

105. Raviglione MC, Uplekar MW. WHO's new Stop TB Strategy. Lancet 2006;367(9514):952–5.

106. Migliori GB, Sotgiu G, Jaramillo E. Development of a standardized multidrug-resistant/extensively drug-resistant assessment and monitoring tool. Int J Tuberc Lung Dis 2009;13:1305–8.

107. Gillespie SH. Evolution of drug resistance in Mycobacterium tuberculosis: clinical and molecular perspective. Antimicrobial Agents Chemother 2002;46(2):267–74.

108. Coker RJ. Review: multidrug-resistant tuberculosis: public health challenges. Trop Med Int Health 2004;9(1):25–40.

109. International Standards for Tuberculosis Care (ISTC) and The Patients' Charter for Tuberculosis Care. Available at: http://www.who.int/tb/publications/2006/istc/en/index.html. Accessed September 18, 2009.

110. Donald PR, van Helden PD. The global burden of tuberculosis—combating drug resistance in difficult times. N Engl J Med 2009;360(23):2393–5.

111. Hillemann D, Rüsch-Gerdes S, Richter E. Feasibility of the GenoType MTBDRsl assay for fluoroquinolone, amikacin-capreomycin, and ethambutol resistance testing of Mycobacterium tuberculosis strains and clinical specimens. J Clin Microbiol 2009;47(6):1767–72.

112. Diacon AH, Pym A, Grobusch M, et al. The diarylquinoline TMC207 for multidrug-resistant tuberculosis. N Engl J Med 2009;360(23):2397–405.

113. Mitnick CD, Castro KG, Harrington M, et al. Randomized trials to optimize treatment of multidrug-resistant tuberculosis. PLoS Med 2007; 4(11):e292.

114. Fauci AS, NIAID Tuberculosis Working Group. Multidrug-resistant and extensively drug-resistant tuberculosis: the National Institute of Allergy and Infectious Diseases Research agenda and recommendations for priority research. J Infect Dis 2008; 197(11):1493–8.

115. Wilkinson RJ, Lange C. Vitamin D and tuberculosis: new light on a potent biologic therapy? Am J Respir Crit Care Med 2009;179(9):740–2.

Multidrug- and Extensively Drug-resistant Tuberculosis in Africa and South America: Epidemiology, Diagnosis and Management in Adults and Children

H. Simon Schaaf, MMed Paed, DCM, MD Paed[a],*,
Anthony P. Moll, BSc, MBChB[b], Keertan Dheda, MBBCh, PhD[c,d,e]

KEYWORDS

- Multidrug-resistant • Extensively drug-resistant
- Tuberculosis • Adults • Children
- Clinical presentation • Management

Africa, and mainly sub-Saharan Africa, have a high incidence of tuberculosis (TB) and the highest prevalence of human immunodeficiency virus (HIV) in the world. In addition, Africa is experiencing an increase in multidrug-resistant TB (MDR-TB) (ie, resistance to at least isoniazid [INH] and rifampicin [RMP]), with 14% of the global burden of new MDR-TB cases occurring in Africa,[1,2] and early warnings of extensively drug-resistant TB (XDR-TB; ie, MDR plus resistance to the fluoroquinolones and 1 of 3 second-line injectable agents), especially in South Africa.[3] Until recently, many African countries treated TB with a 2-month 4-drug intensive Phase including INH and RMP, and a 7-month continuation Phase of INH and ethambutol, excluding RMP. This regimen, together with the lack of second-line anti-TB drugs, protected many poorly resourced countries from developing high rates of MDR-TB, and especially prevented XDR-TB.[2] National TB programs, together with nongovernmental organizations such as the Green Light Committee and other technical and financial partners, are currently rolling out TB treatment to include second-line MDR-TB treatment to many of these countries,[4] and it is of utmost importance that this should be done responsibly to avoid the development of additional drug resistance. Special attention needs to be given to identifying drug resistance patterns in communities, treatment regimens with

[a] Desmond Tutu TB Centre, Department of Paediatrics and Child Health, Faculty of Health Sciences, Stellenbosch University, and Tygerberg Children's Hospital, PO Box 19063, Tygerberg 7505, South Africa
[b] Church of Scotland Hospital, Tugela Ferry, PO Box 195, KwaZulu-Natal 3010, South Africa
[c] Division of Pulmonology and UCT Lung Institute, Department of Medicine, Lung Infection and Immunity Unit, University of Cape Town, J Floor Old Main Building, Groote Schuur Hospital, Observatory, Cape Town 7925, South Africa
[d] Institute of Infectious Diseases and Molecular Medicine, University of Cape Town, Observatory 7925, South Africa
[e] Centre for Infectious Diseases and International Health, Department of Infection, UCL, 43 Cleveland Street, London, W1T 4JF, UK
* Corresponding author.
E-mail address: hss@sun.ac.za (H.S. Schaaf).

Clin Chest Med 30 (2009) 667–683
doi:10.1016/j.ccm.2009.08.019
0272-5231/09/$ – see front matter © 2009 Elsevier Inc. All rights reserved.

an optimal number of drugs to which patients' isolates are susceptible or naive, and supply of and adherence to treatment.

EPIDEMIOLOGY

The World Health Organization (WHO) estimates that 511,000 new cases of MDR-TB occurred in 2007, 4.9% of all TB cases[5]; of these 40,000 (6.6%) are estimated to be XDR-TB.[6,7] Few national surveys have been reported for Africa from 2002 to 2007, but, with available data, Africa together with the Americas and western and central Europe reported the lowest prevalence of MDR-TB.[4] Few MDR-TB hotspots (ie, MDR-TB >3% of TB cases) have been reported in Africa; these include Mozambique, Cote d'Ivoire, and, more recently, Rwanda[8] and Democratic Republic of Congo.[9] However, taking into account the number of TB cases in sub-Saharan Africa, this region is still responsible for 14% of the total MDR-TB burden, with South Africa in first place with more than16,000 new cases per year. Nine African countries rate among the 27 high-burden MDR-TB countries: South Africa (4th), Nigeria (9th), Democratic Republic of Congo (13th), Ethiopia (16th), Kenya (20th), Mozambique (21st), Zimbabwe (23rd), Cote d'Ivoire (25th), and Sudan (26th).[5] In South America, Peru and Ecuador are the only MDR-TB hotspots, with Peru 22nd among the 27 MDR-TB high-burden countries,[5] but Brazil, which has almost one-third of the region's TB cases, is also responsible for a high number of MDR-TB cases.[7] Surveys of anti-TB drug resistance in Africa and South America reported between 2002 and 2007 are summarized in **Table 1**.[4]

Few surveys of drug resistance are done amongst childhood TB cases, yet they usually reflect the currently circulating strains in the community, as more than 90% of children who develop disease after infection will do so within a year of infection. Children usually have transmitted drug resistance; they rarely develop drug resistance because of the paucibacillary nature of their disease. **Table 2** summarizes results of drug resistance surveys in children reported since 2000.

CLINICAL PRESENTATION OF MDR/XDR-TB

Clinical features and chest radiographic changes are not helpful in distinguishing MDR/XDR-TB and drug-susceptible TB, and are not discussed here.[10,11] However, a previous history of TB treatment, particularly combined with a history of non-adherence to TB treatment or substance abuse

problems, exposure to known source cases of MDR- and XDR-TB, failure to culture-convert by month 5 to 6 while on MDR treatment (or month 2 while on first-line therapy for presumed drug-susceptible TB), and relapse soon after treatment completion should prompt suspicion of MDR- or XDR-TB.[12] Molecular epidemiologic methods have shown that transmission of drug-resistant strains is common, and is probably responsible for more than half of MDR/XDR-TB cases.[13–17] However, in another study of 270 South African XDR-TB patients, almost 90% had a history of previous anti-TB treatment, and molecular genotyping confirmed the predominance of secondary, rather than primary, drug resistance.[18] Even in some areas with low TB incidence, transmission may be responsible for most MDR-TB cases.[19] In children, although not confirmed with molecular epidemiology, more than 90% of drug resistance is likely due to transmission from adult source cases.[20,21]

HIV coinfected patients are more susceptible to TB, and progression in this group may be rapid. The only available XDR-TB outcome data from Africa to date indicate that, in a setting of probable nosocomially transmitted XDR-TB, almost all patients were infected with HIV and died at a median of 2 weeks after sputum collection for culture and drug susceptibility testing (DST).[3] Hence, a widely held view is that XDR-TB in Africa occurs predominantly in individuals infected with HIV who are more susceptible to infection.[22] By contrast, a recent study based on 270 South African patients with XDR-TB showed that a large proportion (55%) of XDR-TB patients are not infected with HIV.[18,23]

DIAGNOSIS OF MDR- AND XDR-TB

Drug-resistant TB is a microbiologic diagnosis. Most TB diagnosis in adults in Africa is by sputum smear microscopy for acid-fast bacilli (AFB), and TB in children is diagnosed by a constellation of history of contact with an infectious case, chronic symptoms, tuberculin skin test, chest radiography, and, rarely, by smear or culture. Until recently, only a few African countries had laboratory facilities for culture and DST.[2] Currently there is a strong international drive for the upgrade of laboratories in resource-limited countries to include culture and DST facilities. Although no African country will be able to do culture and DST in all suspected TB cases soon, it will be important to identify patients at risk of drug resistance, such as relapse, retreatment, and chronic TB cases, individuals infected with HIV, those not responding to adherent first-line anti-TB treatment, and close contacts,

Table 1
Surveys of anti-TB drug resistance in Africa and South America 2002 to 2007

	Number of Patients Tested	Any Resistance n (%, SD)	Resistance to INH n (%, SD)	MDR n (%, SD)
African region, year				
Cote d'Ivoire, 2006	N = 320	76 (23.8, 19.2–28.8)	39 (12.2, 8.8–16.3)	8 (2.5, 1.1–4.9)
	P = ND			
Ethiopia, 2005	N = 804	216 (26.9, 23.4–30.7)	62 (7.7, 5.9–9.9)	13 (1.6, 0.9–2.8)
	P = 76	37 (48.7, 37.0–60.4)	19 (25.0, 15.8–36.3)	9 (11.8, 5.6–21.3)
Madagascar, 2007	N = 810	51 (6.3, 4.7–8.3)	37 (4.6, 3.2–6.3)	4 (0.5, 0.1–1.3)
	P = 51	6 (11.8, 4.4–23.9)	5 (9.8, 3.3–21.4)	2 (3.9, 0.5–13.5)
Rwanda, 2005	N = 616	64 (10.4, 8.0–13.3)	38 (6.2, 4.4–8.5)	24 (3.9, 2.5–5.8)
	P = 85	19 (22.4, 14.0–32.7)	9 (10.6, 5.0–19.2)	8 (9.4, 4.2–17.7)
Senegal, 2006	N = 237	25 (10.5, 6.9–15.2)	10 (4.2, 2.0–7.6)	5 (2.1, 0.7–4.9)
	P = 42	13 (31.0, 17.6–47.1)	10 (23.8, 12.1–39.5)	7 (16.7, 7.0–31.4)
South American region, year				
Argentina, 2005	N = 683	68 (10.0, 7.7–12.6)	39 (5.7, 4.1–7.8)	15 (2.2, 1.2–3.6)
	P = 136	34 (25.0, 18.0–33.1)	25 (18.4, 12.3–25.9)	21 (15.4, 9.8–22.6)
Paraguay, 2001	N = 235	26 (11.1, 7.4–15.8)	15 (6.4, 3.6–10.3)	5 (2.1, 0.7–4.9)
	P = 51	10 (19.6, 9.8–33.1)	6 (11.8, 4.4–23.9)	2 (3.9, 0.5–13.5)
Peru, 2006	N = 1809	420 (23.2, 21.0–25.5)	209 (11.6, 10.0–13.2)	95 (5.3, 4.2–6.4)
	P = 360	150 (41.7, 36.5–46.9)	109 (30.3, 25.6–35.3)	85 (23.6, 19.3–28.3)
Uruguay, 2005	N = 335	7 (2.1, 0.8–4.3)	4 (1.2, 0.3–3.0)	0 (0, 0–0.9)
	P = 33	3 (9.1, 1.9–24.3)	2 (6.1, 0.7–20.2)	2 (6.1, 0.7–20.2)

Abbreviations: N, new tuberculosis cases; P, previously treated tuberculosis cases; SD, standard deviation.
Data from Wright A, Zignol M, van Deun A, et al. Epidemiology of antituberculosis drug resistance 2002–2007: an updated analysis of the Global Project on Anti-Tuberculosis Drug Resistance Surveillance. Lancet 2009;373:1861–73.

Schaaf et al

Table 2
Results of anti-TB drug resistance surveys amongst childhood TB cases reported after 2000

Country and Region	Time of Survey	Number of Children	Any Drug Resistance (%)	INH Resistance (%)	Multidrug Resistance (%)
Central African Republic, Bangui[91]	Apr 1998–Jun 2000	190 (DST done in 165)	25 (15.2)	15 (9.1)	1 (0.6)
Egypt[92]		150 (DST done in 73)	18 (24.7)	4 (5.4)	2 (2.7)
Greece[93]	1994–2004	77	16 (20.8)	12 (15.6)	3 (3.9)
India, TB Research Center[94]	1996	201	NA	NA (10)	NA (3.5)
Madagascar, Antananarivo[95]	1997–2000	97	1 (1)	1 (1)	0
South Africa, Western Cape[20]	March 2003–Feb 2005	320	41 (12.8)	41 (12.8)	19 (5.9)
South Africa, Western Cape[21]	March 2005–Feb 2007	291 (DST done in 285)	43 (15.1), only INH and RMP	41 (14.4)	19 (6.7)

Abbreviation: NA, not available.

including children, of drug-resistant source cases. In countries, such as South Africa, where this has been the policy, culture and DST were often neglected, leading to longer duration of infectiousness and transmission of drug-resistant TB. The current strategy of improved hospital-based confirmation of MDR/XDR-TB by DST, and improved infection control measures, is not going to be sufficient to curtail the XDR-TB epidemic in some areas.[13] In countries with high TB incidence and high rates of MDR/XDR-TB and HIV, it has been shown that more aggressive case finding, especially identifying drug-resistant cases at initial TB diagnosis by rapid diagnostic methods and active contact tracing, is necessary to reduce MDR/XDR-TB rates.[13,24,25]

High mortality and transmission rates in MDR/XDR-TB patients, especially in those infected with HIV, have made rapid diagnosis of drug resistance essential. Although liquid broth culture methods and DST are considerably faster than using solid media, they are expensive and still take 2 to 6 weeks. Because of the risk of infectiousness and the risk of acquiring further drug resistance with incorrect treatment regimens, development of more rapid diagnostic methods for drug resistance is receiving much attention.

The nucleic acid amplification tests (NAATs), the line-probe assays, are a major advance in rapid diagnostic methods of drug-resistant TB. These genotypic evaluation assays are used either for detection of *Mycobacterium tuberculosis* directly from clinical samples or for identification of mycobacteria from culture. The major advantages of the nucleic acid–based assays are speed (results available within 48 hours for smear-positive specimens) and ease of interpretation. The tests are still expensive, and laboratory infrastructure is needed, but a large study in a laboratory in Cape Town, South Africa, with a high throughput of specimens has shown this test to be reliable and practicable. The GenoType MTBDR*plus* (Hain Lifescience, Nehren, Germany; **Fig. 1**A) for the diagnosis of MDR-TB is probably the best known of these assays. The kit can be used to detect *M tuberculosis* directly from clinical samples, or for identification of mycobacteria from culture. The underlying principle involves multiplex amplification of extracted mycobacterial DNA by polymerase chain reaction (PCR), with subsequent hybridization of the biotin-labeled amplicons to oligonucleotide probes bound to a membrane strip (line probe). This test can simultaneously identify most RMP and INH resistance; identification is done by evaluation of the resultant banding pattern. The kits have been shown to have excellent correlation with conventional methods, usually more than 95%.[26] One disadvantage of the test is that it does not identify INH resistance other than *inh*A promoter region or *kat*G gene mutations, which may lead to over diagnosis of RMP monoresistance and a proportion of INH-resistant strains may be missed. This disadvantage may potentially lead to a pool of INH-monoresistant cases incorrectly treated as drug-susceptible cases, which may lead to these

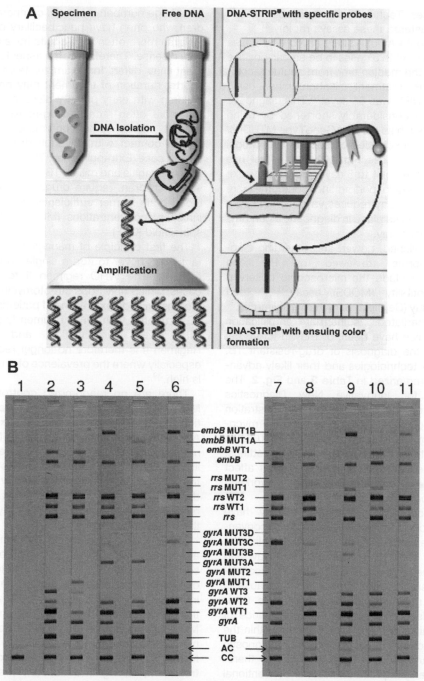

Fig. 1. (A) The Hain GenoType MTBDR*plus* assay. The MTBDR*plus* assay, through PCR amplification of extracted TB DNA and reverse hybridization of the amplicons to membrane-bound probes, confirms a diagnosis of TB and rapidly identifies resistance to rifampicin and isoniazid. (B) GenoType MTBDR*sl* version showing readouts on the hybridization strip. The MTBDR*sl* version identifies additional resistance to fluoroquinolones, aminoglycosides, capreomycin, and ethambutol. Because this is an open-tube system, there are concerns about contamination and false-positive results if used on a wide scale in high-volume clinical laboratories.

becoming MDR-TB cases. All RMP-monoresistant TB cases diagnosed by the line-probe method only should be managed as MDR-TB cases. Another line-probe assay is INNO-LiPA Rif.TB

(Innogenetics, Zwijndrecht, Belgium), which identifies only RMP resistance; with more than 90% of RMP-resistant strains being MDR, patients identified as RMP-resistant are treated as

MDR-TB cases. Technicians in developing countries have mastered these assays rapidly.[27]

A recent South African study of XDR-TB cases found only 16% of 270 cases to be smear-positive for AFB, and the median time from sputum acquisition to XDR treatment initiation, when using conventional DST, was 65 days.[18] This diagnostic delay may be considerably shortened by using rapid NAATs such as the new GenoType MTBDRs/ assay (Hain Lifescience for second-line drugs, Nehren, Germany; see **Fig. 1**B).[28] This test has a turnaround time of 4 to 5 days. However, unlike MDR-TB, for which performance outcomes are excellent,[29] the assay requires validation in larger field studies, and its place in diagnostic algorithms requires further study.

Other established, newer, and emerging diagnostic platforms (reviewed by Pai and colleagues)[30] include the microscopic observed drug susceptibility (MODS) assay,[31,32] Xpert MTB/RIF assay (Cepheid, Sunnyvale, California),[33] and loop-mediated isothermal amplification (LAMP),[34] which have been, or may in future be, adapted for the diagnosis of drug-resistant TB. These newer technologies and their likely advantages are summarized in **Table 3** and **Fig. 2**. The Foundation for Innovative New Diagnostics (FIND) is undertaking large-scale demonstration projects for diagnosis and DST, using the mycobacterial growth indicator tube (MGIT) 960 liquid culture platform,[35] in high-burden settings. However, the newer technologies will not affect diagnostic delay for patients and health workers, which may be considerable.[36]

Most resource-poor settings, if they have access to laboratory facilities, will still use conventional culture and DST techniques to establish the diagnosis of XDR-TB (reviewed by Whitelaw and Sturm).[37] The lack of standardization of second-line DST remains problematic,[12,22] because 2 laboratories may provide conflicting results. Clinicians will also be familiar with the presence of multiple strain types and DST patterns within the same individual.[38] This may cause diagnostic confusion, and patients with XDR-TB may therefore temporarily improve on MDR or conventional anti-TB treatment. The authors tend to interpret laboratory results within the clinical context and treat for XDR-TB if there is any doubt. Further drug resistance may evolve while awaiting DST results.

PRINCIPLES OF MANAGEMENT OF MDR- AND XDR-TB

The basic principles of MDR/XDR-TB management in adults and children are the same. Adults usually have large numbers of bacilli compared with children who often have paucibacillary disease, and children more often than adults have extrapulmonary disease. Therefore some aspects of management may differ; for example, fewer drugs and shorter duration of treatment may be required in children with early primary disease, and children will more often receive drug-resistant treatment without microbiologic confirmation, because of known contact with an adult drug-resistant TB source case. Extrapulmonary TB, such as tuberculous meningitis and miliary TB, which is common in young children, require drugs that penetrate the blood-brain barrier sufficiently to reach minimal inhibitory concentrations (MICs) in the cerebrospinal fluid (CSF).

The first principle of managing any drug-resistant TB is never to add a single drug to a failing regimen. The WHO regimen II for retreatment cases, which only adds streptomycin in the first 2 months, may do exactly that if patients were previously treated with WHO regimen I, consisting of INH, RMP, pyrazinamide, and ethambutol. Regimen II is therefore no longer recommended, especially where the prevalence of drug resistance is high.[39]

There are no randomized controlled trials of MDR-TB treatment and, therefore, recommendations are based on case series and expert opinion. A recent meta-analysis of existing MDR-TB treatment literature pointed out the discrepancies and limitations of current studies, and concluded that treatment success was associated with treatment durations of more than 18 months and patient receipt of directly observed therapy throughout the treatment course.[40]

MDR-TB treatment could be standardized (ie, a regimen with a set number of first- and second-line drugs, preferably reflecting the most common drug resistance pattern in the region), individualized (ie, a regimen built according to the DST result of the patient), or empirical (ie, if MDR-TB has not been confirmed, but the treatment regimen is changed because of a known MDR-TB contact or failure to respond to adherent treatment, taking into account previous drugs used).

Treatment of MDR or XDR-TB should be daily and directly observed. If at all possible, second-line DST should be carried out immediately in any patient with MDR-TB to exclude pre-XDR (MDR plus resistance to the fluoroquinolones or one of the second-line injectable agents) or XDR-TB. WHO guidelines recommend a treatment regimen with 4 or more drugs to which the patient's isolate is susceptible or naive (ie, no previous treatment with the drug). Drug groups

Table 3
Summary of established, newer, and novel technologies for the diagnosis of drug-resistant (MDR and XDR) TB and their performance outcomes

Type of Assay	Status of Technology; Comments	Sensitivity (%)	Specificity (%)
Nucleic acid amplification tests (NAATs)			
GenoType MTBDR*plus* assay (Hain Lifescience)[29]	Established, WHO-approved and commercially available. Evaluates resistance to rifampicin (R) and isoniazid (H). Risk of contamination and false-positive results owing to open-tube method	R = 98[a] H = 84[a]	R = 99[a] H = 100[a]
GenoType MTBDR*sl* (Hain Lifescience)[28]	Newer and commercially available but not well validated. Evaluates resistance to FQ, AG, CM, and E. Used in conjunction with the MTBDR*plus* assay to diagnose XDR-TB	FQ = 89 (n = 9) AM = 75 (n = 7) CM = 88 (n = 7) E = 39 (n = 26)	100
INNO-LiPA Rif.TB (Innogenetics)[96]	Established and commercially available line-probe assay. Evaluates resistance to R	R = 80 to 100[a]	R = 100[a]
Xpert MTB/RIF (Cepheid)[33]	Newer and ongoing validation, now commercially available. Evaluates resistance to R and H using real-time PCR	100 (n = 42)	100 (n = 224)
Non-nucleic acid amplification tests (non-NAATs)			
MODS[31]	Established; low cost; but no standardized version currently available	R = 100 H = 85 E = 63 SM = 66	R = 100 H = 100 E = 99 SM = 99
TLA[b,33]	Established; low cost; but no standardized version currently available[b]	No data available[b]	No data available[b]
NRA[a,97]	Established; low cost; no standardized version currently available	R = 88–100	R = 100
Bacteriophage assays[98]	Standardized version (FASTPlaque) commercially available	86–100	99
HRM assays[99,100]	Novel (uses DNA melting temperature during PCR to scan for mutations). Still in development	Close to 100 in culture isolates	Close to 100 in culture isolates

The figures quoted apply to the clinical sputum samples used, and not culture isolates, unless otherwise specified.

Abbreviations: AM, amikacin; CM, capreomycin; E, ethambutol; H, isoniazid; HRM, high resolution melt; MODS, microscopic observation drug susceptibility assay; NRA, nitrate reductase assay; R, rifampicin; SM, streptomycin; TLA, thin layer agar.

[a] Results of meta-analyses rather than individual studies.

[b] A standardized colorimetric version is currently in development with FIND (see **Fig. 2**) for which no data are currently available.

that can be used are summarized in **Table 4**. Health workers should take into account possible cross-resistance and adverse effects of drugs when building a treatment regimen.[41]

Treatment of children who have known contact with infectious adult MDR/XDR-TB cases should be guided by the isolate DST result of the adult source cases (empirical treatment) if no *M tuberculosis* isolate is obtained from the child. However, every effort should be made to confirm the diagnosis by culture in the child, as, in high incidence areas, approximately 20% of these children may have drug-suscep-tible TB.[21]

Adherence to treatment is essential and is one of the cornerstones of treatment. Patients and care-givers need support by regular counseling about adverse effects, treatment duration, and impor-tance of adherence. The need for psychological and socioeconomic support in adults and children cannot be overemphasized. Failure of adherence urgently needs further studies.

Clinical, radiologic, and culture response to treatment should be carefully monitored, with cultures done at least monthly until negative, as treatment duration is based on the first negative culture. Thereafter monthly or bimonthly cultures can be done.

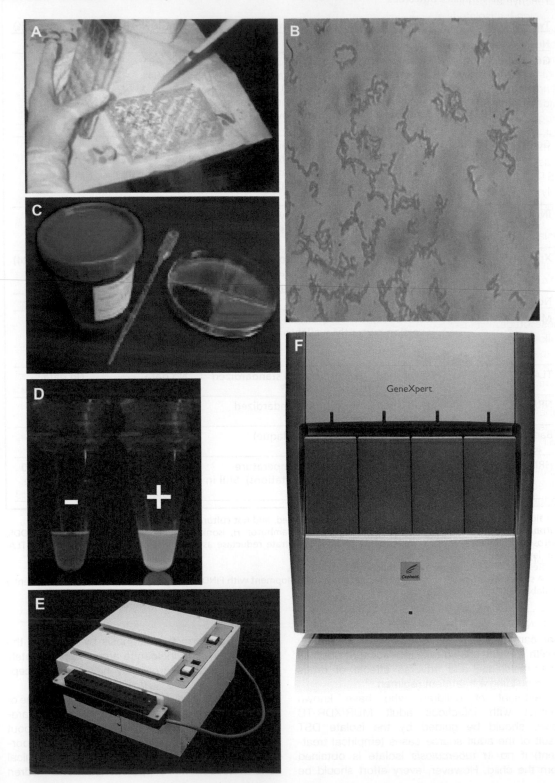

TREATMENT

In children with early primary TB such as uncomplicated hilar lymphadenopathy or primary lung parenchymal (Ghon) focus, 3 bactericidal drugs to which the isolate is susceptible should be sufficient, but in more extensive or complicated pulmonary or disseminated extrapulmonary disease, 4 or more active drugs should be included in the regimen, as with adults. If either the child or the source case had previous treatment with pyrazinamide or ethambutol for more than 1 month, these drugs could be used if DST shows susceptibility, but, because of the difficulty of performing pyrazinamide DST and high resistance rates in MDR-TB cases,[42] and the unreliability of some phenotypic DST methods for ethambutol, they should count only as additional drugs.[41,43] In a surveillance study among children in the Western Cape, 12 of 24 (50%) children with MDR-TB had phenotypic resistance to ethambutol.[44] In building an MDR/XDR-TB treatment regimen, 1 drug each from groups 2 (second-line injectables) and 3 (fluoroquinolones), and 1 or more drugs from group 4 (other proven second-line drugs) should be included in the regimen according to DST or nonexposure to these drugs. If these groups are not sufficient to build an acceptable regimen of 4 active drugs, drugs from group 5 could be added.[41]

In the South African experience in the public sector, where only DST to RMP, INH, ethambutol, streptomycin, ethionamide, terizidone, amikacin/kanamycin, and ofloxacin are available, XDR-TB patients are usually commenced, notwithstanding DST, on a backbone of capreomycin and para-aminosalicylic acid (PAS), and ethambutol (if susceptible) and cycloserine/terizidone are then added. The value of pyrazinamide, although frequently used, is of uncertain significance (see earlier discussion), and frequently amoxicillin/clavulanate and clarithromycin, and sometimes dapsone, are added. Although the latter drugs are of arguable value, little else is available.[11,41]

Linezolid and moxifloxacin are not available in the public sector in most developing countries. Recent data indicate that moxifloxacin is a key predictor of favorable outcome[18,23] and may explain the more favorable outcomes seen in the Peruvian cohort.[45] The mycobactericidal effects of the different fluoroquinolones is likely to be drug specific.[46] The authors believe that moxifloxacin should be made available in resource-poor settings.

INH at high-dose (15–20 mg/kg daily), especially when given in combination with ethionamide where MICs for INH and ethionamide DST are not routinely available, may be beneficial as, depending on which mutation causes INH resistance, the patient may have low-level INH resistance (mainly inhA promoter region mutation), but could then be resistant to ethionamide.[47] Studies have shown low-level INH resistance in 80% of children with INH-resistant TB[48] and, in an adult randomized controlled trial in India, the addition of high-dose INH to a standard MDR-TB treatment regimen, compared with normal dose (5 mg/kg daily) or no INH, found earlier sputum conversion and improvement in chest radiographs in the high-dose INH study group.[49]

TB of the central nervous system needs drugs that penetrate the blood-brain barrier. INH, pyrazinamide, ethionamide, and cycloserine/terizidone penetrate the CSF well. The fluoroquinolones reach reasonable CSF concentrations, whereas the second-line injectables only penetrate the blood-brain barrier during acute inflammation.

Our data indicate substantially improved outcomes in XDR-TB patients coinfected with HIV and on highly active antiretroviral therapy (HAART), which is generally well tolerated with second-line drugs.[18] All XDR-TB patients coinfected with HIV should be commenced on HAART after a run-in period on XDR treatment, irrespective of CD4 count.

Although the optimal duration of treatment of MDR- and XDR-TB is not known, a minimum of

Fig. 2. Newer technologies for the diagnosis of drug-resistant TB. MODS assay (*A, B*) relies on recognition of the characteristic cording pattern (*B*) of *M tuberculosis* using an inverted microscope; simultaneous susceptibility testing is performed, and results are available within a median time of 7 days. The technology is cheap but labor-intensive. (*C*) Thin-layer agar (TLA) relies on early detection of microcolonies by conventional microscopy not only for identification of *M tuberculosis* but also for the simultaneous detection of resistance to rifampicin and INH directly from sputum. FIND is currently working with investigators to develop a standardized version suitable for high-burden countries. MODS and TLA plates remain sealed in plastic wrapping/bags for biosafety purposes. LAMP (*D, E*) does not require a thermal cycler, is a closed tube system, results are available within an hour, and the fluorescence-based readout does not require a microscope. This technology could in future be adapted for the diagnosis of drug-resistant TB (With the permission of Eiken Chemical Co. Ltd, Japan). TB Xpert MTB/RIF (Cepheid) (*F*) GeneXpert System module is a real-time PCR user-friendly detection system that uses a cartridge into which the unprocessed sputum sample is placed.

Table 4
Drug groups for MDR- and XDR-TB treatment regimens for adults and children

Drug Group	Drug Name	Daily Dosage for Children (mg/kg)	<33 kg Dose in mg/kg	33–50 kg	51–70 kg	>70 kg (also Maximum Dose)
				Daily Dosage for Adults (mg)		
[a]Group 1: oral first-line drugs to which the organism shows in vitro susceptibility by DST	Ethambutol	20–25	25	800–1200	1200–1600	1600–2000
	Pyrazinamide	30–40	30–40	1000–1750	1750–2000	2000–2500
[b]Group 2: second-line injectable agents (streptomycin is a first-line drug, not for use in MDR/XDR-TB)	Amikacin	15–22.5	15–20	500–750	750–1000	1000
	Kanamycin	15–30	15–20	500–750	750–1000	1000
	Capreomycin	15–30	15–20	500–750	750–1000	1000
[b]Group 3: fluoroquinolones	Ofloxacin	15–20	15–20	800	800	800–1000
	Levofloxacin	7.5–10	7.5–10	750	750	750–1000
	Moxifloxacin	7.5–10	7.5–10	400	400	400
[c]Group 4: second-line oral bacteriostatic agents	Ethionamide (or prothionamide)	15–20	15–20	500	750	750–1000
	Cycloserine (or terizidone)	10–20	10–20	500	750	750–1000
				600	600	900
	para-Aminosalicylic acid (PAS)	150	150	8 g	8 g	8–12 g
[d]Group 5: drugs of unclear use in drug-resistant TB treatment	High-dose INH	15–20	16–20			
	Linezolid	10 twice daily	600 mg twice daily, but recent data suggest 300 mg twice daily, or 600 mg or 300 mg once daily (see text – New drugs)			
	Amoxicillin/clavulanate	30–40 amoxicillin	Dosage for DR-TB not well defined. Normal adult dose 875/125 mg twice daily or 500/125 mg 3 times daily. Higher dose limited by adverse effects			
	Clarithromycin	7.5–15 twice daily	500 mg twice daily			
	Thioacetazone	3–4	150 mg daily (contraindicated in patients infected with HIV)			
	Imipenem/cilastatin	Only IV	Usual adult dose 500–1000 mg IV 6-hourly			

Linezolid dosage for TB is still uncertain. Thioacetazone should NOT be used in patients infected with HIV.

a Cannot rely on DST; use as additional drug if DST not done, or if the result is susceptible on solid media culture.
b Choose 1 in each of these groups; amikacin is preferred to kanamycin in children.
c Choose 1 or more of these drugs to make up total of 4 new drugs.
d Consider using these drugs if there were insufficient drugs to build an acceptable regimen with previous groups. Data from World Health Organization. Guidelines for the programmatic management of drug-resistant tuberculosis. Emergency update 2008. WHO, Geneva, Switzerland. WHO/HTM/TB/2008.402.

18 months after the first negative culture (or 24 months for XDR-TB) is usually recommended.[41] In general, treatment of MDR/XDR-TB in children should also be 18 months after the first negative culture, but children with early primary (uncomplicated) disease without cavitary lung disease or extrapulmonary dissemination could probably be treated for 12 months only.[50]

MDR/XDR-TB patients are often hospitalized during the intensive Phase of treatment or, in the case of XDR-TB, until they become culture negative. The extent of disease or the clinical condition of the patient may require admission in some patients. The authors usually admit children for the time that they receive second-line injectable drugs, and, if social circumstances and the clinical condition of the child permit, the rest of the treatment is given at primary health care level as daily directly observed therapy. However, with the increasing number of adult patients, this is no longer possible, and while patients are waiting for admission, transmission of infection continues. Community-based diagnosis and early ambulatory treatment of patients has become essential, and studies in Peru on patients not infected with HIV have shown home-based, directly observed treatment to be effective.[13,45,51,52] Community-based treatment programs in patients who are coinfected are needed in high prevalence areas,[53] and some are in progress.[54,55] Community-based strategies, if shown to be effective in this population, carry the benefit of decreasing the risk of nosocomial transmission.

NEW DRUGS

The armamentarium of anti-TB drugs specifically for XDR-TB is limited. According to some investigators, the later-generation fluoroquinolones (eg, moxifloxacin) seem to have activity against some of the ofloxacin-resistant M tuberculosis strains and could be included in XDR-TB regimens,[56,57] but this is not confirmed by other studies.[58] Linezolid, one of a new class of antibiotics, the oxazolidinones, has shown good activity against MDR and XDR M tuberculosis strains in case series, but serious adverse effects, such as partially irreversible peripheral neuropathy, optic neuritis, and severe myelosuppression, and cost has prevented more frequent use.[59–61] The initial 600 mg twice daily dose of linezolid has been reduced to a half dose (300 mg twice daily), and to as low as 300 mg daily to find an optimal dose at which it is still effective but has fewer adverse effects.[62–64] At 300 mg daily, linezolid was still effective, myelosuppression was prevented, but some cases of peripheral

neuropathy still occurred.[64] Yew and Leung[65] have also suggested using linezolid only in the intensive Phase of treatment (2–3 months) to reduce adverse effects. A single case study in a young child with XDR-TB treated with 10 mg/kg 12-hourly showed an excellent response with no serious adverse effects.[66]

Although several potentially good drugs are being developed, none are soon to be marketed. The diarylquinoline Tibotec Medical Compound 207 (TMC207), which has a unique mode of action inhibiting mycobacterial ATP synthase, showed delayed bactericidal activity in early bactericidal activity (EBA) studies in new TB patients, with no serious TMC207-related adverse effects.[67] A recent, randomized, controlled, Phase 2 study in MDR-TB patients receiving either TMC207 (400 mg daily for 2 weeks and 200 mg daily for 6 weeks) or placebo in addition to a 5-drug standard second-line MDR-TB regimen, found a significant reduction in time to sputum smear-negative conversion and conversion to sputum culture negative at the end of 2 months treatment. This result was achieved with only mild to moderate adverse effects, with only vomiting more common than in the placebo group.[68] Other promising bactericidal and potentially sterilizing compounds currently evaluated in Phase 1 trials and EBA studies are the 2 nitroimidazoles, PA-824 (nitroimidazo-oxazine) and OPC-67683 (dihydroimidazo-oxazole), sudoterb (pyrrole LL-3858), and an ethambutol derivative (diamine SQ109).[69–71]

Of the available drugs, the combination of meropenem and clavulanate, which are Food and Drug Administration-approved drugs, could potentially be used to treat patients with currently untreatable TB, as it has shown potent in vitro activity against M tuberculosis.[72] Recently Forgacs and colleagues,[73] after observing clinical improvement on trimethoprim-sulfamethoxazole in a patient, showed that 43 of 44 M tuberculosis isolates tested in vitro were susceptible to trimethoprim-sulfamethoxazole at 1 μg/mL or less of trimethoprim and 19 μg/mL of sulfamethoxazole. Both these drug combinations need further evaluation.

ROLE OF SURGERY IN THE MANAGEMENT OF MDR- AND XDR-TB

The role of surgery in MDR/XDR-TB remains controversial. In conditions such as lymph node obstruction of airways in young children, draining of pericardial effusion, insertion of ventriculoperitoneal shunt for noncommunicating hydrocephalus and some other procedures, the need for surgery is the same as for drug-susceptible cases.

Thoracic resectional surgery (eg, lobectomy or pneumonectomy) and, in some cases, collapse therapy, has proven to be a useful adjunct to MDR-TB drug treatment in adults infected with strains resistant to most drugs.[74–76] Given the poor outcomes of XDR-TB, it is reasonable to embark on surgical intervention in patients with localized unilateral or bilateral disease who are fit for surgery. Trivial contralateral disease (eg, small nodules) are not a contraindication to surgery. These patients should have prior drug treatment to minimize the risk to theater staff, and strict infection control measures should be observed in the operating room. The results of surgical intervention in patients with XDR-TB patients are encouraging.[77,78] These procedures are not without complications. Stump breakdown with bronchopleural fistulas, empyemas, bleeding, and even death may occur; therefore patients should be carefully selected.

ADVERSE EFFECTS OF SECOND-LINE ANTI-TB DRUGS

Second-line anti-TB drugs cause more adverse effects than first-line drugs, and these are usually underestimated. Adults and children, although the latter seem to have fewer adverse effects, need to be monitored carefully. Adverse effects such as hypothyroidism can be asymptomatic, but some children present with a goiter. Important adverse effects to monitor, and how to monitor them, are summarized in **Table 5**. Adverse effects should be treated early, because neglecting to do so could lead to poor adherence or even irreversible problems such as hearing loss and peripheral neuropathy, or death (eg, acute renal failure in capreomycin). Adverse effects of first-line dugs and antiretroviral drugs in patients infected with HIV often have overlapping adverse effects with second-line anti-TB drugs, such as gastrointestinal disturbance (almost all), hepatitis (INH, pyrazinamide, nevirapine, efavirenz, and all protease inhibitors), peripheral neuropathy (INH, d4T, ddI),

Table 5
Important adverse effects of second-line drugs, and tests to monitor them

Second-Line Drug	Adverse Effect[a]	Tests to Monitor
Amikacin Kanamycin	Ototoxicity (cumulative dose important)	Audiology (hearing test). Monthly, if possible
Capreomycin	Nephrotoxicity	Serum creatinine and potassium levels. Monthly; high-risk patients more often
Fluoroquinolones	Gastrointestinal disturbance Insomnia	Clinical observation
	Arthralgia	Serum uric acid if used with pyrazinamide
Ethionamide (or protionamide)	Gastrointestinal disturbance	Clinical observation. Prevent by initially splitting dose or increasing dose (drug ramping)
	Hepatotoxicity	Jaundice. Serum alanine transferase and bilirubin
	Hypothyroidism	Thyroid-stimulating hormone levels (free T4). At least 6-monthly
Cycloserine (or terizidone)	Psychosis, seizures, parasthesia, depression	Clinical observation. All patients to receive preventive pyridoxine
para-Aminosalicylic acid (PAS)	Gastrointestinal disturbance	Clinical observation
	Hypothyroidism	Thyroid stimulating hormone levels (free T4). At least 6-monthly
Linezolid	Myelosuppression	Full blood count. Weekly at first, then monthly
	Lactic acidosis	Serum lactate level
	Peripheral neuropathy	Clinical observation
	Pancreatitis (abdominal pain)	Clinical and serum amylase as indicated
	Optic neuritis	Vision testing

[a] Adverse effects of first-line dugs and antiretroviral drugs in patients infected with HIV often have overlapping adverse effects (see discussion of adverse effects in the text).

central nervous system effects (INH, efavirenz), pancreatitis (d4T, ddI), and lactic acidosis (d4T, ddI, AZT, 3TC).[41]

OUTCOME OF MDR- AND XDR-TB

Long-term outcomes of MDR-TB in adults have improved markedly in recent years, with between 33% and 96% long-term cure or treatment completion with good clinical response.[79]

Treatment of XDR-TB shows varying results.[80–82] Data from Estonia suggest poor outcomes associated with resistance to capreomycin.[83] In contrast, limited data from Peru are encouraging in that 60% of XDR-TB patients completed treatment or were cured with intensive multidrug therapy.[45] An initial report from South Africa indicated a 98% mortality and a median survival of 16 days among patients coinfected with XDR-TB and HIV.[3] In a recent South African XDR-TB study of 270 patients, the overall culture-conversion rate was 17.8% (36/202 who initiated treatment), and, of those, 25/36 (69%) culture-converted within 6 months of treatment initiation.[18] Those with a body weight of less than 50 kg were significantly less likely to convert ($P = .009$). Overall and 12-month mortality rates were 44% (103/234) and 35.9% (84/234), respectively; 25.7% (26/103) of all deaths occurred before treatment initiation. Patients infected with HIV had a higher mortality (12-month mortality of 50% vs 35%; $P = .04$), but culture-converted at the same rate as uninfected patients. Patients infected with HIV and treated with HAART had lower mortality than untreated patients (12-month mortality of 35% vs 75%; $P = .02$). In Cox multivariate regression models, HIV status, treatment with a fluoroquinolone or INH, and radiographic unilateral cavitation were independent predictors of survival. Thus, in South Africa, despite intensive, directly observed, multidrug treatment, the prognosis of XDR-TB, regardless of HIV status, remains poor. Survival, however, in patients infected with HIV is better than previously reported, and substantially improved with HAART. These data have implications for improving case-finding strategies, streamlining diagnostic algorithms, and intensifying the urgent development of XDR-TB–related immunotherapeutic interventions for high HIV-prevalence environments.[18,23]

Few outcome studies are available for children with MDR/XDR-TB. In Peru, cure or probable cure was obtained in 36 of 38 (95%) MDR-TB cases.[52] A South African study of 39 culture-confirmed childhood MDR-TB cases had 4 (10%) deaths and most of the children clinically cured.[50] More data are needed to compare cure rates of children with and without HIV infection with MDR-TB and specific types of TB. In general, MDR tuberculous meningitis has a high mortality.[84] Only case reports of XDR-TB in children are available.[66]

MANAGEMENT OF CONTACTS OF MDR OR XDR-TB

All close contacts of infectious TB cases should be evaluated for TB disease. Once TB disease has been excluded, WHO guidelines recommend that all children less than 5 years old and all patients infected with HIV, irrespective of age, should receive preventive therapy (chemoprophylaxis).[85] In developed countries with low TB incidence, older age groups and all patients infected with HIV will also be advised to take preventive therapy. However, in the case of drug-resistant contacts, no randomized controlled trials for preventive therapy have been conducted. In the case of MDR-TB, the WHO recommends INH preventive therapy only, not to prevent MDR-TB but because, in high TB incidence areas, the patient may have been infected by a drug-susceptible source case.[86] Several failures of INH or INH/RMP combination preventive therapy for MDR-TB child contacts have been documented.[87]

For MDR-TB contacts there is no universally accepted regimen. The WHO does not recommend the use of second-line drugs for preventive therapy for MDR-TB contacts, and recommends only regular follow-up for a minimum of 2 years.[86] However, one study has shown that giving a combination of 2 drugs to which the source case's isolate is susceptible or naive prevents the development of disease in high-risk child contacts.[88] This is also the current recommendation of the American Academy of Pediatrics.[89] The authors prefer a combination of a fluoroquinolone, ethambutol (if DST shows susceptibility), or ethionamide plus high-dose INH for 6 months in high-risk cases such as young children (<3 years) or patients infected with HIV.

There is no effective preventive therapy for XDR-TB contacts. Regular follow-up as for MDR-TB contacts is the only option, with early treatment once disease occurs.

INFECTION CONTROL

No discussion of TB is complete without the mention of proper infection control measures. In developing countries, good ventilation (>6 air changes per hour) by opening windows and doors is the most important and easily implemented measure, other than diagnosing and treating infectious cases early and effectively, and separating suspected cases, especially from children and patients infected with HIV. A recent modeling study of infection control outcomes estimated that half of anticipated XDR-TB cases could be averted by the application of a combination of available strategies in developing countries.[90] In the case of children presenting with possible TB, the adult accompanying the child may be the source case, and therefore it is important that a history of TB should be obtained from the adult or they should be screened, if they are symptomatic, to prevent possible transmission of disease in the health care setting.

REFERENCES

1. Zignol M, Hosseini MS, Wright A, et al. Global incidence of multidrug-resistant tuberculosis. J Infect Dis 2006;194:479–85.
2. World Health Organization. Anti-tuberculosis drug resistance in the world. Report no. 4. Geneva (Switzerland): WHO; 2008. WHO/HTM/TB/2008.394.
3. Gandhi NR, Moll A, Sturm AW, et al. Extensively drug-resistant tuberculosis as a cause of death in patients co-infected with tuberculosis and HIV in a rural area of South Africa. Lancet 2006;368:1575–80.
4. Wright A, Zignol M, van Deun A, et al. Epidemiology of antituberculosis drug resistance 2002–2007: an updated analysis of the Global Project on Anti-Tuberculosis Drug Resistance Surveillance. Lancet 2009;373:1861–73.
5. World Health Organization. Global tuberculosis control: epidemiology, strategy, financing. report. Geneva (Switzerland). WHO/HTM/TB/2009:411
6. Kliiman K, Altraja A. Predictors of extensively drug-resistant pulmonary tuberculosis. Ann Intern Med 2009;150:766–75.
7. Wells CD, Cegielski JP, Nelson LJ, et al. HIV infection and multidrug-resistant tuberculosis – the perfect storm. J Infect Dis 2007;196(Suppl 1):S86–107.
8. Umubyeyi AN, Vandebriel G, Gasana M, et al. Results of a national survey on drug resistance among pulmonary tuberculosis cases in Rwanda. Int J Tuberc Lung Dis 2007;11:189–94.
9. Kabedi MJ, Kashongwe M, Kayembe JM, et al. [Primary resistance of Mycobacterium tuberculosis to anti-tuberculosis drugs in Kinshasa, (DRC)]. Bull Soc Pathol Exot 2007;100:275–6 [French].
10. Schaaf HS, Gie RP, Beyers N, et al. Primary drug-resistant tuberculosis in children. Int J Tuberc Lung Dis 2000;4(12):1149–55.
11. Moll AP, Friedland G, Gandhi N, et al. Extensively drug-resistant tuberculosis (XDR-TB). In: Schaaf HS, Zumla AI, editors. Tuberculosis: a comprehensive clinical reference. 1st edition. St Louis (MO): Saunders Elsevier; 2009. p. 551–7.
12. Yew WW, Leung CC. Management of multidrug-resistant tuberculosis: update 2007. Respirology 2008;13:21–46.
13. Basu S, Friedland GH, Medlock J, et al. Averting epidemics of extensively drug-resistant tuberculosis. Proc Natl Acad Sci U S A 2009;106:7672–7 [Epub 2009 Apr 13].
14. Zhao M, Li X, Xu P, et al. Transmission of MDR and XDR tuberculosis in Shanghai, China. PLoS One 2009;4(2):e4370 [Epub 2009 Feb 3].
15. Andrews JR, Gandhi NR, Moodley P, et al. Tugela Ferry Care and Research Collaboration. Exogenous reinfection as a cause of multidrug-resistant and extensively drug-resistant tuberculosis in rural South Africa. J Infect Dis 2008;198:1582–9.
16. Van Rie A, Warren R, Richardson M, et al. Classification of drug-resistant tuberculosis in an epidemic area. Lancet 2000;356:22–5.
17. Streicher EM, Warren RM, Kewley C, et al. Genotypic and phenotypic characterization of drug-resistant Mycobacterium tuberculosis isolates from rural districts of the Western Cape Province of South Africa. J Clin Microbiol 2004;42:891–4.
18. Dheda K, Shean K, Zumla A, et al. Early treatment outcomes of extensively drug-resistant tuberculosis in South Africa are poor regardless of HIV status. European Respiratory Society Meeting. Vienna, Austria: European Respiratory Society; September, 2009.
19. Vázquez-Gallardo R, Anibarro L, Fernández-Villar A, et al. Multidrug-resistant tuberculosis in a low-incidence region shows a high rate of transmission. Int J Tuberc Lung Dis 2007;11:429–35.
20. Schaaf HS, Marais BJ, Hesseling AC, et al. Childhood drug-resistant tuberculosis in the Western Cape Province of South Africa. Acta Paediatrica 2006;95:523–8.
21. Schaaf HS, Marais BJ, Hesseling AC, et al. Surveillance of antituberculosis drug resistance amongst children from the Western Cape Province of South Africa – an upward trend. Am J Public Health 2009;99:1486–90.
22. LoBue P. Extensively drug-resistant tuberculosis. Curr Opin Infect Dis 2009;22:167–73.
23. Dheda K, Shean K, Badri M. Extensively drug-resistant tuberculosis. N Engl J Med 2008;359:2390 [author reply 2391].
24. Uys PW, Warren R, van Helden PD, et al. Potential of rapid diagnosis for controlling drug-susceptible and drug-resistant tuberculosis in communities where Mycobacterium tuberculosis infections are highly prevalent. J Clin Microbiol 2009;47:1484–90.
25. Dowdy DW, Chaisson RE, Maartens G, et al. Impact of enhanced tuberculosis diagnosis in South Africa: a mathematical model of expanded culture and drug susceptibility testing. Proc Natl Acad Sci U S A 2008;105:11293–8.

26. Barnard M, Albert H, Coetzee G, et al. Rapid molecular screening for multidrug-resistant tuberculosis in a high-volume public health laboratory in South Africa. Am J Respir Crit Care Med 2008; 177:787–92.

27. Quezada CM, Kamanzi E, Mukamutara J, et al. Implementation validation performed in Rwanda to determine whether the INNO-LiPA Rif.TB line probe assay can be used for detection of multidrug-resistant Mycobacterium tuberculosis in low-resource countries. J Clin Microbiol 2007;45:3111–4.

28. Hillemann D, Rusch-Gerdes S, Richter E. Feasibility of the genotype MTBDRsl assay for fluoroquinolone, amikacin-capreomycin, and ethambutol resistance testing of Mycobacterium tuberculosis strains and clinical specimens. J Clin Microbiol 2009;47:1767–72.

29. Ling DI, Zwerling AA, Pai M. Genotype MTBDR assays for the diagnosis of multidrug-resistant tuberculosis: a meta-analysis. Eur Respir J 2008;32:1165–74.

30. Pai M, Kalantri S, Dheda K. New tools and emerging technologies for the diagnosis of tuberculosis: part II. Active tuberculosis and drug resistance. Expert Rev Mol Diagn 2006;6:423–32.

31. Moore DA, Evans CA, Gilman RH, et al. Microscopic-observation drug-susceptibility assay for the diagnosis of tuberculosis. N Engl J Med 2006;355:1539–50.

32. Oberhelman RA, Soto-Castellares G, Caviedes L, et al. Improved recovery of Mycobacterium tuberculosis from children using the microscopic observation drug susceptibility method. Pediatrics 2006; 118:100–6.

33. O'Brien R. New diagnostic methods for tuberculosis. APHL 5th National Conterence on Laboratory Aspects of Tuberculosis San Diego 11–13 August. Available at: http://www.aphl.org/profdev/conferences/proceedings/Documents/2008TBconference/2009-OBrien.pdf; 2008.

34. Boehme CC, Nabeta P, Henostroza G, et al. Operational feasibility of using loop-mediated isothermal amplification for diagnosis of pulmonary tuberculosis in microscopy centers of developing countries. J Clin Microbiol 2007;45:1936–40.

35. Kruuner A, Yates MD, Drobniewski FA. Evaluation of MGIT 960-based antimicrobial testing and determination of critical concentrations of first- and second-line antimicrobial drugs with drug-resistant clinical strains of Mycobacterium tuberculosis. J Clin Microbiol 2006;44:811–8.

36. Storla DG, Yimer S, Bjune GA. A systematic review of delay in the diagnosis and treatment of tuberculosis. BMC Public Health 2008;8:15.

37. Whitelaw AC, Sturm WA. Microbiological testing for Mycobacterium tuberculosis. In: Schaaf HS, Zumla AI, editors. Tuberculosis a comprehensive clinical reference. 1st edition. St Louis (MO): Saunders Elsevier; 2009. p. 169–78.

38. Van Rie A, Victor TC, Richardson M, et al. Reinfection and mixed infection cause changing Mycobacterium tuberculosis drug-resistance patterns. Am J Respir Crit Care Med 2005;172:636–42.

39. Mak A, Thomas A, del Granado M, et al. Influence of multidrug resistance on tuberculosis treatment outcomes with standardized regimens. Am J Respir Crit Care Med 2008;178:306–12.

40. Orenstein EW, Basu S, Shah NS, et al. Treatment outcomes among patients with multidrug-resistant tuberculosis: systematic review and meta-analysis. Lancet Infect Dis 2009;9:153–61.

41. World Health Organization. Guidelines for the programmatic management of drug-resistant tuberculosis. Emergency update. 2008. WHO. Geneva (Switzerland). WHO/HTM/TB/2008.402.

42. Mphahlele M, Syre H, Valvatne H, et al. Pyrazinamide resistance among South African multidrug-resistant Mycobacterium tuberculosis isolates. J Clin Microbiol 2008;46:3459–64.

43. Johnson R, Jordaan AM, Pretorius L, et al. Ethambutol resistance testing by mutation detection. Int J Tuberc Lung Dis 2006;10:68–73.

44. Hoek KGP, Schaaf HS, Gey van Pittius NC, et al. Resistance to pyrazinamide and ethambutol compromises MDR/XDR-TB treatment. S Afr Med J, in press.

45. Mitnick CD, Shin SS, Seung KJ, et al. Comprehensive treatment of extensively drug-resistant tuberculosis. N Engl J Med 2008;359:563–74.

46. Kam KM, Yip CW, Cheung TL, et al. Stepwise decrease in moxifloxacin susceptibility amongst clinical isolates of multidrug-resistant Mycobacterium tuberculosis: correlation with ofloxacin susceptibility. Microb Drug Resist 2006;12:7–11.

47. Schaaf HS, Victor TC, Venter A, et al. Ethionamide cross- and co-resistance in children with isoniazid-resistant tuberculosis. Int J Tuberc Lung Dis, in press.

48. Schaaf HS, Victor TC, Engelke E, et al. Minimal inhibitory concentration of isoniazid in isoniazid-resistant Mycobacterium tuberculosis isolates from children. Eur J Clin Microbiol Infect Dis 2007;26:203–5. DOI: 10.1007/s10096-007-0257-9.

49. Katiyar SK, Bihari S, Prakash S, et al. A randomized controlled trial of high-dose isoniazid adjuvant therapy for multidrug-resistant tuberculosis. Int J Tuberc Lung Dis 2008;12:139–45.

50. Schaaf HS, Shean K, Donald PR. Culture-confirmed multidrug-resistant tuberculosis in children: diagnostic delay, clinical features, response to treatment and outcome. Arch Dis Child 2003; 88:1106–11.

51. Mitnick CD, Appleton SC, Shin SS. Epidemiology and treatment of multidrug resistant tuberculosis. Semin Respir Crit Care Med 2008;29:499–524.

52. Drobac PC, Mukherjee JS, Joseph JK, et al. Community-based therapy for children with

multidrug-resistant tuberculosis. Pediatrics 2006; 117:2022–9.

53. Padayatchi N, Friedland G. Decentralised management of drug-resistant tuberculosis (MDR-and XDR-TB) in South Africa: an alternate model of care. Int J Tuberc Lung Dis 2008;12:978–80.

54. Brust JCM, Moll AP, Scott M, et al. Community-based treatment of multidrug-resistant tuberculosis (MDR TB) and HIV in rural KwaZulu-Natal. XVII International AIDS Conference Mexico City, 3–8 August, 2008.

55. Scott M, Brust JCM, Moll AP, et al. Community-based treatment of MDR-TB and HIV in rural KwaZulu-Natal. Int J Tuberc Lung Dis 2008;12(Suppl 2):S305.

56. Sulochana S, Rahman F, Paramasivan CN. In vitro activity of fluoroquinolones against Mycobacterium tuberculosis. J Chemother 2005;17:169–73.

57. Matrat S, Veziris N, Mayer C, et al. Functional analysis of DNA gyrase mutant enzymes carrying mutations at position 88 in the A subunit found in clinical strains of Mycobacterium tuberculosis resistant to fluoroquinolones. Antimicrob Agents Chemother 2006;50:4170–3.

58. Devasia RA, Blackman A, May C, et al. Fluoroquinolone resistance in Mycobacterium tuberculosis: an assessment of MGIT 960, MODS and nitrate reductase assay and fluoroquinolone cross-resistance. J Antimicrob Chemother 2009;63:1173–8.

59. Fortún J, Martín-Dávila P, Navas E, et al. Linezolid for the treatment of multidrug-resistant tuberculosis. J Antimicrob Chemother 2005;56:180–5.

60. Von der Lippe B, Sandven P, Brubakk O. Efficacy and safety of linezolid in multidrug resistant tuberculosis (MDR-TB) – a report of ten cases. J Infect 2006;52:92–6.

61. Condos R, Hadjiangelis N, Leibert E, et al: Case series report of a linezolid-containing regimen for extensively drug-resistant tuberculosis. Chest 2008;134:187–92.

62. Park IN, Hong SB, Oh YM, et al. Efficacy and tolerability of daily-half dose linezolid in patients with intractable multidrug-resistant tuberculosis. J Antimicrob Chemother 2006;58:701–4.

63. Nam HS, Koh WJ, Kwon OJ, et al. Daily half-dose linezolid for the treatment of intractable multidrug-resistant tuberculosis. Int J Antimicrob Agents 2009;33:92–3.

64. Koh WJ, Kwon OJ, Gwak H, et al. Daily 300 mg dose of linezolid for the treatment of intractable multidrug-resistant and extensively drug-resistant tuberculosis. J Antimicrob Chemother 2009, in press.

65. Yew WW, Leung CC. How should we treat "difficult" multidrug-resistant tuberculosis? Chest 2009;135: 587–8.

66. Schaaf HS, Willemse M, Donald PR. Long-term linezolid treatment in a young child with extensively drug-resistant tuberculosis. Pediatr Infect Dis J 2009;28:748–50.

67. Rustomjee R, Diacon AH, Allen J, et al. Early bactericidal activity and pharmacokinetics of the diarylquinoline TMC207 in treatment of pulmonary tuberculosis. Antimicrob Agents Chemother 2008; 52:2831–5.

68. Diacon AH, Pym A, Grobusch M, et al. The diarylquinoline TMC207 for multidrug-resistant tuberculosis. N Engl J Med 2009;360:2397–405.

69. Hu Y, Coates AR, Mitchison DA. Comparison of the sterilising activities of the nitroimidazopyran PA-824 and moxifloxacin against persisting Mycobacterium tuberculosis. Int J Tuberc Lung Dis 2008;12:69–73.

70. Saliu OY, Crismale C, Schander SK, et al. Bactericidal activity of OPC-67683 against drug-tolerant Mycobacterium tuberculosis. J Antimicrob Chemother 2007;60:994–8.

71. Doi N. [New horizons of next generation chemotherapy for mycobacteriosis]. Kekkaku 2009;84: 133–40 [in Japanese].

72. Hugonnet JE, Tremblay LW, Boshoff HI, et al. Meropenem-clavulanate is effective against extensively drug-resistant Mycobacterium tuberculosis. Science 2009;323:1215–8.

73. Forgacs P, Wengenack NL, Hall L, Tuberculosis and trimethoprim-sulfamethoxazole 2009, in press.

74. Takeda S, Maeda H, Hayakawa M, et al. Current surgical intervention for pulmonary tuberculosis. Ann Thorac Surg 2005;79:959–63.

75. Mohsen T, Zeid AA, Haj-Yahia S. Lobectomy or pneumonectomy for multidrug-resistant tuberculosis can be performed with acceptable morbidity and mortality: a seven-year review of a single institution's experience. J Thorac Cardiovasc Surg 2007;134:194–8.

76. Wang H, Lin H, Jiang G. Pulmonary resection in the treatment of multidrug-resistant tuberculosis: a retrospective study of 56 cases. Ann Thorac Surg 2008;86:1640–5.

77. Somocurcio JG, Sotomayor A, Shin SS, et al. Surgery for patients with drug-resistant tuberculosis: report of 121 cases receiving community-based treatment in Lima, Peru. Thorax 2007;62:416–21.

78. Dravniece G, Cain KP, Holtz TH, et al. Adjunctive resectional lung surgery for extensively drug-resistant tuberculosis. Eur Respir J 2009;34:180–3.

79. Chan ED, Iseman MD. Multidrug-resistant and extensively drug-resistant tuberculosis: a review. Curr Opin Infect Dis 2008;21:587–95.

80. Chan ED, Strand MJ, Iseman MD. Treatment outcomes in extensively resistant tuberculosis. N Engl J Med 2008;359:657–9.

81. Kwon YS, Kim YH, Suh GY, et al. Treatment outcomes for HIV-uninfected patients with multidrug-resistant and extensively drug-resistant tuberculosis. Clin Infect Dis 2008;47:496–502.

82. Keshavjee S, Gelmanova IY, Farmer PE, et al. Treatment of extensively drug-resistant tuberculosis in Tomsk, Russia: a retrospective cohort study. Lancet 2008;372:1403–9.

83. Migliori GB, Lange C, Centis R, et al. Resistance to second-line injectables and treatment outcomes in multidrug-resistant and extensively drug-resistant tuberculosis cases. Eur Respir J 2008;31:1155–9.

84. Padayatchi N, Bamber S, Dawood H, et al. Multidrug-resistant tuberculous meningitis in children in Durban, South Africa. Pediatr Infect Dis J 2006;25:147–50.

85. World Health Organization. Guidance for national tuberculosis programmes on the management of tuberculosis in children. 2006. WHO, Geneva (Switzerland). WHO/HTM/TB/2006.371

86. World Health Organization. Guidelines for the programmatic management of drug-resistant tuberculosis. Geneva (Switzerland). WHO/HTM/TB/2006.361.

87. Sneag DB, Schaaf HS, Cotton MF, et al. Failure of chemoprophylaxis with standard anti-tuberculosis agents in child contacts of multidrug-resistant tuberculosis cases. Pediatr Infect Dis J 2007;26:1142–6.

88. Schaaf HS, Gie RP, Kennedy M, et al. Evaluation of young children in contact with adult multidrug-resistant pulmonary tuberculosis: a 30-month follow-up. Pediatrics 2002;109:765–71.

89. American Academy of Pediatrics. Tuberculosis. In: Pickering LJ, Baker CJ, Long SS, et al, editors. Red book; 2006 report of the committee on infectious diseases. 27th edition. Elk Grove Village (IL): American Academy of Pediatrics; 2006. p. 678–704.

90. Basu S, Andrews J, Poolman E, et al. Prevention of nosocomial transmission of extensively drug-resistant tuberculosis in rural South African district hospitals: an epidemiological modelling study. Lancet 2007;370:1500–7.

91. Kassa-Kelembho E, Bobossi-Serengbe G, Takeng EC, et al. Surveillance of drug-resistant tuberculosis in Bangui, Central African Republic. Int J Tuberc Lung Dis 2004;8:574–8.

92. Morcos W, Morcos M, Doss S, et al. Drug-resistant tuberculosis in Egyptian children using Etest. Minerva Pediatr 2008;60:1385–92.

93. Kanavaki S, Mantadakis E, Nikolaou E, et al. Antimicrobial resistance of mycobacterial tuberculosis isolates from children in Greece, 1994–2004. Int J Tuberc Lung Dis 2007;11:424–8.

94. Rekha B, Swaminathan S. Childhood tuberculosis – global epidemiology and the impact of HIV. Pediatr Respir Rev 2007;8:99–106.

95. Rasolofo Razanamparany V, Ramarokoto H, Clouzeau J, et al. [Tuberculosis in children less than 11 years old: primary resistance and dominant genetic variants of *Mycobacterium tuberculosis* in Antananarivo]. Arch Inst Pasteur Madagascar 2002; 68(1–2):41–3 [in French].

96. Morgan M, Kalantri S, Flores L, et al. A commercial line probe assay for the rapid detection of rifampicin resistance in *Mycobacterium tuberculosis*: a systematic review and meta-analysis. BMC Infect Dis 2005;5:62.

97. Martin A, Panaiotov S, Portaels F, et al. The nitrate reductase assay for the rapid detection of isoniazid and rifampicin resistance in *Mycobacterium tuberculosis*: a systematic review and meta-analysis. J Antimicrob Chemother 2008;62: 56–64.

98. Pai M, Kalantri S, Pascopella L, et al. Bacteriophage-based assays for the rapid detection of rifampicin resistance in *Mycobacterium tuberculosis*: a meta-analysis. J Infect 2005;51: 175–87.

99. Hoek KG, Gey van Pittius NC, Moolman-Smook H, et al. Fluorometric assay for testing rifampin susceptibility of *Mycobacterium tuberculosis* complex. J Clin Microbiol 2008;46:1369–73.

100. Pietzka AT, Indra A, Stoger A, et al. Rapid identification of multidrug-resistant *Mycobacterium tuberculosis* isolates by rpoB gene scanning using high-resolution melting curve PCR analysis. J Antimicrob Chemother 2009;63:1121–7.

Antiretroviral Therapy for Control of the HIV-associated Tuberculosis Epidemic in Resource-Limited Settings

Stephen D. Lawn, MD[a,b,*], Katharina Kranzer, MD[a,b], Robin Wood, FCP MMed[a]

KEYWORDS

- HIV • Tuberculosis • Antiretroviral
- Disease control • Mortality

HIV-ASSOCIATED TUBERCULOSIS EPIDEMIC

Tuberculosis (TB) remains a major challenge to global public health and has proved particularly difficult to control in regions with high HIV prevalence. Of the estimated global burden of 9.3 million new TB cases in 2007, 1.37 million (14.8%) were associated with HIV.[1,2] TB remains a major cause of mortality, with an estimated 1.3 million deaths among individuals who are not infected with HIV and a further 0.5 million TB deaths among people who have HIV. The latter accounted for almost 25% of global AIDS-related mortality.

HIV was a key factor underlying the approximately 1% annual increase in global TB incidence rates between 1990 and 2004. Sub-Saharan Africa has borne the brunt of this co-epidemic, accounting for 79% of cases of the global burden of HIV-associated TB in 2007. Here TB notification rates have increased three- to fivefold in many countries, especially in the south of the continent where HIV prevalence is highest. As a result, TB incidence rates in the region far exceed those observed in most other parts of the world (**Fig. 1**). Elsewhere, South and East Asia account for 11% of the global burden of HIV-associated TB and the combined epidemics of HIV and drug resistant TB are undermining TB control in Eastern Europe.[1]

MILLENNIUM DEVELOPMENT GOALS FOR TUBERCULOSIS CONTROL

The Millennium Development Goals (MDG) TB control targets are to halt and start to reverse the rising incidence of TB and to halve the 1990 prevalence and death rates by 2015.[3] Although the absolute number of TB cases occurring worldwide continued to increase in 2007, it was largely the result of global population growth. Global TB incidence rates are actually thought to have peaked in 2004 at 142 cases per 100,000 population and to have started to slowly decrease thereafter.[1,2]

This recent downward trend in global TB incidence was preceded by a sustained decrease in

S. D. Lawn and K. Kranzer are funded by the Wellcome Trust, London, UK. R. Wood is funded in part by the National Institutes of Health through a CIPRA grant 1U19AI53217–01 and RO1 grant (A1058736–01A1).

[a] The Desmond Tutu HIV Centre, Institute of Infectious Disease and Molecular Medicine, Faculty of Health Sciences, University of Cape Town, Anzio Road, Observatory 7925, Cape Town, South Africa
[b] Department of Infectious and Tropical Diseases, Clinical Research Unit, London School of Hygiene and Tropical Medicine, London, UK
* Corresponding author. The Desmond Tutu HIV Centre, Institute of Infectious Disease and Molecular Medicine, Faculty of Health Sciences, University of Cape Town, Anzio Road, Observatory 7925, Cape Town, South Africa.
E-mail address: stevelawn@yahoo.co.uk (S.D. Lawn).

Clin Chest Med 30 (2009) 685–699
doi:10.1016/j.ccm.2009.08.010

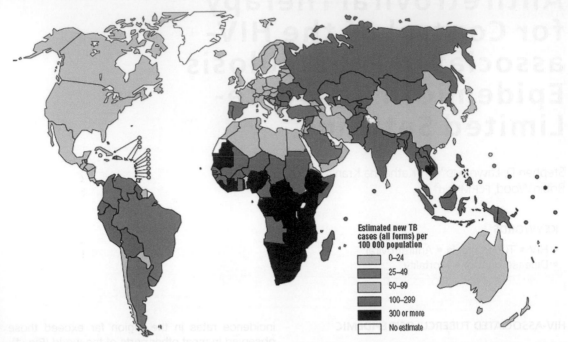

Fig. 1. Estimated TB incidence rates by country for 2006. (*Reproduced from* World Health Organization. Global Tuberculosis Control. Surveillance, planning, and financing. WHO/HTM/TB/2008.393. Geneva (Switzerland): World Health Organization; 2008; with permission.)

global TB prevalence since 1990.[1] Rates of TB mortality (HIV-associated and non-HIV–associated) are also estimated to have peaked around the year 2000 and have since decreased.[1] Despite these encouraging overall trends, however, the global MDG TB control target of halving the 1990 TB prevalence and death rates by 2015 will not be achieved with current rates of progress.[3] Targets are projected to be missed in the regions of sub-Saharan Africa and Eastern Europe where the TB and HIV epidemics intersect. Concerted international public health action is needed.

INTERNATIONAL PUBLIC HEALTH RESPONSE

Since the World Health Organization (WHO) declaration in 1993 that TB was a global emergency, the directly observed treatment, short-course (DOTS) strategy has served as the key public health intervention that has been widely implemented to effect global TB control.[4] This strategy prioritizes the detection of patients who are sputum smear-positive presenting to health facilities with symptoms and aims to achieve high cure rates using short-course rifampicin-containing chemotherapy. Although this has been effective in most parts of the world, contributing to the sustained downward trend in global TB prevalence, it has nevertheless been comparatively ineffective in countries with high HIV prevalence.[1,2,5,6] Although the DOTS strategy remains the foundation for TB control programs in high HIV-prevalence settings, it is clear that additional interventions are needed.

Under the leadership of the WHO and the Stop-TB Partnership, TB-HIV guidelines,[7] a TB-HIV strategic framework,[8] and an interim TB-HIV policy[9] were published between 2002 to 2004 to address the challenge of HIV-associated TB in severely affected countries. The aim of these interventions is to reduce the burden of TB in people who are HIV-infected through use of TB prevention strategies, such as isoniazid preventive therapy, intensified case finding, infection control, and antiretroviral therapy (ART). A further aim is to reduce the impact of HIV in patients who have TB through HIV testing and use of trimethoprim-sulfamethoxazole prophylaxis and ART.

Great progress has been made over the past few years in HIV testing in patients who have TB[1] and in the scale-up of ART.[10] More than 3 million people in resource-limited settings were estimated to have started ART by the end of 2007 and 2 million of these were in sub-Saharan Africa.[10] However, little is known about what impact this massive public health intervention will have on the HIV-associated TB epidemic or how ART might be used to best effect TB control. This article provides an in-depth review of these issues.

TUBERCULOSIS INCIDENCE RATES IN ANTIRETROVIRAL TREATMENT COHORTS

Data from 12 observational studies that included over 32,000 participants living in high-income countries (seven studies) and resource-limited countries (five studies) are shown in **Table 1**. In two of these studies, TB rates were simply compared before and after 1995 when triple-drug ART was introduced, whereas in the remaining studies TB rates were determined according to person-time of exposure to ART. All but two of these studies found a statistically significant reduction in TB risk during ART.

In nine studies, the reductions in TB risk associated with use of antiretrovirals are expressed as hazard ratios adjusted for covariates, such as baseline patient characteristics and antiretroviral regimen. Triple-drug ART was associated with a risk reduction of more than 70% in the majority of these studies (n = 6) with a range of 54% to 92% (see **Table 1**). This protective effect against TB was seen in countries with low-TB burden, such as the United States,[11] and South Africa,[12] which has the highest burden of HIV-associated TB in the world.[2] The benefits of ART are seen across a broad range of degrees of baseline immunodeficiency and clinical stage of disease, although the absolute reduction in TB rates is greatest in those with the most advanced HIV disease (**Fig. 2**).

TB incidence rates in 14 ART cohorts are shown in **Table 2**. The observed rates are heterogeneous and are likely to vary according to the local TB incidence rates, the baseline degree of immunodeficiency, and the duration of ART. Several studies report rates stratified according to duration of ART and these are shown in **Fig. 3**. The figure illustrates the major differences between TB rates in various settings and the rapidity of the beneficial impact of ART. All of these studies show time-dependent reductions in TB rates, with most of the benefit occurring within the first 2 years of ART.[13–19] Although reductions in TB incidence in high- and low-TB burden settings are proportionately similar,[15] the greatest absolute reductions in TB risk of course occur in high-TB prevalence settings.

Baseline risk factors for incident TB during ART in resource-limited settings included low-CD4 cell count,[12–15] advanced WHO stage of disease,[12,14] younger age,[14,15] low socioeconomic status,[12] past history of TB,[20] and male sex.[15] In high-income countries, baseline risk factors for TB included low-baseline CD4 count and HIV transmission category.[15,18] However, the risk of TB decreased as CD4 cell counts rose (**Fig. 4**). Thus, with increasing duration of treatment, the immunologic response to ART, rather than baseline

patients' characteristics, emerges as the dominant predictor of TB risk.[13] The strong relationship between TB rates and updated CD4 cell counts during ART is shown in **Fig. 5**.[19]

Data are scarce concerning TB rates among those with optimum immune recovery. However, in a study in South Africa, subjects achieving CD4 cell counts of greater than 500 cells/μL retained a TB rate that was approximately two-fold higher than that in subjects who were non-HIV–infected living in the same community.[19] These data suggest that recovery of TB-specific immune function during ART may be incomplete even at high CD4 cell counts.

ANTIRETROVIRALS AND TUBERCULOSIS INCIDENCE AT A COMMUNITY LEVEL

Despite the extensive data that have arisen from observational cohort studies, empiric data regarding the impact of ART on TB incidence rates at the community level are lacking. This is a difficult issue to study. In-depth observational studies of sentinel communities with high TB and HIV prevalence during scale-up of ART are needed. Outcome measures should include the impact of ART scale-up on TB incidence and prevalence, TB transmission, and TB-associated mortality. However, trends in TB incidence and mortality over time will inevitably be confounded by other variables, such as the natural evolution of the HIV epidemic, changes over time in socio-economic factors, and the efficiency of TB control programs. Ecological studies comparing settings differing in the rapidity and coverage of ART scale-up may provide further insights.

LIKELY LIMITED IMPACT OF ANTIRETROVIRALS AT COMMUNITY LEVEL

Despite the major beneficial impact of ART on TB rates in observational cohorts, mathematical modeling studies suggest that the impact of ART on TB rates at a population level will be limited.[21] Various observations suggest that this conclusion is likely to be true[22] and are discussed in full in **Box 1**.

Risk of Tuberculosis Before Starting Antiretroviral Treatment

Following HIV seroconversion, risk of TB doubles and continues to increase as CD4 cell counts decline.[12,23–25] Patients, therefore, typically remain at a high risk of TB for many years before eligibility for ART. Further compounding this, HIV infection is often only diagnosed once patients

Table 1
Studies (n = 12) reporting the impact of antiretroviral therapy on tuberculosis incidence rates in observational cohorts

Study	Setting	N	Study Period	Study Design	Impact of ART on TB Incidence Rates	Adjusted Hazards Ratio (95%CI)
Studies comparing TB rates in cohorts before and after introduction of ART						
Brodt et al, 1997[57]	Germany	1003	1992–1996	Cohort of homosexual men 1992–1996	No change in overall cohort incidence rates (range, 2.1–2.7 cases/100 PY)	–
Kirk et al, 2000[58]	Europe	6,972	1994–1999	EuroSIDA multicenter cohort 1994–1999	Overall rate in cohort decreased from 1.8 cases/100 PY to 0.3 cases/100 PY	–
Studies comparing TB rates in patients receiving or not receiving ART						
Ledergerber et al, 1999[17]	Switzerland	2410	1995–1997	Swiss HIV Cohort Study	Rate 0.78 cases/100 PY pre-ART and 0.22 cases/100 PY during first 15 months ART	0.2 (0.1–0.5)
Jones et al, 2000[11]	United States	–	1992–1998	Multicenter cohort Adult/ Adolescent Spectrum of HIV Disease project	Steep decreases in TB incidence rates	–
Girardi et al, 2000[59]	Italy	1360	1995–1996	Multicenter cohort	Not stated	0.08 (0.01–0.88)
Santoro-Lopes et al, 2002[60]	Brazil	255	1991–1998	Prospective cohort	Not stated	0.2 (0.04–1.13)
Badri et al, 2002[12]	South Africa	1034	1992–2001	Rates compared in separate prospective observational cohorts receiving or not receiving ART	Markedly lower TB rates across a broad spectrum of baseline CD4 counts and WHO stage	0.19 (0.09–0.38)

Study	Location	N	Years	Study type	Description	Value
Golub et al, 2007[40]	Brazil	11,026	2003–2005	Multicenter retrospective cohort	Rates among those receiving and not receiving ART were 1.9 and 4.0 cases/100 PY, respectively	0.46 (0.33–0.63)
Miranda et al, 2007[61]	Brazil	463	1995–2001	Multicenter retrospective study	Rates among those receiving and not receiving ART were 1.2 and 13.4 cases/100 PY, respectively	0.2 (0.1–0.6)
Muga et al, 2007[62]	Spain	2238	1980s–2004	Multicenter seroconverter cohort	Marked reduction in rates after 1995 in all HIV transmission categories	0.31 (0.17–0.54)
Moreno et al, 2008[63]	Spain	4268	1997–2003	Multicenter hospital-based cohort	Rates among those receiving and not receiving ART were 0.5 and 1.6 cases/100 PY, respectively	0.26 (0.16–0.40)
Golub et al, 2009[64]	South Africa	2778	2003–2007	Retrospective data from two study sites	Rates among those receiving and not receiving ART were 4.6 and 7.1 cases/100 PY, respectively	0.36 (0.25–0.51)

Abbreviation: PY, person-years.

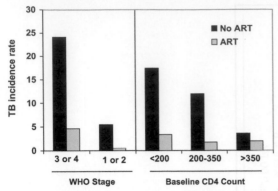

Fig. 2. TB incidence (cases per 100 person-years) among patients who were HIV-infected in Cape Town, South Africa, who were or were not receiving antiretroviral therapy. Patients were stratified according to baseline CD4 cell count and WHO stage of disease. Overall, TB rates were approximately 80% lower among those receiving ART, which was observed across a broad spectrum of baseline immunodeficiency. (*Data from* Badri M, Wilson D, Wood R. Effect of highly active antiretroviral therapy on incidence of tuberculosis in South Africa: a cohort study. Lancet 2002;359(9323):2059–64).

present to medical services with advanced immunodeficiency and either have active TB or high risk of developing TB in the short term.[26]

In addition to TB occurring before enrollment for ART, a substantial burden of prevalent TB may be diagnosed in ART services during screening before starting treatment.[13,16,27,28] The proportion detected may vary according to the intensity of investigation and availability of mycobacterial culture. In two studies from South Africa, 20% to 25% of adults referred for ART who did not already have a TB diagnosis were found to have sputum culture-positive TB, the majority of which was smear-negative.[27,28]

The overall cumulative risk of TB before initiating ART may therefore be very high. In one ART service in Cape Town, this represented two thirds of adult patients.[13] Thus, ART is frequently implemented too late in the course of HIV progression to prevent much of the overall burden of HIV-associated TB.

Incidence of Tuberculosis During Antiretroviral Therapy

In addition to TB occurring pre-ART, TB incidence rates during ART persist at rates substantially higher than background (see **Table 2**). During the initial months of treatment, a proportion of TB cases present as a result of the unmasking of subclinical TB during ART-induced restoration of TB-specific immune responses.[19,29,30] Through

this mechanism, the risk of TB during ART may actually increase in the short term after starting ART. However, the size of this effect will be highly dependent on the efficiency with which patients are screened for clinical and subclinical TB before commencing ART. Unmasking TB was estimated to account for more than one third of the TB cases presenting during the first 4 months of ART in a treatment service in South Africa.[19]

In the longer term, TB rates during ART appear to be largely dependent on changes in the CD4 cell count over time. With CD4 cell counts less than 200 cells/μL, TB rates exceeded 9.0 cases/100 person-years (PY) in the same study from South Africa.[19] Rates at higher CD4 counts were substantially lower, but nevertheless remained more than five-fold higher than rates in individuals who were non-HIV-infected living in the same community.[13,19]

Persistence of high TB rates in ART cohorts is likely to reflect the fact that most patients spend prolonged periods at CD4 cell counts less than 500 cells/μL. In addition, immunologic studies also suggest that defects in functional TB-specific immune responses may persist despite ART,[31] leaving patients vulnerable to TB long-term. This may be compounded by high rates of nosocomial exposure to TB within overcrowded ART services where infection control procedures are often lacking.[32,33]

Despite high early mortality risk,[34] long-term survival after the first year of ART is likely to be good in patients who are in treatment programs in sub-Saharan Africa. In light of the persistence of high rates of TB during ART, the life-time cumulative risk of TB in survivors will inevitably be high. It is not yet clear whether this is reduced compared with the cumulative life-time risk in patients who are HIV-infected in the pre-ART era.

A further critical factor affecting the magnitude of the impact of ART on community TB rates is the coverage of ART. In mathematical modeling studies, high coverage with ART was needed to impact TB rates.[21] However, coverage in sub-Saharan Africa was only approximately one third of those estimated to be in need at the end of 2007.[10] In most countries, rates of HIV-testing are low and only a small proportion of individuals who are HIV-infected know their HIV status.

The magnitude of any impact of ART on TB transmission is unknown. It has been generally assumed that patients who are HIV-infected are not the key drivers of TB transmission in the community in view of their comparatively low infectivity. If true then ART is unlikely to have a major impact on community TB transmission. Conversely, however, patients receiving ART survive longer and remain at

Table 2
Studies (n = 14) reporting tuberculosis incidence rates during antiretroviral therapy

Study	Setting	N	Median / Mean Follow-up (Months)	Median Baseline CD4 Cell Count (Cells/μL)	TB Cncidence, Cases/ 100 PY (Months of ART)	Estimated National TB Incidence Rate (Per 100 Population)[a]
High-income countries						
Girardi et al, 2005[18]	Germany, Switzerland, France, Netherland, UK, Canada, United States	17,142	25.8	280	1.31 (0–3) 0.78 (4–6) 0.46 (7–12) 0.33 (13–24) 0.15 (25–36)	0.005–0.016
Brinkhof et al, 2007[15]	Europe, North America	22,217	11.0	234	1.7 (0–3) 1.0 (4–6) 0.6 (7–12)	<0.015
Moreno et al, 2008[63]	Spain	4268	46.0	324	0.5	0.035
Resource-limited settings						
Badri et al, 2002[12]	South Africa	1034	16.8	254	2.4	0.406
Santoro-Lopes et al, 2002[60]	Brazil	284	22.0	–	8.4	0.071
Lawn et al. 2005[14]	South Africa	346	40.0	242	3.35 (0–12) 1.56 (13–24) 1.36 (25–36) 0.90 (37–48) 1.01 (49–60)	0.576
Seyler et al, 2005[20]	Côte d'Ivoire	129	26.0	125	4.8	0.368
Lawn et al, 2006[13]	South Africa	1002	0.9	96	23.0 (0–3) 10.7 (4–6) 7.0 (7–12) 3.7 (13–24)	0.898

(continued on next page)

Table 2
(continued)

Study	Setting	N	Median / Mean Follow-up (Months)	Median Baseline CD4 Cell Count (Cells/µL)	TB Cncidence, Cases/ 100 PY (Months of ART)	Estimated National TB Incidence Rate (Per 100 Population)[a]
Bonnet et al, 2006[65]	Kenya	3151	3.7	–	17.6	0.419
	Malawi		6.7		14.3	0.416
	Cameroon		11.1		4.8	0.194
	Thailand		3.7		10.4	0.142
	Cambodia		7.3		7.6	–
Golub et al, 2007[40,64]	Brazil	11,026	17.0	–	1.90	0.053
Miranda et al, 2007[61]	Brazil	245	–	–	1.2	0.064
Brinkhof et al, 2007[15]	Botswana, Brazil, Côte d'Ivoire, India, Kenya, Nigeria, Malawi, Morocco, Senegal, South Africa, Thailand, Uganda	4540	9.6	107	10.7 (0–3) 7.5 (4–6) 5.2 (7–12)	0.055–0.852
Moore et al, 2007[16]	Uganda	1044	17.0	127	3.9 (overall) 7.5 (0–6) 2.4 (7–12) 1.9 (13–18)	0.385
Walters et al, 2008[66]	South Africa	290 (pediatric)	–	–	6.4	0.898

Abbreviation: PY, person-years.

[a] National TB incidence estimates at the midpoint of the study duration; data sourced from World Health Organization. Global tuberculosis control: epidemiology, strategy, financing. Geneva (Switzerland): World Health Organization; 2009. WHO/HTM/TB/2009.411.

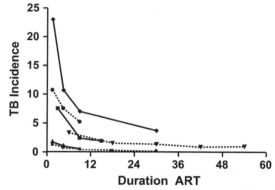

Fig. 3. TB incidence rates during ART. The graph shows data from studies included in (see **Table 2**) in which changing TB incidence rates were calculated according to increasing duration of ART. The two lowest curves present data from studies conducted in high-income countries.[15,18] The remaining four studies are from South Africa (diamonds[13] and inverted triangles[14]), a range of resource-limited countries (circles[15]), and Uganda (squares[16]).

substantial risk of TB that may be more likely to be sputum smear-positive as immune function improves. However, transmission risk among such patients remains undefined.

Perhaps the most important issue relating to TB transmission is that occurring between individuals who are HIV-infected in health care settings.[33] This issue was exemplified by the outbreak of multi-drug-resistant and extensively drug-resistant TB in a hospital-based ART service in rural South Africa from 2005 to 2006.[32] Although ART may serve as a potent preventive therapy for TB, ART

services without adequate infection-control measures may nevertheless be sites associated with high risk of nosocomial TB transmission and outbreaks.

ENHANCING THE IMPACT OF ANTIRETROVIRALS ON TUBERCULOSIS CONTROL

Earlier Initiation of Antiretroviral Therapy

It is likely that ART could be used much more effectively as a TB-prevention strategy (**Box 2**). ART should be initiated much earlier in the course of disease than is currently being done. In sub-Saharan Africa, the median CD4 cell count at baseline in ART programs is often in the range of 100 to 150 cells/μL[34] and many patients have already had TB before starting ART. Earlier HIV diagnosis would permit more timely initiation of ART, thereby enhancing its role as a preventive intervention. Consideration should be given to revision of ART eligibility guidelines in countries, such as South Africa, where treatment is restricted to patients who have WHO stage 4 disease or blood CD4 cell counts of less than 200 cells/μL.[35] A randomized controlled trial of early (CD4 200–350 cells/μL) versus late (CD4 <200 cells/μL) initiation of ART in Haiti was discontinued in 2009 following interim analysis.[36] In the delayed initiation group, the mortality was fourfold higher and the TB incidence rate was twofold higher than in the early initiation group, clearly demonstrating the benefits to be derived from earlier treatment.

A mathematical modeling study explored the potential impact of a test and treat strategy

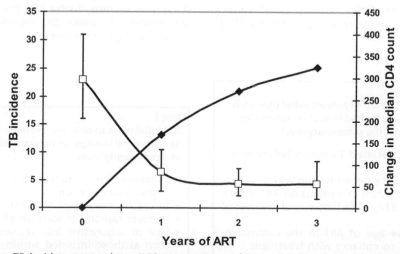

Fig. 4. Decreasing TB incidence rates (cases/100 person-years, white squares) and rising median CD4 cell counts (cells/μL, black diamonds) during the first 3 years of ART. These data are from a community-based ART cohort in a township in Cape Town, South Africa. (*Data from* Refs.[13,19,56]).

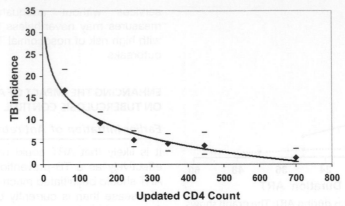

Fig. 5. Relationship between updated CD4 cell-count measurements made every 4 months during 4.5 years of ART in a treatment cohort in a township in Cape Town, South Africa. Observed rates are shown as diamonds together with 95% confidence intervals indicated by bars. A logarithmic trend line is overlaid ($R^2 = 0.97$). TB incidence rates are seen to fall substantially as CD4 cell counts increase during ART. (*Data from* Lawn SD, Myer L, Edwards D, et al. Short-term and long-term risk of tuberculosis associated with CD4 cell recovery during antiretroviral therapy in South Africa. AIDS 2009;23(13):1717–25.)

whereby all patients who are diagnosed with HIV are immediately offered ART irrespective of the blood CD4 cell count.[38] Although interest has primarily focused on the potential of such a strategy for HIV prevention, this also has the potential to impact TB control. The rapidity of scale-up of ART may also be an important variable that affects not only the numbers of deaths averted by ART[39] but also the number of TB cases averted.

Adjunctive Interventions

Because TB rates do not decrease to background levels during long-term ART, use of concurrent adjunctive interventions is needed. Three key interventions are encompassed within the WHO 3I's strategy launched in April 2008.[37] This three-pronged strategy includes intensified case finding, isoniazid preventive therapy, and infection control.

Intensified case finding is needed in ART services as this designates patients as either having active TB (and in need of treatment) or being TB-free and potentially benefitting from isoniazid preventive therapy. Initiation of TB treatment in those who have disease also plays a critical role in reducing the risk of nosocomial TB transmission. Observational data have examined the potential role of isoniazid preventive therapy concurrently with ART in Brazil. Although isoniazid alone was not associated with significant reductions in TB risk compared with the nonintervention group, it was suggested that concurrent isoniazid preventive therapy during ART provided an additive benefit.[40] However, this requires confirmation by randomized controlled trials.

Box 1
Reasons why scale-up of antiretroviral therapy is likely to have only limited impact on tuberculosis incidence rates at the community level

- Much HIV-associated TB occurs before initiation of ART
- High rates of TB persist during ART
- Prolonged survival of patients on ART is associated with a high life-time cumulative risk of TB
- Limited coverage of ART in the community and limited compliance with treatment
- Impact of ART on TB transmission in the community is suspected to be low

---

Box 2
Potential ways to enhance the impact of antiretroviral therapy on tuberculosis prevention at a community level

- Diagnose HIV earlier and initiate ART at higher CD4 cell counts
- Increase coverage of ART in the community
- Increase rapidity of scale-up of ART
- Use of adjunctive interventions with ART, such as those included within the WHO 3I's strategy (intensified case finding, isoniazid preventive therapy and infection control)[37]

Table 3
Observational cohort studies (n=8) showing the impact of antiretroviral therapy on mortality among patients who have HIV-associated tuberculosis

Study	Country	Study Design	Outcome
Dheda et al, 2004[67]	United Kingdom	Retrospective study of patients who had HIV-TB (n = 99) treated in pre-ART era and in ART era	Adjusted hazards of death or new AIDS-defining illness was 0.34 (95%CI, 0.18–0.63) during ART era
Manosuthi et al, 2006[68]	Thailand	Retrospective cohort study (n = 1003) comparing mortality in a historic natural- history cohort with rates in an ART cohort	The adjusted hazards of death associated with use of ART was 0.05 (95%CI, 0.02–0.12).
Akksilp et al, 2007[69]	Thailand	Prospective cohort (n = 329) comparing patients receiving and not receiving ART	Adjusted hazards of death was 0.2 (95%CI, 0.1–0.4)
Zachariah et al, 2007[43]	Malawi	Retrospective observational cohort in which a proportion of patients started ART during the continuation phase of TB treatment (n = 658)	No difference in mortality between patients who chose or did not choose to receive ART, but potential allocation bias according to degree of immunodeficiency and most deaths occurred pre-ART during intensive phase
Nahid et al, 2007[49]	United States	Retrospective observational cohort (n = 264) 1990–2001 spanning pre-ART and ART era	Use of ART protected against mortality compared with patients who did not receive ART (hazard ratio 0.36, 95% CI 0.14–0.91)
Haar et al, 2007[42]	Netherlands	Retrospective observational study of national data 1993–2001 spanning pre-ART and ART era	Compared with 1993–1995, adjusted odds of death during 1999–2001 was 0.46 (95%CI, 0.24–0.89), whereas no such change was observed among patients who had TB and were not infected with HIV
Varma et al, 2009[70]	Thailand	Prospective multicenter observational study (n = 667) comparing patients receiving and not receiving ART	Adjusted hazards of death among those who received ART was 0.16 (95%CI, 0.07–0.36)
Velasco et al, 2009[71]	Spain	Retrospective observational cohort 1987–2004 (n = 313) comparing patients receiving and not receiving ART	Compared with no ART, initiation of ART within the first 2 months of TB treatment was associated with an adjusted hazards of death of 0.37 (95%CI, 0.17–0.66)

IMPACT OF ANTIRETROVIRALS ON MORTALITY RISK

TB case fatality rates (the proportion of patients dying while receiving antituberculosis treatment) in Africa are 16% to 35% among patients who are infected with HIV and not receiving ART and 4% to 9% among individuals who were not infected with HIV.[41] The authors identified observational studies (n = 8) that provided information on the impact of ART on survival of patients who have HIV-associated TB (**Table 3**). Of these, half were from high-income countries and half were from resource-limited settings.

One study using national data from The Netherlands found a 54% reduction in risk of death of patients who had HIV-associated TB treated in the ART era compared with in the pre-ART era.[42] Of seven further studies, six found that use of ART was associated with significant reductions in mortality risk of 64% to 95% in adjusted analyses (see **Table 3**). The remaining study from Malawi found no such association but analyses were not adjusted for CD4 cell counts and ART was not commenced during the intensive phase of TB treatment when most deaths occurred.[43]

A key issue that remains to be resolved regarding the clinical management of patients who have HIV-associated TB is the optimal time to start ART during TB treatment. Early mortality rates are extremely high among patients waiting to start ART in resource-limited settings.[44,45] However, early initiation of ART in those who have HIV-associated TB increases the risk of TB immune reconstitution disease.[46] This increase is associated with mortality risk in a small proportion of patients[46,47] but may be greater in those who have neurologic involvement.[48] Overall, the risk/benefit ratio is likely to favor initiation of ART in the initial weeks of TB treatment, but the outcome of randomized controlled trials are awaited.

ANTIRETROVIRALS AND TUBERCULOSIS TREATMENT OUTCOMES

Data concerning the impact of ART on TB treatment outcomes other than death are scarce. A large retrospective observational cohort study in San Francisco reported that use of ART was associated with significant shortening of the time to smear and culture conversion.[49] A systematic review of 32 studies[50] and recently published data from Rio de Janeiro, South African gold mines, and San Francisco[49,51,52] confirm that patients who have HIV-associated TB are at increased risk of recurrent disease, especially those who have low CD4 cell counts. Various

strategies can be used to address high recurrence rates, including prolongation of the duration of TB therapy[49,53] and use of secondary isoniazid prophylaxis.[54,55] However, more recent data from a study in Brazil have now shown that recurrence rates were halved in patients who had TB who received ART.[51] It remains to be determined whether combining ART and isoniazid has an additive effect.

SUMMARY

The HIV-associated TB epidemic is undermining progress toward TB control and additional interventions must be used in combination with the DOTS strategy in resource-limited settings. Observational cohort studies in a wide range of settings have demonstrated that the use of ART is associated with a 54% to 92% reduction in TB incidence rates and a halving of the risk of TB recurrence. ART is also a potent means of improving the survival of those who have HIV-associated TB, reducing mortality rates by 64% to 95%. Thus, ART confers huge benefits to individual patients.

However, limited data are available concerning the effects of ART on TB rates at a population level. Mathematical modeling and a range of empiric observations suggest that this may be limited, largely because of the high burden of TB that occurs before ART initiation and the persistence of TB rates several-fold higher than background rates during long-term ART. Thus, ART is likely to have limited impact on lifetime cumulative risk of TB. To enhance the impact on community TB control, it is likely that ART will need to be implemented with high-population coverage and at much higher CD4 cell counts than is currently the case. Adjunctive interventions, such as those included in the 3I's policy, may help reduce rates further.

Despite the likely limited impact on TB rates at a community level, ART nevertheless transforms the prognosis of patients who have HIV-associated TB. By reducing mortality rates, ongoing ART scale-up may accelerate progress toward the MDG TB control target of halving the 1990 mortality rate by 2015.

REFERENCES

1. World Health Organization. Global tuberculosis control: epidemiology, strategy, financing. Geneva (Switzerland): World Health Organization; 2009. WHO/HTM/TB/2009.411.

2. Lawn SD, Churchyard G. Epidemiology of HIV-associated tuberculosis. Curr Opin HIV AIDS 2009;4:325–33.

3. United Nations. The millennium development goals report 2008. Available at: http://www.un.org/millenniumgoals. Accessed June 8, 2009.

4. Frieden TR, Munsiff SS. The DOTS strategy for controlling the global tuberculosis epidemic. Clin Chest Med 2005;26(2):197–205.

5. De Cock KM, Chaisson RE. Will DOTS do it? A reappraisal of tuberculosis control in countries with high rates of HIV infection. Int J Tuberc Lung Dis 1999; 3(6):457–65.

6. Lawn SD, Bekker LG, Middelkoop K, et al. Impact of HIV infection on the epidemiology of tuberculosis in a peri-urban community in South Africa: the need for age-specific interventions. Clin Infect Dis 2006; 42(7):1040–7.

7. World Health Organization. Guidelines for implementing collaborative TB and HIV programme activities. Available at: http://www.who.int/tb/publications/2003/en/index1.html http://www.who.int/hiv/pub/prev_care/pub31/en/. Accessed February 20, 2008.

8. World Health Organization. Strategic framework to decrease the burden of TB/HIV. Available at: http://www.who.int/tb/publications/who_cds_tb_2002_296/en/index.html. Accessed August 1, 2009.

9. World Health Organization. Interim policy on collaborative TB/HIV activities 2004. Available at: http://whqlibdoc.who.int/hq/2004/WHO_HTM_TB_2004.330_eng.pdf. Accessed August 1, 2009.

10. World Health Organization. Towards universal access. Scaling up priority HIV/AIDS interventions in the health sector. Progress report 2008. Available at: http://www.who.int/entity/hiv/pub/towards_universal_access_report_2008.pdf. Accessed August 1, 2009.

11. Jones JL, Hanson DL, Dworkin MS, et al. HIV-associated tuberculosis in the era of highly active antiretroviral therapy. The Adult/Adolescent Spectrum of HIV Disease Group. Int J Tuberc Lung Dis 2000; 4(11):1026–31.

12. Badri M, Wilson D, Wood R. Effect of highly active antiretroviral therapy on incidence of tuberculosis in South Africa: a cohort study. Lancet 2002; 359(9323):2059–64.

13. Lawn SD, Myer L, Bekker LG, et al. Burden of tuberculosis in an antiretroviral treatment programme in sub-Saharan Africa: impact on treatment outcomes and implications for tuberculosis control. AIDS 2006;20(12):1605–12.

14. Lawn SD, Badri M, Wood R. Tuberculosis among HIV-infected patients receiving HAART: long term incidence and risk factors in a South African cohort. AIDS 2005;19(18):2109–16.

15. Brinkhof MW, Egger M, Boulle A, et al. Tuberculosis after initiation of antiretroviral therapy in low-income and high-income countries. Clin Infect Dis 2007; 45(11):1518–21.

16. Moore D, Liechty C, Ekwaru P, et al. Prevalence, incidence and mortality associated with tuberculosis in HIV-infected patients initiating antiretroviral therapy in rural Uganda. AIDS 2007;21(6):713–9.

17. Ledergerber B, Egger M, Erard V, et al. AIDS-related opportunistic illnesses occurring after initiation of potent antiretroviral therapy: the Swiss HIV Cohort Study. JAMA 1999;282(23):2220–6.

18. Girardi E, Sabin CA, d'Arminio MA, et al. Incidence of tuberculosis among HIV-infected patients receiving highly active antiretroviral therapy in Europe and North America. Clin Infect Dis 2005; 41(12):1772–82.

19. Lawn SD, Myer L, Edwards D, et al. Short-term and long-term risk of tuberculosis associated with CD4 cell recovery during antiretroviral therapy in South Africa. AIDS 2009;23(13):1717–25.

20. Seyler C, Toure S, Messou E, et al. Risk factors for active tuberculosis after antiretroviral treatment initiation in Abidjan. Am J Respir Crit Care Med 2005; 172(1):123–7.

21. Williams BG, Dye C. Antiretroviral drugs for tuberculosis control in the era of HIV/AIDS. Science 2003; 301(5639):1535–7.

22. Lawn SD, Wood R. Tuberculosis control in South Africa–will HAART help? S Afr Med J 2006;96(6): 502–4.

23. Sonnenberg P, Glynn JR, Fielding K, et al. How soon after infection with HIV does the risk of tuberculosis start to increase? A retrospective cohort study in South African gold miners. J Infect Dis 2005; 191(2):150–8.

24. Glynn JR, Murray J, Bester A, et al. Effects of duration of HIV infection and secondary tuberculosis transmission on tuberculosis incidence in the South African gold mines. AIDS 2008;22(14):1859–67.

25. Holmes CB, Wood R, Badri M, et al. CD4 decline and incidence of opportunistic infections in Cape Town, South Africa: implications for prophylaxis and treatment. J Acquir Immune Defic Syndr 2006; 42(4):464–9.

26. Lawn SD, Wood R. How can earlier entry of patients into antiretroviral programs in low-income countries be promoted? Clin Infect Dis 2006;42(3):431–2.

27. Lawn SD, Edwards SD, Kranzer K, et al. Urine lipoarabinomannan assay for tuberculosis screening prior to ART: diagnostic yield and association with immune reconstitution disease. AIDS 2009;23(14): 1875–80.

28. Bassett I, Chetty S, Wang B, et al. Intensive TB screening for HIV-infected patients ready to start ART in Durban, South Africa: limitations of WHO guidelines [Abstract #779]. Program and Abstracts of the 16th Conference on Retroviruses and Opportunistic Infections. Montreal (Canada), February, 2009.

29. Breen RA, Smith CJ, Cropley I, et al. Does immune reconstitution syndrome promote active tuberculosis in patients receiving highly active antiretroviral therapy? AIDS 2005;19(11):1201–6.

30. Lawn SD, Wilkinson RJ, Lipman MC, et al. Immune reconstitution and "unmasking" of tuberculosis during antiretroviral therapy. Am J Respir Crit Care Med 2008;177(7):680–5.

31. Lawn SD, Bekker LG, Wood R. How effectively does HAART restore immune responses to Mycobacterium tuberculosis? Implications for tuberculosis control. AIDS 2005;19(11):1113–24.

32. Gandhi NR, Moll A, Sturm AW, et al. Extensively drug-resistant tuberculosis as a cause of death in patients co-infected with tuberculosis and HIV in a rural area of South Africa. Lancet 2006; 368(9547):1575–80.

33. Bock NN, Jensen PA, Miller B, et al. Tuberculosis infection control in resource-limited settings in the era of expanding HIV care and treatment. J Infect Dis 2007;196(Suppl 1):S108–13.

34. Lawn SD, Harries AD, Anglaret X, et al. Early mortality among adults accessing antiretroviral treatment programmes in sub-Saharan Africa. AIDS 2008;22(15):1897–908.

35. Lawn SD, Wood R. National adult antiretroviral therapy guidelines in South Africa: concordance with 2003 WHO guidelines? AIDS 2007;21(1):121–2.

36. NIAID. The CIPRA HT 001 clinical trial. Available at: http://www3.niaid.nih.gov/news/QA/CIPRA_HT01_qa.htm. Accessed June 10, 2009.

37. World Health Organization. WHO three I's meeting. Report of a joint WHO HIV/AIDS and TB department meeting 2008. Available at: http://www.who.int/hiv/pub/meetingreports/WHO_3Is_meeting_report.pdf. Accessed August 1, 2009.

38. Granich RM, Gilks CF, Dye C, et al. Universal voluntary HIV testing with immediate antiretroviral therapy as a strategy for elimination of HIV transmission: a mathematical model. Lancet 2009;373(9657): 48–57.

39. Walensky RP, Wood R, Weinstein MC, et al. Scaling up antiretroviral therapy in South Africa: the impact of speed on survival. J Infect Dis 2008;197(9): 1324–32.

40. Golub JE, Saraceni V, Cavalcante SC, et al. The impact of antiretroviral therapy and isoniazid preventive therapy on tuberculosis incidence in HIV-infected patients in Rio de Janeiro, Brazil. AIDS 2007;21(11):1441–8.

41. Mukadi YD, Maher D, Harries A. Tuberculosis case fatality rates in high HIV prevalence populations in sub-Saharan Africa. AIDS 2001;15(2):143–52.

42. Haar CH, Cobelens FG, Kalisvaart NA, et al. HIV-related mortality among tuberculosis patients in The Netherlands, 1993–2001. Int J Tuberc Lung Dis 2007;11(9):1038–41.

43. Zachariah R, Fitzgerald M, Massaquoi M, et al. Does antiretroviral treatment reduce case fatality among HIV-positive patients with tuberculosis in Malawi? Int J Tuberc Lung Dis 2007;11(8): 848–53.

44. Lawn SD, Myer L, Orrell C, et al. Early mortality among adults accessing a community-based antiretroviral service in South Africa: implications for programme design. AIDS 2005;19(18):2141–8.

45. Fairall LR, Bachmann MO, Louwagie GM, et al. Effectiveness of antiretroviral treatment in a South african program: a cohort study. Arch Intern Med 2008;168(1):86–93.

46. Lawn SD, Myer L, Bekker LG, et al. Tuberculosis-associated immune reconstitution disease: incidence, risk factors and impact in an antiretroviral treatment service in South Africa. AIDS 2007;21(3):335–41.

47. Manosuthi W, Kiertiburanakul S, Phoorisri T, et al. Immune reconstitution inflammatory syndrome of tuberculosis among HIV-infected patients receiving antituberculous and antiretroviral therapy. J Infect 2006;53(6):357–63.

48. Pepper DJ, Marais S, Maartens G, et al. Neurologic manifestations of paradoxical tuberculosis-associated immune reconstitution inflammatory syndrome: a case series. Clin Infect Dis 2009;48(11):e96–107.

49. Nahid P, Gonzalez LC, Rudoy I, et al. Treatment outcomes of patients with HIV and tuberculosis. Am J Respir Crit Care Med 2007;175(11):1199–206.

50. Panjabi R, Comstock GW, Golub JE. Recurrent tuberculosis and its risk factors: adequately treated patients are still at high risk. Int J Tuberc Lung Dis 2007;11(8):828–37.

51. Golub JE, Durovni B, King BS, et al. Recurrent tuberculosis in HIV-infected patients in Rio de Janeiro, Brazil. AIDS 2008;22(18):2527–33.

52. Charalambous S, Grant AD, Moloi V, et al. Contribution of reinfection to recurrent tuberculosis in South African gold miners. Int J Tuberc Lung Dis 2008; 12(8):942–8.

53. Perriens JH, St Louis ME, Mukadi YB, et al. Pulmonary tuberculosis in HIV-infected patients in Zaire. A controlled trial of treatment for either 6 or 12 months. N Engl J Med 1995;332(12):779–84.

54. Fitzgerald DW, Desvarieux M, Severe P, et al. Effect of post-treatment isoniazid on prevention of recurrent tuberculosis in HIV-1-infected individuals: a randomised trial. Lancet 2000;356(9240):1470–4.

55. Churchyard GJ, Fielding K, Charalambous S, et al. Efficacy of secondary isoniazid preventive therapy among HIV-infected Southern Africans: time to change policy? AIDS 2003;17(14):2063–70.

56. Lawn SD, Little F, Bekker LG, et al. Changing mortality risk associated with CD4 cell response to antiretroviral therapy in South Africa. AIDS 2008;23:335–42.

57. Brodt HR, Kamps BS, Gute P, et al. Changing incidence of AIDS-defining illnesses in the era of antiretroviral combination therapy. AIDS 1997; 11(14):1731–8.

58. Kirk O, Gatell JM, Mocroft A, et al. EuroSIDA Study Group JD. Infections with *Mycobacterium tuberculosis* and *Mycobacterium avium* among HIV-infected patients after the introduction of highly active antiretroviral therapy. Am J Respir Crit Care Med 2000; 162(3 Pt 1):865–72.

59. Girardi E, Antonucci G, Vanacore P, et al. Impact of combination antiretroviral therapy on the risk of tuberculosis among persons with HIV infection. AIDS 2000;14(13):1985–91.

60. Santoro-Lopes G, de Pinho AM, Harrison LH, et al. Reduced risk of tuberculosis among Brazilian patients with advanced human immunodeficiency virus infection treated with highly active antiretroviral therapy. Clin Infect Dis 2002;34(4):543–6.

61. Miranda A, Morgan M, Jamal L, et al. Impact of antiretroviral therapy on the incidence of tuberculosis: the Brazilian experience, 1995–2001. PLoS One 2007;2(9):e826.

62. Muga R, Ferreros I, Langohr K, et al. Changes in the incidence of tuberculosis in a cohort of HIV-seroconverters before and after the introduction of HAART. AIDS 2007;21(18):2521–7.

63. Moreno S, Jarrin I, Iribarren JA, et al. Incidence and risk factors for tuberculosis in HIV-positive subjects by HAART status. Int J Tuberc Lung Dis 2008; 12(12):1393–400.

64. Golub JE, Pronyk P, Mohapi L, et al. Isoniazid preventive therapy, HAART and tuberculosis risk in HIV-infected adults in South Africa: a prospective cohort. AIDS 2009;23(5):631–6.

65. Bonnet MM, Pinoges LL, Varaine FF, et al. Tuberculosis after HAART initiation in HIV-positive patients from five countries with a high tuberculosis burden. AIDS 2006;20(9):1275–9.

66. Walters E, Cotton MF, Rabie H, et al. Clinical presentation and outcome of tuberculosis in human immunodeficiency virus infected children on anti-retroviral therapy. BMC Pediatr 2008;8:1.

67. Dheda K, Lampe FC, Johnson MA, et al. Outcome of HIV-associated tuberculosis in the era of highly active antiretroviral therapy. J Infect Dis 2004; 190(9):1670–6.

68. Manosuthi W, Chottanapand S, Thongyen S, et al. Survival rate and risk factors of mortality among HIV/tuberculosis-coinfected patients with and without antiretroviral therapy. J Acquir Immune Defic Syndr 2006;43(1):42–6.

69. Akksilp S, Karnkawinpong O, Wattanaamornkiat W, et al. Antiretroviral therapy during tuberculosis treatment and marked reduction in death rate of HIV-infected patients, Thailand. Emerg Infect Dis 2007; 13(7):1001–7.

70. Varma JK, Nateniyom S, Akksilp S, et al. HIV care and treatment factors associated with improved survival during TB treatment in Thailand: an observational study. BMC Infect Dis 2009;9:42.

71. Velasco M, Castilla V, Sanz J, et al. Effect of simultaneous use of highly active antiretroviral therapy on survival of HIV patients with tuberculosis. J Acquir Immune Defic Syndr 2009;50(2):148–52.

Novel and Improved Technologies for Tuberculosis Diagnosis: Progress and Challenges

Madhukar Pai, MD, PhD[a],*, Jessica Minion, MD[a],
Hojoon Sohn, MPH[a,b], Alice Zwerling, MSc[a], Mark D. Perkins, MD[b]

KEYWORDS

- Tuberculosis • Diagnostics • New tools
- Sensitivity and specificity

Despite substantial success in implementing standardized care and improving rates of cure in recent years, the global burden of tuberculosis (TB) remains enormous. Lack of rapid and accurate diagnosis and case detection are major obstacles to TB control. TB diagnosis, even today, continues to rely heavily on tools such as direct smear microscopy, solid culture, chest radiography, and tuberculin skin testing: tools that often perform poorly, and require infrastructure frequently unavailable in the periphery of the health system where patients first seek care. The limitations of the existing diagnostics toolbox have been exposed by the human immunodeficiency virus (HIV) epidemic[1,2] and by the emergence of multidrug-resistant TB (MDR-TB) and extensively drug-resistant TB (XDR-TB). Diagnostic delays and health system failures often result in missed or late diagnoses, with serious consequences for TB patients.[3]

In the past few years, there has been an unprecedented level of interest and activity focused on the development of new tools for TB diagnosis, largely because of agencies such as the Foundation for Innovative New Diagnostics (FIND), the Stop TB Partnership's New Diagnostics Working Group (NDWG), the Global Laboratory Initiative (GLI) (another Stop TB Partnership Working Group), the World Health Organization (WHO), and the Special Program for Research and Training in Tropical Diseases (TDR).[2,4–6] Funding agencies such as the Bill & Melinda Gates Foundation, the Global Fund to Fight AIDS, TB and Malaria (GFATM), and UNITAID have provided the much-needed resources and impetus to push the new tools agenda, in keeping with the Global Plan to Stop TB.[7]

This article reviews the existing evidence base of TB diagnostics, describes new technologies and the progress made in their development and

Financial and competing interests disclosure: Madhukar Pai, Hojoon Sohn and Mark Perkins are affiliated with the Foundation for Innovative New Diagnostics (FIND), Geneva. FIND is a nonprofit agency that works with several industry partners in developing and evaluating new diagnostics for neglected infectious diseases. Madhukar Pai and Mark Perkins are core group members of the Stop TB Partnership's New Diagnostics Working Group. The authors have no financial involvement with any organization or entity with a financial interest in or financial conflict with the subject matter or materials discussed in this article apart from those disclosed. This work was supported in part by Canadian Institutes for Health Research (CIHR) grant MOP-89,918 and MOP-81,362, and European Commission grant TBSusgent (FP7-HEALTH-2007-B). Madhukar Pai is supported by a CIHR New Investigator Award. These funding agencies had no role in the development of this article.

[a] Department of Epidemiology, Biostatistics & Occupational Health, McGill University, 1020 Pine Avenue West, Montreal, H3A 1A2, Canada
[b] Foundation for Innovative New Diagnostics, Avenue de Budé, 161202 Geneva, Switzerland
* Corresponding author.
E-mail address: madhukar.pai@mcgill.ca (M. Pai).

Clin Chest Med 30 (2009) 701–716
doi:10.1016/j.ccm.2009.08.016

evaluation, and ends with a review of cost-effectiveness and modeling studies of the potential impact of new diagnostics in TB control.

THE EVIDENCE BASE OF TB DIAGNOSIS

Although primary diagnostic trials are performed to generate data on test accuracy and operational performance, systematic reviews and meta-analyses provide the best synthesis of current evidence on any given diagnostic test. In the past few years, more than 30 systematic reviews and meta-analyses have been published on various TB tests.[8] These reviews have synthesized the results of more than 1000 primary studies and have provided useful insights into the diagnostic accuracy and role of various tests (**Table 1**).[8] They have also played a key role in recent policy statements and guidelines on TB diagnostics.[9] However, much of the existing evidence base is focused on test accuracy (ie, sensitivity and specificity). There are limited data on outcomes such as accuracy of diagnostic algorithms (rather than single tests) and their relative contributions to the health care system, incremental value of new tests, effect of new tests on clinical decision-making and therapeutic choices, cost-effectiveness in routine programmatic settings, and effect on patient-centered outcomes.[8] Recently, NDWG launched a comprehensive Web site resource "Evidence-based tuberculosis diagnosis," available at http://www.tbevidence.org/ (**Fig. 1**). This Web site is the most comprehensive single source of evidence syntheses, policies, guidelines, and research agendas on TB diagnosis.

IMPROVED AND NEW TECHNOLOGIES: WHAT'S IN THE PIPELINE?

New diagnostics pipeline for TB is rapidly expanding. In 2008, the Stop TB Partnership's Retooling Task Force (RTF) and NDWG produced a detailed brochure on diagnostic tools in the pipeline, mainly to provide guidance to National TB Programs (NTPs), and for funding and technical agencies that may wish to support the development, evaluation, or implementation of new tools.[10] **Fig. 2** shows the pipeline; the tools are stratified as "WHO-endorsed," "Tools in late-stage development/evaluation," or "Tools in early phase development." The figure not only describes the various tests but also provides some information on the commercial kits available, training requirements, and estimated costs.[10] A more exhaustive list of various TB technologies was published by Perkins and Cunningham.[1] Some of the technologies are described in greater detail in subsequent sections.

OPTIMIZED SMEAR MICROSCOPY

Although much work is being done to develop new diagnostics, in most resource-limited countries direct sputum smear microscopy remains the primary means for diagnosis of TB. Given the known limitations of smear microscopy, considerable effort has been given to identifying methods that can optimize the yield and accuracy of smear microscopy.[11–14] These include light-emitting diode (LED)-based fluorescence microscopy (FM), use of sputum processing methods, and optimization of specimen collection for same-day diagnosis[15] (ie, front-loaded microscopy). **Fig. 3** provides an overview of the major commercial LED technologies for microscopy.[16] Although published data are limited (reviewed by Minion and colleagues[16]), LED technologies seem to be promising in settings in which FM has not been feasible, and a WHO policy on LED microscopy is expected in November 2009. Mobile phone-based microscopy[17] and automated detection systems using image processing[18] are other novel approaches that have been proposed, although the use of these approaches is yet to be adequately validated.

IMPROVED AND NEWER CULTURE METHODS
Automated Liquid Cultures

Automated liquid culture systems such as BacT/ALERT MP (bioMerieux Inc, Durham, NC, USA) and BD BACTEC MGIT (Becton Dickinson, Sparks, MD, USA) are currently considered the gold-standard approach for isolating mycobacteria. Meta-analyses have shown that liquid systems are more sensitive for detection of mycobacteria and may increase the case yield by 10% compared with solid media.[19,20] They also reduce the delays in obtaining results to days rather than weeks. Use of liquid media for drug susceptibility results in even greater time savings. However, liquid systems are prone to contamination and require stringent quality assurance systems and training standards. In addition, they are more expensive and require equipment investments, though MGIT can also be used as a manual system. Traditionally, liquid culture has always been used in tandem with solid media to maximize yield and allow examination of colony morphology. FIND projects demonstrated the feasibility of using liquid culture as a stand-alone method if rapid species confirmation is possible through the use of rapid antigen detection tests for speciation.

There are currently 3 manufacturers of these rapid tests, which detect the TB-specific protein MPT64 in a lateral flow format (eg, Capilia-TB, TAUNS, Numazu, Japan).[21] In 2007, WHO released a policy statement on the use of liquid culture systems and on species confirmation through antigen detection.[22] The WHO policy recommends phased implementation of these systems as a part of a country-specific comprehensive plan for laboratory capacity strengthening, and addresses key issues, including biosafety, customer support, staff training, maintenance of infrastructure and equipment, specimen transport, and reporting of results.[22]

Unconventional and Newer Culture Methods

Because commercial automated liquid cultures are expensive and may require sophisticated instrumentation, several researchers have proposed unconventional and novel culture-based approaches for TB diagnosis and drug resistance testing. These approaches include microscopic observation drug-susceptibility test (MODS),[23] thin-layer agar (TLA),[24] and the direct nitrate reductase assay (NRA),[25] also known as the Griess method. Recent reviews have summarized their characteristics and potential role.[26–28] Although these methods are promising as they allow the use of inexpensive materials and give turnaround times similar to liquid culture, these tests are not well standardized, and require extensive training and optimization before routine clinical use. These methods all require routine specimen processing, the most burdensome component of mycobacterial culture, before direct inoculation with sputum.

As for all culture-based methods, quality assurance is critical to minimize contamination and to ensure biosafety standards are followed. Appropriate quality-control systems are often lacking, recommended equipment (such as biosafety cabinets) may be unavailable, and strict adherence to infection control practices is infrequently enforced in resource-limited settings. Some of these novel culture-based assays have attempted to address laboratory safety issues inherent in the culturing of *Mycobacterium tuberculosis* by sealing the inoculated cultures in transparent plates or tubes, and relying on visual inspection of typical colony morphology (MODS and TLA) or color changes (Griess) to identify TB growth. Although disposal of the biohazardous material remains a concern, minimizing the need for direct handling and manipulation of mycobacterial cultures by laboratory technologists is an important advantage.

MOLECULAR TESTS

Nucleic acid amplification tests (NAATs) have been in use for many years, although their use has been largely restricted to high-income countries. For example, the 2009 updated guideline on use of NAATs by the US Centers for Disease Control and Prevention (CDC) states that "NAA testing be performed on at least one respiratory specimen from each patient with signs and symptoms of pulmonary TB for whom a diagnosis of TB is being considered but has not yet been established, and for whom the test result would alter case management or TB control activities, such as contact investigations."[29] Clearly, this recommendation is focused on high-income settings that have the resources to implement these guidelines.

As demonstrated in several meta-analyses, existing NAATs have high specificity, but modest and variable sensitivity, especially in smear-negative and extrapulmonary TB.[30–33] Several newer NAATs have been developed recently, including 2 technologies codeveloped with FIND, the loop-mediated isothermal amplification (Eiken Chemical Co Ltd, Tokyo, Japan), a simplified manual NAAT designed for peripheral laboratory facilities,[34] and the Xpert MTB/RIF assay (Cepheid, Sunnyvale, CA, USA), a fully automated NAAT platform that can detect TB and rifampin resistance.[35] Both of these tests are formatted for use outside reference centers, to replace or supplement microscopy at health centers and district hospitals. These tests have shown great promise in early studies, although published evidence is still limited. FIND is currently evaluating these tests in high-burden countries. The Xpert MTB/RIF assay has recently been CE marked with package insert data showing greater than 95% detection of all TB patients.

Line probe assays (LPAs) have recently been introduced in many countries for molecular detection of drug resistance from smear-positive specimens. Two commercial LPAs are available: the INNO-LiPA Rif.TB (Innogenetics NV, Gent, Belgium) and GenoType MTBDR*plus* (Hain Lifescience GmbH, Nehren, Germany). Meta-analyses have shown that LPAs are highly accurate, and the GenoType assay, in particular, performs well for rapid detection of rifampin resistance in smear-positive sputum specimens.[36,37] In 2009, a newer assay (GenoType MTBDRs*l* assay) became available.[38] This assay allows the simultaneous detection of the *M tuberculosis* complex and resistance to fluoroquinolones or aminoglycosides/cyclic peptides or ethambutol from smear-positive pulmonary specimens or culture isolates. Thus, the combined use of GenoType MTBDR*plus* and

Table 1
Summary of findings from several systematic reviews on TB diagnostic tests

Diagnostic Test	Disease/Site	Major Findings/Results of Systematic Reviews
Diagnosis of active TB		
Sputum smear microscopy	Pulmonary TB	▪ FM is on average 10% more sensitive than conventional microscopy. Specificity of FM and conventional microscopy is similar. FM is associated with improved time efficiency ▪ Centrifugation and overnight sedimentation preceded by any of several chemical methods (including bleach) are more sensitive than direct microscopy; specificity is unaffected by sputum-processing methods ▪ When serial sputum specimens are examined, the mean incremental yield or increase in sensitivity from examination of third sputum specimen ranges between 2% and 5%
NAATs	Pulmonary and extrapulmonary TB	NAATs have high specificity and positive predictive value. However, they have lower (and highly variable) sensitivity and negative predictive value for all forms of TB, especially in smear-negative and extrapulmonary disease. In-house ("home brew") NAATs produce highly inconsistent results compared with commercial, standardized NAATs
Commercial serologic antibody detection tests	Pulmonary and extrapulmonary TB	Serologic tests for pulmonary and extrapulmonary TB produce inconsistent estimates of sensitivity and specificity; none of the assays performs well enough to replace microscopy
ADA	TB pleuritis, pericarditis, peritonitis	Measurement of ADA levels in pleural, pericardial, and ascitic fluid has high sensitivity and specificity for extrapulmonary TB
IFN-γ	TB pleuritis	Pleural fluid IFN-γ determination is a sensitive and specific test for the diagnosis of TB pleuritis
Phage amplification assays	Pulmonary TB	Phage-based assays have high specificity but lower and variable sensitivity. Their performance characteristics are similar to sputum microscopy
Automated liquid cultures	Pulmonary TB	Automated liquid cultures are more sensitive than solid cultures; time to detection is more rapid than solid cultures

(continued on next page)

Table 1
(continued)

Diagnostic Test	Disease/Site	Major Findings/Results of Systematic Reviews
Diagnosis of latent TB		
TST	Latent TB infection	■ Individuals who have received BCG vaccination are more likely to have a positive TST; the effect of BCG on TST results is less after 15 years; positive TST with indurations of greater than 15 mm are more likely to be the result of TB infection than of BCG vaccination ■ The effect on TST of BCG received in infancy is minimal, especially 10 years after vaccination. BCG received after infancy produces more frequent, more persistent, and larger TST reactions. NTM infection is not a clinically important cause of false-positive TST, except in populations with a high prevalence of NTM sensitization and a low prevalence of TB infection
T-cell–based IGRAs	Latent TB infection	IGRAs have excellent specificity (higher than the TST), and are unaffected by prior BCG vaccination
Diagnosis of drug resistance		
Phage amplification assays	Rapid detection of rifampicin resistance	When used on culture isolates, phage assays have high sensitivity, but variable and lower specificity. In contrast, evidence is lacking about the accuracy of these assays when they are directly applied to sputum specimens
LPAs: INNO-LiPA Rif.TB (LiPA) and GenoType MTBDR assays	Rapid detection of rifampicin resistance	LiPA is a highly sensitive and specific test for the detection of rifampicin resistance in culture isolates. The test has lower sensitivity when used directly on clinical specimens. The GenoType MTBDR assays have excellent sensitivity and specificity for rifampicin resistance even when directly used on clinical specimens
Colorimetric redox-indicator methods and NRAs	Rapid detection of rifampicin and isoniazid resistance	Colorimetric methods and NRAs are highly sensitive and specific for the rapid detection of rifampicin and isoniazid resistance in culture isolates

Abbreviations: ADA, adenosine deaminase; NTM, nontuberculous mycobacterial.
Adapted from Pai M, Ramsay A, O'Brien R. Evidence-based tuberculosis diagnosis. PLoS Med 2008;5(7):e156.

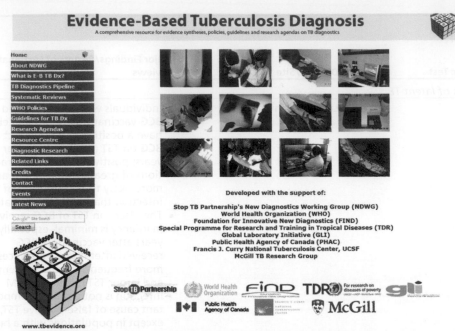

Fig. 1. Home page of the Web site "Evidence-based TB Diagnosis," http://www.tbevidence.org. (*Courtesy of* the Stop TB Partnership's New Diagnostics Working Group; with permission. Available at: http://www.tbevidence.org.)

GenoType MTBDRs/ allows the rapid detection of XDR-TB. LPAs currently require routine specimen processing, DNA extraction, and conventional polymerase chain reaction analysis in a multiroom facility, and are thus limited to use in reference laboratories.

In 2008, WHO endorsed the use of LPAs for rapid detection of MDR-TB at the country level.[39] In 2009, UNITAID approved funding for a program called EXPAND-TB that will supply MDR-TB diagnostics to high-burden countries.[40] With a new grant of US\$61,482,085, the project, led

Summary of technologies				Estimated costs		
Technology	Description	Product	Training[1]	Infrastructure[2]	Equip.[2]	Consumables
WHO-endorsed tools (2006-2008)						
Liquid culture	Commercial broth-based culture systems detect TB bacteria (manual and automated systems are available); can be configured for DST.	BacT/ALERT 3D; MGIT	Extensive (3 weeks)	■■■	High	High
Molecular line probe assay	Strip test simultaneously detects TB bacteria and genetic mutations that indicate isoniazid and/or rifampicin resistance.	GenoType® MTBDR and MTBDRplus; INNO-LiPA Rif.TB	Moderate (3 days)	■■ to ■■■	High	High
Strip speciation	Strip speciation test detects a TB-specific antigen from positive liquid or solid cultures to confirm the presence of TB bacteria in culture samples.	Capilia TB Rapid Diagnostic Test	Minimal (1 day)	■■■	Low	Medium
Tools in late-stage development/evaluation						
Automated detection and MDR screening	Device allows automated sample processing, DNA amplification and detection of M. tuberculosis and screening for rifampicin resistance.	Cepheid GeneXpert device and Xpert MTB cartridge	Minimal	■	High	High
Colorimetric redox indicators	Technique detects isoniazid and rifampicin resistance in culture samples after incubation with redox dyes.	Non-commercial method (Resazurin)	Extensive	■■■	Low	Medium
Front-loaded smear microscopy	Based on 2 or 3 specimens but aims to examine specimens on the day that patient presents to the health service (thus identifying 95% of TB cases).	n/a	Minimal	■	Low	Low
Interferon gamma release assay	Blood test detects specific cellular immune responses indicating TB infection.	QuantiFERON®-TB Gold In Tube; T-SPOT.TB®	Moderate	■	Low	High
LED fluorescence microscopy	Robust fluorescence microscopy (FM) systems based on light-emitting diodes (LEDs) that could allow the advantages of FM at levels of the health system where conventional FM would be impractical.	Fraen	Moderate	■	Medium	Low
		LW Scientific	Moderate	■	Medium	Low
		Zeiss	Moderate	■	Medium	Low
Microscopic Observation Drug Susceptibility (MODS)	Manual liquid culture technique uses basic laboratory equipment (incl. an inverted light microscope) and microscopy skills to detect TB bacteria.	Non-commercial method	Extensive	■■ to ■■■	Medium	Medium
New solid culture methods	Solid culture technique measures nitrate reduction to indicate isoniazid and rifampicin resistance.	Non-commercial method (Nitrate reductase assay)	Moderate	■■ to ■■■	Low	Medium
	Solid culture technique simultaneously detects TB bacteria and indicate isoniazid and rifampicin resistance.	Non-commercial method (Thin layer agar culture)	Extensive	■■ to ■■■	Low	Medium
Tools in early phase of development						
Tool		Level of health system	Tool			Level of health system
Breathalyser screening test		Community or point-of-care	Sodium hypochlorite (bleach) microscopy			Peripheral laboratory
First-generation loop-mediated isothermal amplification technology platform (LAMP)		Peripheral laboratory	Sputum filtration			Peripheral laboratory
Lipoarabinomannan (LAM) detection in urine		Peripheral laboratory	TB Patch Test			Health post
Phage-based tests		Reference laboratory	Vital fluorescent staining of sputum smears			Peripheral laboratory

[1]Key   Description

■   Basic laboratory*; no specialized biosafety equipment.

■■   Biosafety level 2. Specialized biosafety equipment required, such as biosafety cabinet.

■■■   Biosafety level 3. Biosafety cabinet and other primary safety equipment required. Controlled ventilation system that maintains a directional airflow into the laboratory required.

⑧ [1]Estimates assume that technicians are already trained in existing TB diagnostic techniques (such as smear microscopy and culturing) and the necessary laboratory safety precautions.
[2]Product prices may vary depending on geographical location and terms of supply. Ranges are indicative only. Low (minimum-2000 US\$); Medium (2001-7000 US\$); high (7001+ US\$).
*Detailed information available in the WHO Laboratory Biosafety Manual: http://www.who.int/csr/delibepidemics/WHO_CDS_CSR_LYO_2004_11/en/.

Fig. 2. Summary of new technologies by the RTF and NDWG. (*From* World Health Organization & Stop TB Partnership. New laboratory diagnostic tools for tuberculosis control. Geneva: World Health Organization; 2008; with permission.)

Commercial LED products currently available for TB diagnostics

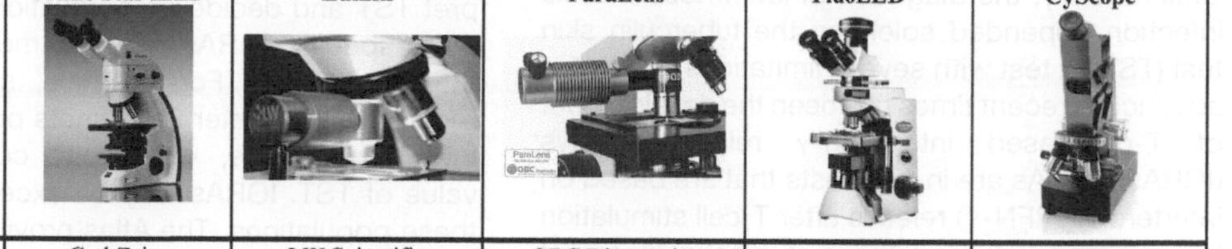

	Primo Star iLED	Lumin	ParaLens	FluoLED	CyScope
Manufacturer	Carl Zeiss Oberkochen, Germany	LW Scientific Lawrenceville, GA, USA	QBC Diagnostics Philipsburg, PA, USA	Fraen Settimo Milanese, Italy	Partec Gorlitz, Germany
Stand-alone microscope	Yes	No	No	No	Yes
Attachment	NA	Objective Lens Replacement (20X, 40X, 60X, 100X oil)	Objective Lens Replacement (40X, 60X oil, 100X oil)	Adaptor Attached to Base and Filter Installed on Head of Microscope	NA
Light Transmission	Epifluorescent	Epifluorescent	Epifluorescent	Transfluorescent	Epifluorescent
Battery Power	Yes	Yes	Yes	Yes	Yes
Weight	9.5kg	448g	1.27kg	5kg	2.7kg

Fig. 3. Commercial LED products currently available for TB diagnostics. (*Adapted from* Minion J, Sohn H, Pai M. Light emitting diode technologies for TB diagnosis: what's on the market? Expert Rev Med Devices 2009;6(4):341–45; with permission. Images have been reproduced with permission from the respective companies.)

by the GLI in close collaboration with FIND and the Global Drug Facility, will expand the use of LPAs for rapid MDR-TB diagnosis.[40] A key component of this initiative will be the strengthening of laboratories in countries where LPAs will be introduced in a phased manner, through collaboration between various partners. Strengthening of laboratory capacity is critical for the success of this program, and indeed, for the successful implementation of any new TB technology.

IMMUNE-BASED TESTS
Serologic, Antibody Detection Tests

Systematic reviews have reported strong evidence that existing commercial serologic tests are of little clinical value because of suboptimal accuracy and high inconsistent results.[41,42] This was reaffirmed in a recent study of 19 commercial tests by TDR/WHO, which showed suboptimal performance of all the rapid tests evaluated.[43] A more recent systematic review examined the accuracy of various in-house, purified antigens for serodiagnosis.[44] Although no antigen achieved sufficient sensitivity to replace sputum smear microscopy, this review helped identify several promising potential candidate antigens for an antibody detection test for pulmonary TB in patients infected and uninfected with HIV. This comprehensive review also showed that combinations of select antigens provided higher sensitivities than single antigens.[44] Several industry and academic

groups are currently working on developing improved serodiagnostic tests, especially for point-of-care (POC) use.

Antigen Detection Tests

Antigen detection has the potential to overcome some of the well-recognized problems with antibody detection assays, especially in populations infected with HIV. Although several antigen detection assays have been evaluated, detection of urinary lipoarabinomannan (LAM) (a heat-stable lipoglycan in the mycobacterial cell wall) was considered a particularly good candidate, based on early studies, especially in individuals infected with HIV.[45] Early proof-of-principle data and the attractiveness of a simple urine-based TB test led to rapid commercialization of this test, initially by Chemogen Inc (Portland, ME, USA), and subsequently by Inverness Medical Innovations (Waltham, MA, USA), which marketed the test as Clearview TB enzyme-linked immunosorbent assay (ELISA). Subsequent field studies in high-burden settings have shown LAM performance to be variable and suboptimal, with lower sensitivity than expected.[46,47] However, some emerging data suggest that LAM may perform better in HIV-positive individuals with advanced immunosuppression.[48] Work is ongoing to improve and optimize the performance of LAM detection assays.

Interferon-γ Release Assays

Until recently, the diagnosis of latent tuberculosis infection depended solely on the tuberculin skin test (TST), a test with several limitations.[49] A major advance in recent times has been the development of T-cell-based interferon-γ release assays (IGRAs). IGRAs are in vitro tests that are based on interferon-γ (IFN-γ) release after T-cell stimulation by antigens (such as early secreted antigenic target 6 [ESAT6] and culture filtrate protein 10 [CFP10]) that are more specific to M tuberculosis than the purified protein derivative (PPD). Two IGRAs are currently available as commercial kits that are approved by the US Food and Drug Administration (FDA) and CE marked for use in Europe: the QuantiFERON-TB Gold In-Tube (QFT) assay (Cellestis Ltd., Carnegie, Australia), and the T-SPOT.TB assay (Oxford Immunotec, Abingdon, UK).

Systematic reviews have reported strong evidence that IGRAs have high specificity that is unaffected by bacille Calmette-Guérin (BCG) vaccination.[50,51] TST, in contrast, has high specificity in populations who have not been vaccinated with BCG but specificity is modest and inconsistent in populations vaccinated with BCG. In low-incidence settings, IGRA results correlate well with surrogates of TB exposure. The high specificity of IGRAs is proving to be useful in individuals vaccinated with BCG, particularly in countries where TST specificity is compromised by BCG vaccination after infancy or by multiple BCG vaccinations.[49] A World Atlas of BCG Policies and Practices (**Fig. 4**) has been compiled to help clinicians and public health practitioners better interpret TST and decide on populations in which the more-specific IGRAs may be more appropriate than the TST.[52] For example, some countries recommend booster BCG shots post infancy and into adolescence, which can compromise the value of TST. IGRAs may be excellent options in these populations. The Atlas provides information on current and past policies on vaccination.

Sensitivity of IGRAs and TST is not consistent across tests and populations, but IGRAs seem to be at least as sensitive as the TST (estimated with active TB as the surrogate reference standard).[51] However, as pointed out by several investigators,[53,54] the diagnosis of active TB depends on microbiological detection of M tuberculosis. Immune-based tests, such as IGRAs and TST, do not directly detect M tuberculosis; they merely indicate a cellular immune response to recent or remote sensitization with M tuberculosis. Because IGRAs cannot distinguish between latent and active TB, a positive IGRA result may not necessarily indicate active TB. A negative IGRA result would not conclusively rule out active disease in an individual suspected to have TB (similar to the results of a TST).

The use of IGRAs is steadily increasing in countries with low or intermediate incidence. More than a dozen countries now have at least 1 guideline or statement on the use of IGRAs.[55] These include the United States, Canada, the United Kingdom,

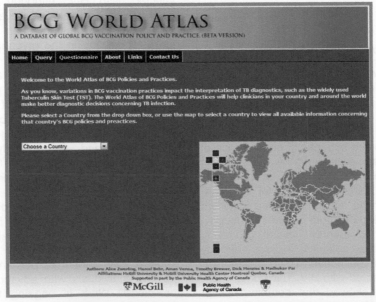

Fig. 4. World Atlas of BCG Policies and Practices, http://www.bcgatlas.org. (*Courtesy of* Alice Zwerling, MSc, Montreal, Canada; with permission.)

Japan, France, Spain, Italy, Germany, Switzerland, Australia, the Netherlands, Denmark, the Czech Republic, the Slovak Republic, Korea, and Norway. In these guidelines, 3 main approaches have been recommended for the use of IGRAs: (1) TST should be replaced by IGRA; (2) either TST or IGRA may be used; (3) 2-step approach with TST first, followed by IGRA. Although the broad approach may follow 1 of these recommendations, some guidelines recommend more than 1 approach, depending on the risk group tested. For example, subgroups such as children and immunocompromised patients often receive different recommendations from other groups. **Table 2** shows the approaches recommended for use of IGRAs in several low-incidence countries.[55] As seen in the table, there is considerable diversity of how various countries currently recommend and use IGRAs. The 2-step approach seems to be the most dominant strategy and this may partly be because of cost considerations.

Despite the large number of publications on IGRAs, evidence is still limited on the prognostic value of these tests, and their added value in TB diagnosis and control.[51,56] There is growing evidence that the performance of IGRAs varies between countries with high and low incidence of TB.[57] Their role, if any, seems to be limited in low-income countries with a high TB burden, although several field evaluations are ongoing, supported by FIND and other agencies.[57]

Improved Skin Tests

A well-recognized limitation of the conventional TST is the lack of specificity of the PPD, a crude mixture with a large number of potentially cross-reacting antigens. Investigators working on this problem have attempted to replace PPD with antigens (such as ESAT6) that are specific to *M tuberculosis*. Small-scale, phase 1 trials of this improved skin test have shown promise, but further validation is needed.[58,59] Despite the limited evidence on these reagents, 1 company (Masterpharm, Russia) is already marketing a commercial product called Diaskintest (based on ESAT6/CFP10).[60] It remains to be seen if this improved skin test reagent can safely replace the conventional PPD.

POC TECHNOLOGIES

The ideal TB diagnostic test is a simple, low-technology, POC test that can be rapidly performed and yield accurate results. In 2009, a group including representatives from Médecins Sans Frontières, Treatment Action Group, Partners in Health, and other agencies, developed minimum technical test specifications that must drive the development of any new POC TB test (**Table 3**).[61] No existing test meets all of these specifications, although the Xpert MTB/RIF assay meets most of them. However, because of growing interest in new tools and biomarkers, and the increased availability of funding and grants, several agencies and groups are working on developing POC tests for TB, including improved serologic assays, detection of volatile organic compounds in breath, hand-held molecular devices, microchip technologies, and tests based on platforms such as proteomics and metabolomics.

Recently, the X PRIZE Foundation received a planning grant from the Bill & Melinda Gates Foundation to develop an X PRIZE for effective diagnosis of TB in the developing world.[62] It remains to be seen if such prize-based competitions foster innovations that deliver the POC test that will revolutionize TB diagnosis. A significant limitation on the effect of a POC test for TB is that TB is a notifiable disease that requires patient

Table 2
Recommendations from various countries that have guidelines on the use of IGRAs[a]

General Testing Approach	Countries
TST should be replaced by IGRA (ie, only IGRA is used)	Germany (anti-TNF-α therapy), Switzerland (anti-TNF-α therapy), Denmark (anti-TNF-α therapy, BCG-vaccinated contacts/adults)
Either TST or IGRA may be used	United States, France, Australia (refugees), Japan (QFT preferred in all groups except in children <5 years), Denmark (child contacts)
Two-step approach: TST first, followed by IGRA (either to improve specificity or sensitivity)	Canada, United Kingdom, Italy, Spain, Australia, the Slovak Republic, Germany (contacts), Switzerland (contacts), the Netherlands (contacts, immigrants), Norway, Korea (contacts)

[a] Some guidelines recommend more than 1 approach, depending on the risk group tested (eg, contacts, immunocompromised patients, children). The subgroups are indicated in parentheses.

Table 3
Proposed minimum set of specifications for the design of any new POC diagnostic test for TB

Test Specification	Minimum Required Value
Medical decision	Treatment initiation
Sensitivity: adults (for pulmonary TB only; regardless of HIV status)	Pulmonary TB: - 95% for smear-positive, culture-positive - (60%–)80%[a] for smear-negative, culture-positive (detection of extrapulmonary TB being a preferred but not a minimal requirement)
Sensitivity: children (including extrapulmonary TB; regardless of HIV status)	- 80% compared with culture of any specimen and - 60% of probable TB (noting problem of lack of a gold standard)
Specificity: adults	95% compared with culture
Specificity: children	- 95% compared with culture - 90% for culture-negative probable TB (noting problem of lack of a gold standard)
Time to results	3 hours maximum (patient must receive results the same day) (desirable would be less than 15 minutes)
Throughput	20 tests/d, minimum, by 1 laboratory staff member
Specimen type	Adults: urine, oral, breath, venous blood, sputum (desired: nonsputum-based sample type and use of finger prick instead of venous blood) Children: urine, oral, capillary blood (finger/heel prick)
Sample preparation	- 3 steps maximum - Safe: biosafety level 1 - Ability to use approximate volumes (ie, no need for precise pipetting) - Preparation that is not highly time sensitive
Number of samples	One sample per test
Readout	- Easy to read, unambiguous, simple "yes," "no," or "invalid" answer - Readable for at least 1 h
Waste disposal	- Simple burning or sharps disposal; no glass component - Environmentally acceptable disposal
Controls	- Positive control included in test kit - Quality control simpler and easier than with SSM
Reagents	- All reagents in self-contained kit - Kit contains sample collection device and water (if needed)
Storage/stability	- Shelf life of 24 mo, including reagents - Stable at 30°C, and at higher temperatures for shorter time periods (to be defined) - Stable in high humidity environments
Instrumentation	- If instrument needed, no maintenance required - Instrument works in tropical conditions - Acceptable replacement cost - Fits in backpack - Shock resistant
Power requirement	Can work on battery
Training	- 1 d maximum training time - Can be performed by any health worker
Cost	Less than US$10 per test after scale-up

[a] Consensus could not be reached on a definite minimum value. The group could not reach consensus for 3 test specifications: sensitivity in smear-negative adults; 60% versus 80%; diagnosis of extrapulmonary TB in adults as a minimal requirement; rejection of use of sputum as a sample. For extrapulmonary TB diagnosis in adults, the interim decision was to define this specification as highly desirable but not a minimal requirement. Similarly, for exclusion of sputum as an acceptable sample, the interim decision was to define this as highly desirable but not a minimal requirement. The group concluded that further consultation with a broader group of end users and practitioners is required to obtain further confirmation of these specifications.

From Médecins Sans Frontières. Paris Meeting on TB Point-of-Care Test Specifications. URL: http://www.msfaccess.org/TB_POC_Parismeeting/. Paris: Médecins Sans Frontières. 2009; with permission.

education, 6 months of treatment, follow-up, and contact tracing. Thus, POC testing for TB through community health workers would still result only in referral of patients to a health center, and not to direct initiation of treatment.

DIAGNOSTICS FOR CHILDHOOD TB

Childhood TB is a diagnostic challenge and although many new TB diagnostics are in progress, few have been evaluated extensively in children.[63,64] For example, several IGRA studies have been performed in adults, but few large studies exist in children. Despite the lack of strong evidence, many guidelines on IGRAs have suggested that they could be used as an adjunct tool for diagnosing TB in children,[65,66] because evidence of TB infection in children is often used in making a diagnosis of active TB, in addition to symptoms, radiological abnormalities, history of exposure, and microbiological investigations.[67] Although IGRAs may be used as a supplementary diagnostic aid in combination with the TST and other investigations to help support a diagnosis of TB, IGRAs should not be a substitute for, or obviate, appropriate specimen collection for microbiologic diagnosis.[65] Apart from IGRAs, there is a need to validate all new tools under development among children, especially young children and children infected with HIV. The poor performance of reference standard methods makes this a challenging population in which to validate the performance of a new assay.

COST-EFFECTIVENESS AND POTENTIAL IMPACT OF NEW TOOLS

For resource-poor countries with a high TB burden, the cost of introducing new tools, their successful implementation, and long-term sustainability are important concerns. Most existing studies on TB diagnostics focus on the test performance and accuracy. Few studies examine cost-effectiveness, and few model the potential impact of introduction of new diagnostic tests.

Recently, Sohn and colleagues[68] described an approach for computing the costs of TB diagnostic tests, and provided templates for various data elements and parameters that contribute to the costing analysis (**Fig. 5**). The development of a standardized methodology for costing of TB diagnostic tests would enable improved and more generalizable costing analyses, which would then provide a strong foundation for more advanced analyses that evaluate the full economic and epidemiologic impact of the implementation of validated new diagnostics.[68] This in turn should enable evidence-based adoption of new diagnostics, especially in settings with limited resources.

Dowdy and colleagues[69] used a decision-analysis model that suggested that novel diagnostic tests have the potential to be cost-effective tools in TB control. They argued that "to produce a cost-effective tool for public health, the quest for new TB diagnostics should focus on high specificity, affordability and sensitivity for cases missed by existing diagnostic standards."[69]

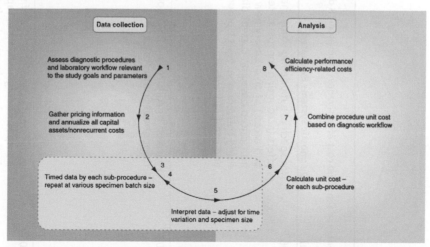

Fig. 5. Major steps involved in cost analyses of TB laboratory diagnostics. This diagram provides a step-by-step plan for cost analysis in evaluating TB diagnostic tests in various study settings. Steps 3, 4, and 5 should be undertaken for all the methods evaluated and relevant subprocedures and repeated to capture data variations caused by specimen loads (or specimen batch size). In step 7, the investigator should consult laboratory experts regarding diagnostic workflow to reflect local laboratory practice in combining procedure unit costs. (*From* Sohn H, Minion J, Albert H, et al. TB diagnostic tests: how do we figure out their costs? Expert Rev Anti Infect Ther 2009;7(6): 723–33; with permission.)

Table 4
Summary of recent modeling and cost-effectiveness studies on TB diagnostics

Study (Reference)	Diagnostic Systems Evaluated	Key Finding(s)
Keeler et al 2006[70]	Not specific: a modeling study that evaluated the effect (accounting for speed, test performance, and access) of an arbitrary new diagnostic test introduced based on current diagnostic capacity using conventional tests (sputum microscopy and chest radiograph)	• More than 400,000 lives can be saved if new innovative TB diagnostic tests can achieve 85% sensitivity for smear-positive and -negative cases, and greater than 97% specificity • New diagnostic tools should be simple, easy to use, and rapid, with results available within 1 h • There is no 1 specific solution (diagnostic tool) in achieving the best health outcome: the need for implementation of "multiple solutions"
Dowdy et al 2008[71]	Expansion of culture and DST capacity throughout South Africa	• Culture and DST on 37% of new cases and 85% of previously treated cases can save approximately 48,000 lives • This is explained as 17.2% reduction in TB mortality, 14.1% reduction in MDR-TB cases (~8000 MDR-TB cases averted) and prevention of close to 47% of MDR-TB related deaths • Expansion of culture and DST capacity can bring significant reduction in overall TB incidences and mortality in South Africa, but additional testing capacity other than culture (molecular and second line drug testing) is needed to address concerns for XDR-TB
Dowdy et al 2006[72]	Five different interventions (2 of which are nonspecific diagnostic tests: rapid molecular testing and mycobacterial culture) and their effect on TB incidence, prevalence, and steady-state population with TB-HIV coinfection problems	• Enhanced diagnostic techniques are projected to reduce TB prevalence and mortality by 20% or more, which is greater than interventions such as case-finding or antiretroviral therapy in HIV-positive patients alone • Improving TB diagnostic techniques can have a substantial effect on TB epidemiology, which in turn will provide improvement in socioeconomic factors

Study	Objective	Findings
Dowdy et al 2008[73]	Comparison of cost-effectiveness of use of 3 different diagnostic strategies in diagnosing TB in HIV patients: (1) smear microscopy only, (2) TB culture with solid media, and (3) TB culture with liquid media	• With smear microscopy as a baseline, solid media culture can potentially avert an estimated 8 TB deaths and 37 DALY at a cost of US$962 per DALY, whereas automated liquid culture can avert 1 additional death (9 deaths) and 8 DALYs at $2751 per DALY • Higher cost per DALY associated with liquid culture is not necessarily caused by actual cost of the diagnostic test (see later discussion) • Cost-effectiveness of introduction of TB culture was more sensitive to the characteristics of the existing TB diagnostic infrastructure (communication of test results and use of these test results for clinical treatment is more important) than the test accuracy or cost
Mueller et al 2008[74]	Comparison of cost and cost-effectiveness of various liquid (automated and manual) and solid (commercially prepared and home-made) culture methodologies	• All methodologies indicate comparable costs per culture (between US$28 and $32) • Cost per M tuberculosis specimen detected were between US$197 and $340, where home-made solid culture method was most expensive • Liquid media brought substantially higher yields with comparable cost-effectiveness to solid culture
Acuna-Villaorduna et al 2008[75]	Comparison of cost and cost-effectiveness of 4 different rapid DST (FASTPlaque-response, direct amplification and reverse hybridization of the rpoB gene [INNO-LiPA], indirect colorimetric minimum inhibitory concentration assay [MTT], and direct proportion method on solid media) methods to conventional culture DST (indirect proportion method on solid media) in the context of a clinical trial	• At 2% MDR-TB prevalence direct proportion method on solid culture and MTT assays were most cost-effective with US$41 and $95 per DALY gained • Other methodologies such as FASTPlaque and INNO-LiPA (US$150 and $163 per DALY) are less cost-effective because of their higher test "kit" costs • Compared with the baseline indirect proportion method on solid culture ($156 per DALY), all rapid methodologies evaluated show comparable cost-effectiveness • Selection of rapid diagnostic technology/techniques should also take consideration of implementation issues (infrastructure capacity to introduce new technology and complexity of methodology)

Abbreviations: DALY, disability-adjusted life years; DST, drug susceptibility testing.

What impact can new diagnostics have on TB control? A few modeling studies have explored this issue (**Table 4**). Keeler and colleagues[70] reported that a rapid and widely available diagnostic for TB with sensitivity greater than 85% for smear-positive and smear-negative cases, and 97% specificity, could save approximately 400,000 lives each year. In another modeling study, Dowdy and colleagues[71] showed that expanding TB culture capacity and drug susceptibility testing in South Africa could substantially reduce TB, and particularly MDR-TB, mortality. These investigators also showed that TB cultures and new diagnostics are potentially effective and cost-effective for HIV-positive patients in diverse resource-constrained settings.[72,73] Other modeling studies have explored the use of solid versus liquid cultures,[74] and cost-effectiveness of rapid drug susceptibility testing methods.[75]

Although modeling studies are heavily dependent on the underlying assumptions and cost estimates used, they are useful for predicting the likely costs versus impact and benefits of new tools. Uncertainty in model parameters can often be addressed using sensitivity analyses. Modeling studies should be followed up with real-world studies in which new tools are introduced, to see if they really make a difference to the lives of TB patients; this is often done in field demonstration studies, as part of routine NTP services. Implementation and operations research are therefore highly desirable whenever new tools and interventions are introduced in programmatic conditions. Indeed, they are essential for evidence-based selection and implementation of diagnostic tools in the global strategy to control TB.

REFERENCES

1. Perkins MD, Cunningham J. Facing the crisis: improving the diagnosis of tuberculosis in the HIV era. J Infect Dis 2007;196(Suppl 1):S15–27.
2. Pai M, O'Brien R. New diagnostics for latent and active tuberculosis: state of the art and future prospects. Semin Respir Crit Care Med 2008;29:560–8.
3. Sreeramareddy CT, Kishore PV, Menten J, et al. Time delays in diagnosis of pulmonary tuberculosis: a systematic review of literature. BMC Infect Dis 2009;9:91.
4. Perkins MD, Roscigno G, Zumla A. Progress towards improved tuberculosis diagnostics for developing countries. Lancet 2006;367:942–3.
5. Perkins MD, Small PM. Partnering for better microbial diagnostics. Nat Biotechnol 2006;24:919–21.
6. Minion J, Zwerling A, Pai M. Diagnostics for tuberculosis: what new knowledge did we gain through the International Journal of Tuberculosis and Lung Disease in 2008? Int J Tuberc Lung Dis 2009;13:691–7.
7. Stop TB Partnership, World Health Organization. The global plan to stop TB 2006–2015. Geneva (Switzerland): World Health Organization; 2006.
8. Pai M, Ramsay A, O'Brien R. Evidence-based tuberculosis diagnosis. PLoS Med 2008;5:e156.
9. World Health Organization. Moving research findings into new WHO policies. Geneva (Switzerland): World Health Organization; 2008. Available at: http://www.who.int/tb/dots/laboratory/policy/en/index4.html. Accessed October 1, 2009.
10. World Health Organization, Stop TB Partnership. New laboratory diagnostic tools for tuberculosis control. In: Geneva (Switzerland): World Health Organization; 2008.
11. Steingart KR, Henry M, Ng V, et al. Fluorescence versus conventional sputum smear microscopy for tuberculosis: a systematic review. Lancet Infect Dis 2006;6:570–81.
12. Steingart KR, Ng V, Henry M, et al. Sputum processing methods to improve the sensitivity of smear microscopy for tuberculosis: a systematic review. Lancet Infect Dis 2006;6:664–74.
13. Steingart KR, Ramsay A, Pai M. Optimizing sputum smear microscopy for the diagnosis of pulmonary tuberculosis. Expert Rev Anti Infect Ther 2007;5:327–31.
14. Mase SR, Ramsay A, Ng V, et al. Yield of serial sputum specimen examinations in the diagnosis of pulmonary tuberculosis: a systematic review. Int J Tuberc Lung Dis 2007;11:485–95.
15. Cambanis A, Yassin MA, Ramsay A, et al. A one-day method for the diagnosis of pulmonary tuberculosis in rural Ethiopia. Int J Tuberc Lung Dis 2006;10:230–2.
16. Minion J, Sohn H, Pai M. Light-emitting diode technologies for TB diagnosis: what's on the market? Expert Rev Med Devices 2009;6(4):341–5.
17. Breslauer DN, Maamari RN, Switz NA, et al. Mobile phone based clinical microscopy for global health applications. PLoS One 2009;4:e6320.
18. Sadaphal P, Rao J, Comstock GW, et al. Image processing techniques for identifying Mycobacterium tuberculosis in Ziehl-Neelsen stains. Int J Tuberc Lung Dis 2008;12:579–82.
19. Dinnes J, Deeks J, Kunst H, et al. A systematic review of rapid diagnostic tests for the detection of tuberculosis infection. Health Technol Assess 2007;11:1–178.
20. Cruciani M, Scarparo C, Malena M, et al. Meta-analysis of BACTEC MGIT 960 and BACTEC 460 TB, with or without solid media, for detection of mycobacteria. J Clin Microbiol 2004;42:2321–5.
21. Ngamlert K, Sinthuwattanawibool C, McCarthy KD, et al. Diagnostic performance and costs of Capilia TB for Mycobacterium tuberculosis complex identification from broth-based culture in Bangkok, Thailand. Trop Med Int Health 2009;14:748–53.

22. World Health Organization. The use of liquid medium for culture and DST. Geneva (Switzerland): World Health Organization; 2007. Available at: http://www.who.int/tb/dots/laboratory/policy/en/index3.html. Accessed October 1, 2009.

23. Moore DA, Evans CA, Gilman RH, et al. Microscopic-observation drug-susceptibility assay for the diagnosis of TB. N Engl J Med 2006;355: 1539–50.

24. Martin A, Munga Waweru P, Babu Okatch F, et al. Implementation of the thin layer agar for the diagnosis of smear-negative pulmonary tuberculosis in a high HIV prevalence setting in Homa Bay, Kenya. J Clin Microbiol 2009;47:2632–4.

25. Shikama ML, Ferro e Silva R, Villela G, et al. Multicentre study of nitrate reductase assay for rapid detection of rifampicin-resistant M. tuberculosis. Int J Tuberc Lung Dis 2009;13:377–80.

26. Palomino JC. Nonconventional and new methods in the diagnosis of tuberculosis: feasibility and applicability in the field. Eur Respir J 2005;26:339–50.

27. Bwanga F, Hoffner S, Haile M, et al. Direct susceptibility testing for multi drug resistant tuberculosis: a meta-analysis. BMC Infect Dis 2009;9:67.

28. Palomino JC. Molecular detection, identification and drug resistance detection in Mycobacterium tuberculosis. FEMS Immunol Med Microbiol 2009;56: 103–11.

29. Centers for Disease Control and Prevention. Updated guidelines for the use of nucleic acid amplification tests in the diagnosis of tuberculosis. MMWR Morb Mortal Wkly Rep 2009;58:7–10.

30. Greco S, Girardi E, Navarra S, et al. The current evidence on diagnostic accuracy of commercial based nucleic acid amplification tests for the diagnosis of pulmonary tuberculosis. Thorax 2006;61:783–90.

31. Ling DI, Flores LL, Riley LW, et al. Commercial nucleic-acid amplification tests for diagnosis of pulmonary tuberculosis in respiratory specimens: meta-analysis and meta-regression. PLoS One 2008;3:e1536.

32. Pai M, Flores LL, Hubbard A, et al. Nucleic acid amplification tests in the diagnosis of tuberculous pleuritis: a systematic review and meta-analysis. BMC Infect Dis 2004;4:6.

33. Pai M, Flores LL, Pai N, et al. Diagnostic accuracy of nucleic acid amplification tests for tuberculous meningitis: a systematic review and meta-analysis. Lancet Infect Dis 2003;3:633–43.

34. Boehme CC, Nabeta P, Henostroza G, et al. Operational feasibility of using loop-mediated isothermal amplification for diagnosis of pulmonary tuberculosis in microscopy centers of developing countries. J Clin Microbiol 2007;45:1936–40.

35. Cepheid announces new diagnostic technology in ongoing efforts to halt the spread of TB. Available at: http://www.finddiagnostics.org/export/sites/default/media/press/090324.html. Foundation for Innovative New Diagnostics, 2009. Accessed June 17, 2009.

36. Morgan M, Kalantri S, Flores L, et al. A commercial line probe assay for the rapid detection of rifampicin resistance in Mycobacterium tuberculosis: a systematic review and meta-analysis. BMC Infect Dis 2005;5:62.

37. Ling DI, Zwerling AA, Pai M. GenoType MTBDR assays for the diagnosis of multidrug-resistant tuberculosis: a meta-analysis. Eur Respir J 2008;32: 1165–74.

38. Hillemann D, Rusch-Gerdes S, Richter E. Feasibility of the GenoType MTBDRsl assay for fluoroquinolone, amikacin-capreomycin, and ethambutol resistance testing of Mycobacterium tuberculosis strains and clinical specimens. J Clin Microbiol 2009;47:1767–72.

39. Policy statement. Molecular line probe assays for rapid screening of patients at risk of multidrug-resistant tuberculosis (MDR-TB). Available at: http://www.who.int/tb/features_archive/policy_statement.pdf. World Health Organization. Accessed October 1, 2009.

40. UNITAID approves over US $61 million to GLI, FIND and GDF for MDR-TB diagnostics. Available at: http://www.finddiagnostics.org/export/sites/default/media/news/090518.html. Foundation for Innovative New Diagnostics, 2009. Accessed June 17, 2009.

41. Steingart KR, Henry M, Laal S, et al. A systematic review of commercial serological antibody detection tests for the diagnosis of extra-pulmonary tuberculosis. Thorax 2007;62:911–8.

42. Steingart KR, Henry M, Laal S, et al. Commercial serological antibody detection tests for the diagnosis of pulmonary tuberculosis: a systematic review. PLoS Med 2007;4:e202.

43. World Health Organization. Diagnostics Evaluation Series No.2. Laboratory-based evaluation of 19 commercially available rapid diagnostic tests for tuberculosis. Geneva (Switzerland): World Health Organization; 2008.

44. Steingart KR, Dendukuri N, Henry M, et al. Performance of purified antigens for serodiagnosis of pulmonary tuberculosis: a meta-analysis. Clin Vaccine Immunol 2009;16:260–76.

45. Boehme C, Molokova E, Minja F, et al. Detection of mycobacterial lipoarabinomannan with an antigen-capture ELISA in unprocessed urine of Tanzanian patients with suspected tuberculosis. Trans R Soc Trop Med Hyg 2005;99:893–900.

46. Daley P, Michael JS, Hmar P, et al. Blinded evaluation of commercial urinary lipoarabinomannan for active tuberculosis: a pilot study. Int J Tuberc Lung Dis 2009;13(8):989–95.

47. Mutetwa R, Boehme C, Dimairo M, et al. Diagnostic accuracy of commercial urinary lipoarabinomannan detection in African TB suspects and patients. Int J Tuberc Lung Dis 2009;13(10):1253–9.

48. Lawn SD, Edwards D, Kranzer K, et al. Urine lipoarabinomannan assay for tuberculosis screening before antiretroviral therapy diagnostic yield and association with immune reconstitution disease. AIDS 2009;23(14):1875–80.

49. Farhat M, Greenaway C, Pai M, et al. False-positive tuberculin skin tests: what is the absolute effect of BCG and non-tuberculous mycobacteria? Int J Tuberc Lung Dis 2006;10:1192–204.

50. Menzies D, Pai M, Comstock G. Meta-analysis: new tests for the diagnosis of latent tuberculosis infection: areas of uncertainty and recommendations for research. Ann Intern Med 2007;146:340–54.

51. Pai M, Zwerling A, Menzies D. T-cell based assays for the diagnosis of latent tuberculosis infection: an update. Ann Intern Med 2008;149:177–84.

52. Zwerling A, Behr M, Brewer T, et al. Which countries are most likely to benefit from highly specific IGRAs? Findings from the World Atlas of BCG Policies and Practices. Am J Respir Crit Care Med 2009;179: A4773.

53. Lange C, Pai M, Drobniewski F, et al. Interferon-gamma release assays for the diagnosis of active tuberculosis: sensible or silly? Eur Respir J 2009; 33:1250–3.

54. Pai M, Menzies D. Interferon-gamma release assays: what is their role in the diagnosis of active tuberculosis? Clin Infect Dis 2007;44:74–7.

55. Pai M. Guidelines on IGRAs: concordant or discordant? In: 2nd Global symposium on IGRAs; May 30–June 1, 2009; Dubrovnik, Croatia: 2009.

56. Pai M, Dheda K, Cunningham J, et al. T-cell assays for the diagnosis of latent tuberculosis infection: moving the research agenda forward. Lancet Infect Dis 2007;7:428–38.

57. Dheda K, Smit RZ, Badri M, et al. T-cell interferon-gamma release assays for the rapid immunodiagnosis of tuberculosis: clinical utility in high-burden vs. low-burden settings. Curr Opin Pulm Med 2009;15:188–200.

58. Arend SM, Franken WP, Aggerbeck H, et al. Double-blind randomized Phase I study comparing rdESAT-6 to tuberculin as skin test reagent in the diagnosis of tuberculosis infection. Tuberculosis 2008;88:249–61.

59. Wu X, Zhang L, Zhang J, et al. Recombinant early secreted antigen target 6 protein as a skin test antigen for the specific detection of Mycobacterium tuberculosis infection. Clin Exp Immunol 2008;152:81–7.

60. Kiselev VI, Baranovsky PM, Rudykh IV, et al. [Clinical trials of the new skin test Diaskintest for the diagnosis of tuberculosis]. Probl Tuberk Bolezn Legk 2009;2:11–6 [in Russian].

61. Paris Meeting on TB Point-of-Care Test Specifications. Available at: http://www.msfaccess.org/TB_POC_Parismeeting/. Médecins Sans Frontières, 2009. Accessed June 17, 2009.

62. X PRIZE Foundation to Help Fight Tuberculosis Worldwide with Gates Foundation Support. URL.http://www.xprize.org/foundation/press-release/x-prize-foundation-to-help-fight-tuberculosis-worldwide-with-gates-foundati. XPrize Foundation, 2008. Accessed June 17, 2009.

63. Marais BJ, Gie RP, Schaaf HS, et al. Childhood pulmonary tuberculosis: old wisdom and new challenges. Am J Respir Crit Care Med 2006;173: 1078–90.

64. Marais BJ, Pai M. New approaches and emerging technologies in the diagnosis of childhood tuberculosis. Paediatr Respir Rev 2007;8:124–33.

65. Updated recommendations on interferon gamma release assays for latent tuberculosis infection. An Advisory Committee Statement (ACS). Can Commun Dis Rep 2008;34:1–13.

66. Mazurek GH, Jereb J, Lobue P, et al. Guidelines for using the QuantiFERON-TB Gold test for detecting Mycobacterium tuberculosis infection, United States. MMWR Recomm Rep 2005;54:49–55.

67. Hopewell PC, Pai M, Maher D, et al. International standards for tuberculosis care. Lancet Infect Dis 2006;6:710–25.

68. Sohn H, Minion J, Albert H, et al. TB diagnostic tests: how do we figure out their costs? Expert Rev Anti Infect Ther 2009;7(6):723–33.

69. Dowdy DW, O'Brien MA, Bishai D. Cost-effectiveness of novel diagnostic tools for the diagnosis of tuberculosis. Int J Tuberc Lung Dis 2008;12: 1021–9.

70. Keeler E, Perkins MD, Small P, et al. Reducing the global burden of tuberculosis: the contribution of improved diagnostics. Nature 2006;444(Suppl 1):49–57.

71. Dowdy DW, Chaisson RE, Maartens G, et al. Impact of enhanced tuberculosis diagnosis in South Africa: a mathematical model of expanded culture and drug susceptibility testing. Proc Natl Acad Sci U S A 2008; 105:11293–8.

72. Dowdy DW, Chaisson RE, Moulton LH, et al. The potential impact of enhanced diagnostic techniques for tuberculosis driven by HIV: a mathematical model. AIDS 2006;20:751–62.

73. Dowdy DW, Lourenco MC, Cavalcante SC, et al. Impact and cost-effectiveness of culture for diagnosis of tuberculosis in HIV-infected Brazilian adults. PLoS One 2008;3:e4057.

74. Mueller DH, Mwenge L, Muyoyeta M, et al. Costs and cost-effectiveness of tuberculosis cultures using solid and liquid media in a developing country. Int J Tuberc Lung Dis 2008;12:1196–202.

75. Acuna-Villaorduna C, Vassall A, Henostroza G, et al. Cost-effectiveness analysis of introduction of rapid, alternative methods to identify multidrug-resistant tuberculosis in middle-income countries. Clin Infect Dis 2008;47:487–95.

Advances in Imaging Chest Tuberculosis: Blurring of Differences Between Children and Adults

Savvas Andronikou, MBBCh, FCRad, FRCR, PhD[a,b,*],
Filip M. Vanhoenacker, MD, PhD[c,d],
Adelard I. De Backer, MD, PhD[e]

KEYWORDS
- Imaging • Children and adults • Chest
- Radiological classification

ROLE OF IMAGING

If there was a reliable, cheap, and fast clinical test to diagnose tuberculosis (TB), then imaging would probably be relegated to looking for complications and providing alternative diagnoses in nonresponders. As things stand however, current clinical signs and tests for diagnosing TB do not do the job well enough, cheaply enough, or quickly enough and imaging continues to play a role in the diagnosis and management of TB. Sputum microscopy (and culture) is specific for diagnosis and may be widely available, however, a large proportion of patients, and children in particular, are found to be smear-negative. Imaging remains useful for diagnosis, detection of complications, monitoring response to therapy, and for evaluating outcome.

Diagnosis using imaging is difficult for several reasons: changing patterns of disease; effects of human immunodeficiency virus (HIV) coinfection and AIDS[1]; inability to identify drug resistance; nonspecific radiographic signs[1]; subjective interpretation with inter- and intraobserver variability of readers[1–3]; possibility of a normal radiograph[1]; problems distinguishing active from inactive disease and infection from disease; imaging is also expensive and often unavailable; radiography is subject to variable quality in technique.

HAS OUR THINKING CHANGED?

The traditional classification of TB into primary and postprimary (reactivation TB) should be avoided[4] as the pathologic differences between these and the corresponding classic imaging patterns characterizing disease in adults and children have blurred. The age-related distinction has changed because primary infection can occur at any age (especially in countries with low TB incidence)[5]; because of exogenous reinfection in endemic areas[4,6–8]; cavitation occurring within 6 months of initial infection (reducing its status as indicator of reactivation),[4] and because HIV infection results in atypical patterns of disease. A radiological classification of disease is more appropriate.

[a] Diagnostic Imaging Working Group, Medecins Sans Frontieres, Plantage middenlaan 14, Amsterdam, The Netherlands
[b] Department of Radiology, University of Cape Town, Anzio Road, Observatory, Cape Town, South Africa
[c] Department of Radiology, Sint-Maarten Hospital, Duffel-Mechelen, Belgium
[d] University Hospital Antwerp, UZA, University of Antwerp, Wilrijkstraat, 10, B-2650, Edegem, Belgium
[e] Department of Radiology, Sint-Lucas Hospital, Groenebriel, 1, B-9000, Ghent, Belgium
* Corresponding author. Department of Radiology, University of Cape Town, Anzio Road, Observatory, Cape Town, South Africa.
E-mail address: docsav@mweb.co.za (S. Andronikou).

Clin Chest Med 30 (2009) 717–744
doi:10.1016/j.ccm.2009.08.022
0272-5231/09/$ – see front matter © 2009 Elsevier Inc. All rights reserved.

RADIOLOGICAL CLASSIFICATION

- Lymph node TB (gangliopulmonary TB)
- Air-space parenchymal TB (consolidation)
- Tuberculoma
- Miliary TB
- Cavities
- Pleural TB
- Fibrosis and destruction

ADDITIONAL FACTORS

Various situations requires different information from the image reader and in turn require more information to be supplied to the reader for an insightful and meaningful interpretation: drug resistance requires the reader to give information on the presence and location of cavities and progression or stability of radiographic findings; HIV coinfection requires a different level of suspicion and a specific differential diagnosis depending on the combination of radiographic findings and clinical information (eg, CD4 count); complications of TB should be looked for, depending on the clinical presentation and previous imaging findings; treatment centers require comment on activity and whether findings indicate infection or disease, which affects management.

NATIONAL OR PROGRAM POLICY

The role, influence, and level of imaging depend on various factors within each country, project, and setting, and may even vary according to current universal attitude or personal experience of individuals. These variations are influenced by the incidence of TB in a community or the world at large, geography, socioeconomic factors, the age of patients, HIV coinfection, drug resistance, and philosophy of the program managers. There are currently active programs that use imaging because: it is mandatory to screen the general population[2]; smear microscopy and culture are unavailable; of the predominant number of smear-negative patients suspected of having TB[1], HIV-infected patients require exclusion of active TB before initiation of highly active antiretroviral therapy (HAART); radiographs are useful to guide a change, continuation, or termination of treatment in patients with drug-resistant TB; only the tuberculin skin test is positive in a patient without symptoms; at the end of treatment it is useful to predict relapse of disease.[9] More advanced programs use: computed tomography (CT) when radiographs are normal or equivocal but there are symptoms of TB; multidetector CT with multiplanar reconstruction in an attempt to replace bronchoscopy in complicated lymphobronchial TB[10]; ultrasound to

diagnose TB lymphadenopathy in children; magnetic resonance imaging (MRI) to detect and differentiate TB lymphadenopathy from other causes of mediastinal widening; positron emission tomography (PET) to differentiate solitary nodules of TB (tuberculoma) from other causes such as malignancy.[11] Conversely, there is no or little use of radiography when services are unavailable, expensive, require referral elsewhere, are poorly performed or interpreted, or when other more specific tests are proving successful.

DIFFERENCES IN IMAGING CHILDREN AND ADULTS

Children are different in size, anatomy, and physiology from adults. The thymus for example confounds interpretation of the mediastinal width on radiographs. Children are also imaged with a different technique to adults (anteroposterior (AP) instead of posteroanterior (PA) with different settings), provide opportunities for alternative imaging (imaging the mediastinum using ultrasound), and require significant considerations with regard to radiation dose.

IMAGING FINDINGS
Lymph Node TB (Gangliopulmonary TB)

TB lymph nodes in the mediastinum and hilar regions drain a primary parenchymal focus of

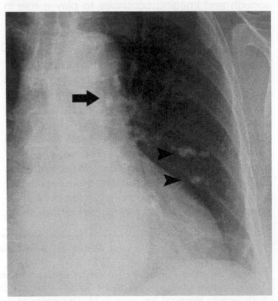

Fig. 1. Calcified Ghon (Ranke) complex. Plain radiograph (detailed view of the left hilum and left lower lobe). Note the presence of multiple calcified parenchymal foci in the lingula and calcified lymph nodes at the left hilum (*arrowhead*) and aortopulmonary window (*black arrow*).

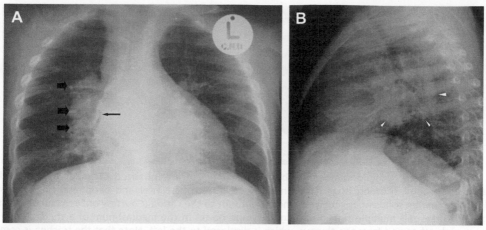

Fig. 2. Hilar lymphadenopathy (gangliopulmonary TB) in a child. (*A*) On the AP radiograph there is a multilobulated mass of lymph nodes projecting beyond the right cardiac margin (*short arrows*). There is resultant compression of the bronchus intermedius (*long arrow*). (*B*) On the lateral radiograph there is an oval dense mass often referred to as a "doughnut" representing a mass of hilar lymphadenopathy (*arrowheads*).

infection. Together the parenchymal focus and lymphadenopathy are known as the "Ghon complex" (**Fig. 1**).[12]

Lymphadenopathy was not a major feature of what was previously termed "postprimary TB" in adults (only 5% of cases),[13] but recently, especially with HIV coinfection, this tendency has reversed. Enlarged TB lymph nodes may cause complications involving the airways and other surrounding structures (see later discussion on complications of lymphobronchial TB).

Chest radiographs (CXR)

Parenchymal abnormality may be small, peripheral, and difficult to identify.[11] In children and immune-suppressed adults, the focal abnormality may not be contained and may present as an air-space process (see later discussion on air-space disease).[14,15] Lymphadenopathy in children is only obvious when it projects beyond the cardiac margins and is less often seen on the left (**Fig. 2**A). Lateral radiographs are useful for detecting lymphadenopathy posterior and inferior to the bronchus intermedius (**Fig. 2**B). Calcification of lymphadenopathy (and the pulmonary focus) represents a healed lesion but is rare in childhood (**Fig. 3**).

CT

Characteristic TB lymphadenopathy shows the "rim sign" on contrast-enhanced studies, with a low density center and an enhancing rim (**Fig. 4**A, B).[16,17] There are other causes for the rim sign including atypical mycobacteria,[18] lymphoma, and carcinoma.[12] More delicate and bizarre enhancement patterns particularly in matted nodes

in children have been described as ghostlike (**Fig. 5**).[14] Calcification is easily detected on CT particularly in adults but is rare in children (**Fig. 6**).[14]

MRI

Lymphadenopathy may have a characteristic low signal on T2-weighted short Tau inversion recovery (STIR) imaging, probably related to free radicals, which are paramagnetic and associated with caseous necrosis (**Fig. 7**A, B). Some TB

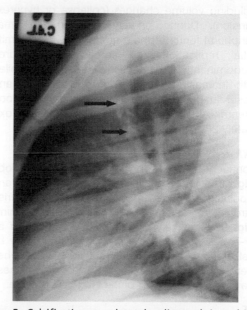

Fig. 3. Calcification on a lateral radiograph in a child. Small calcified foci (*arrows*) representing calcification within TB lymphadenopathy are an unusual finding in children.

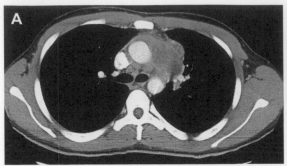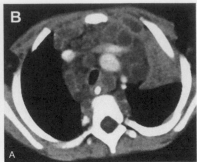

Fig. 4. Lymph node TB (gangliopulmonary tuberculosis). (*A*) Contrast-enhanced CT image at the level of the aortic arch in an adult showing huge lymph nodes with a necrotic center and peripheral rim enhancement. Note also some smaller solid enhancing lymph nodes anterior to the carina (*Courtesy of* Dr. A. Snoeckx, Antwerp, Belgium). (*B*) CT reveals multiple rim-enhancing TB lymph nodes in the mediastinum of a child, clearly demarcated from each other and from the thymus, which is displaced to the left. Note that the trachea is compressed from either side by lymphadenopathy. (*From* Andronikou S, Wieselthaler N. Imaging for tuberculosis in children. In: Schaaf HS, Zumla A, editors. Tuberculosis: a comprehensive clinical reference. Philadelphia: Saunders Elsevier; 2009. p. 266; with permission.)

lymphadenopathy shows solid nodular enhancement, whereas necrotic nodes show rim enhancement (**Fig. 8**A, B).

Air-space Parenchymal Disease (Consolidation)

This pattern is seen with primary infection (especially in children) as a complication of bronchial erosion and resultant bronchogenic spread of disease or as a complication of bronchial compression with distal parenchymal disease including volume changes (collapse or hyperexpansion). During primary infection the small peripheral focus forms a granuloma, which limits initial replication and spread.[15] In children predominantly, the infection is not well controlled with increasing numbers of mycobacteria and dissemination via lymphatics and the blood stream. Air-space disease is seen in approximately 25% of children with TB.[14]

CXR

Confluent areas of opacity often affecting 1 lobe (**Fig. 9**A) and showing air bronchograms and a positive "silhouette sign" (obliterating the crisp cardiac, mediastinal, or diaphragmatic margins) (**Fig. 9**B) are the main features. The edge of an air-space process may be ill defined or may be well defined by a fissure that may bulge when there is volume gain (**Fig. 9**C). In children these may occur in any part of the lung parenchyma.

CT

Lung becomes isodense to muscle and shows air bronchograms. Viable (non-necrotic) lung tissue enhances with contrast and shows enhancing

vessels branching within it (**Fig. 10**), whereas necrosis shows lower density and does not enhance, often losing the vascular detail.

MRI

The signal of air-space disease is isointense to muscle on T1-weighted MR images and hyperintense on T2-weighted imaging (see **Fig. 7**B). The signal enhances with intravenous gadolinium when there is no necrosis (**Fig. 11**). The type of necrosis that may take place can be distinguished using T2-weighted imaging. Liquefactive necrosis

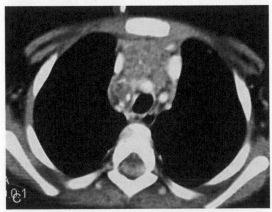

Fig. 5. CT in a child with primary infection shows characteristic ghost like enhancement. The lymph nodes have various shapes with a suggested translucency created by faintly enhancing margins and low density necrotic centers. (*From* Andronikou S, Wieselthaler N. Imaging for tuberculosis in children. In: Schaaf HS, Zumla A, editors. Tuberculosis: a comprehensive clinical reference. Philadelphia: Saunders Elsevier; 2009. p. 266; with permission.)

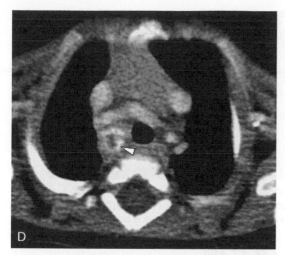

Fig. 6. CT image in a child shows calcification of right paratracheal lymphadenopathy (*arrowhead*) better than plain radiography. (*From* Andronikou S, Wieselthaler N. Imaging for tuberculosis in children. In: Schaaf HS, Zumla A, editors. Tuberculosis: a comprehensive clinical reference. Philadelphia: Saunders Elsevier; 2009. p. 266; with permission.)

has a high T2 signal and caseous necrosis a low T2 signal within the lung, which already has a high T2 signal caused by the air-space process.

Tuberculoma/Parenchymal Nodules

Round or oval lesions involving the lung parenchyma in TB are usually granulomas. By definition, granulomas greater than 1 cm are termed tuberculomas. Tuberculomas may show central necrosis and cavitate. Only calcified lesions should be considered inactive.

CXR

Lesions are round or oval and show smooth, sharply defined margins (**Fig. 12**A). Size varies from 0.4 to 5 cm and the majority are stable in size over time (**Fig. 12**B, C). Calcification is present in 20% to 30% of tuberculomas in adults. In 80% of tuberculomas there are characteristic satellite lesions in the immediate vicinity of the main lesion (see **Fig. 12**B, C).

CT

Lesions are more easily identified (**Fig. 13**) and CT is more sensitive for showing calcification. Some lesions may show central low density in keeping with necrosis.

MRI

Tuberculomas are isointense to muscle on T1-weighted images but on T2-weighted images signal intensity varies according to the stage/type of necrosis (liquefactive necrosis being of high signal and caseous necrosis of low signal intensity (**Fig. 14**).

Miliary Pattern

Miliary nodules result from and indicate hematogenous dissemination of TB bacilli into the lungs and other organs, where innumerable

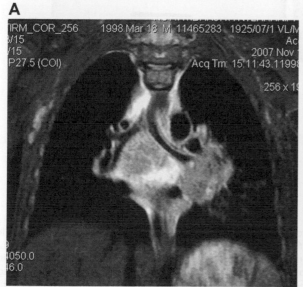

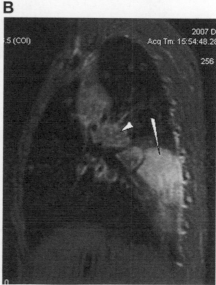

Fig. 7. (*A*) Coronal and (*B*) sagittal STIR MRI images show a characteristic low signal to subcarinal and hilar lymphadenopathy that is believed to result from free radicals. Note how the low signal of the lymphadenopathy (*short arrowhead*) contrasts with the high signal of the consolidated lung (*long arrowhead*) in (*B*).

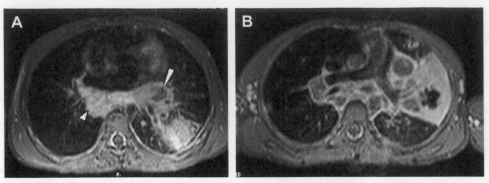

Fig. 8. Axial gadolinium-enhanced MRI reveals nodular (*short arrowhead*) and rim-enhancing (*long arrowhead*) lymphadenopathy in (*A*), and distinctly rim-enhancing lymphadenopathy in (*B*). Note also the enhancing lung parenchyma where there is air-space disease and an area of signal void where there is an air-filled cavity.

granulomas develop. This is classically seen in children in endemic areas (up to one-third of cases)[14] but there is an increasing incidence in adults.

CXR, CT, MRI

Innumerable nodules of similar size (1–4 mm) are scattered randomly and diffusely throughout both lungs (**Fig. 15**A). By definition the nodules, being

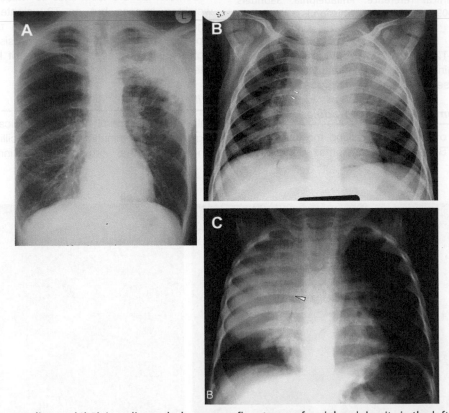

Fig. 9. Air-space disease. (*A*) Plain radiograph shows a confluent area of peripheral density in the left upper lobe of an adult with primary infection. (*Courtesy of* Steve Beningfield, University of Cape Town, South Africa). (*B*) Typical primary infection in a child showing left upper lobe confluent density of an air-space process. In addition there is right hilar lymphadenopathy causing compression of the bronchus intermedius (*arrows*). (*C*) The right-sided air-space process in this child has a bulging inferior margin in keeping with an exudative process. In this case it is caused by compression of the right main bronchus by tuberculous lymphadenopathy (*arrow*). (*From* Andronikou S, Wieselthaler N. Imaging for tuberculosis in children. In: Schaaf HS, Zumla A, editors. Tuberculosis: a comprehensive clinical reference. Philadelphia: Saunders Elsevier; 2009. p. 268; with permission.)

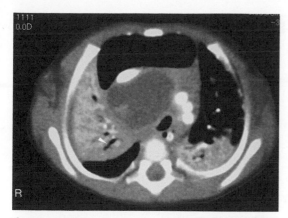

Fig. 10. Air-space disease in a child with primary infection. CT scan shows the imaging characteristics of air-space disease on the right (and less prominent on the left). There is confluent density, which is enhancing, indicating that the lung is viable. There are air bronchograms (*arrowhead*) and visible enhancing vessels. There is also a large necrotic right paratracheal lymph node compressing and displacing the distal trachea.

interstitial, do not coalesce and remain discreetly marginated (**Fig. 15**B). Even though the appearance is easily recognized on CXR, high-resolution CT (HRCT) is ideally suited to showing these and often also shows interlobular septal thickening (**Fig. 15**C).[14,19] A tip for distinguishing nodules from normal vessels for inexperienced observers is to look in the costophrenic angles and the peripheral 1 cm of the lungs where few vessels are expected.

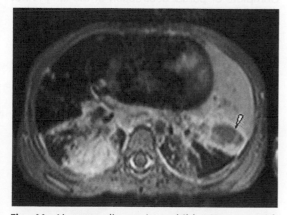

Fig. 11. Air-space disease in a child. MRI scan with intravenous gadolinium contrast shows enhancement (and therefore high signal) involving the dependent portion of the right lung where there is an air-space process. A large confluent area in the left lung is not as brightly enhancing (indicating early necrosis) and shows an oval area where there is low signal in keeping with advanced necrosis (*arrowhead*).

Cavities

These are formed by liquefaction of caseous necrosis and subsequent fibrosis with lung destruction. They are reported to occur in 40% to 50% of adults with a new diagnosis of TB. They also occur in children and should not be considered as an indication of reinfection. Risk of relapse after anti-TB treatment is significantly higher in patients with cavities whether these are present early on during treatment or at the end of treatment.[9] It is also important to recognize cavities and report their position for surgical management when treatment options become limited. There are 4 mechanisms described for cavity formation:

- primary cavitation as early as 6 months after primary infection (**Fig. 16**A)
- reactivation of previous hematogenous spread with confluence of nodular lesions
- bronchial cavities caused by bronchiectasis or bronchial perforation and distal parenchymal cavitation
- Exogenous reinfection[4,6,7]

CXR and CT

Air-filled oval areas within an opacity (**Fig. 16**B) or a nodule (**Fig. 16**C) represent cavitation. "True" cavities have thick walls (3 mm) and may be nodular or smooth, whereas bullae or pneumatocoeles have thin walls and little surrounding opacity (**Fig. 16**D). Air-fluid levels occur within 10% of cavities (**Fig. 16**E) (often caused by superinfection). Bronchiectasis is more difficult to confirm on CXR by identification of "ring shadows" with thick walls and parallel tubular markings ("tram-track sign"). HRCT shows the characteristic "signet-ring sign" of the ectatic thick-walled bronchus (representing the ring portion) adjacent to the smaller blood vessel (representing the "gem" of the ring). Traction bronchiectasis exists within distorted lung parenchyma with elevated fissures or hila and pleural adhesions (**Fig. 16**F).[12]

Pleural TB

Previously, exudative pleuritis was seen mainly in older children and adolescents. It is currently also seen in adults (in countries with a low incidence of TB infection) and younger children. It occurs 3 to 6 months after primary infection and is often unilateral (and asymptomatic). Pleural fluid only yields culture of the organism in 20% to 40% of samples in patients with TB.[20]

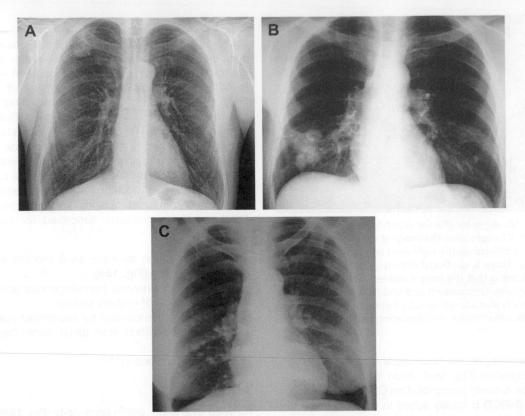

Fig. 12. Tuberculoma. (*A*) A large partially calcified tuberculoma is present in the right upper lobe on a plain radiograph. (*B*) The large tuberculoma in the right lower zone seems to represent a conglomerate predominant lesion with some satellite foci. (*C*) A group of tuberculous parenchymal granulomata in the right lower zone of an adult female. (Images (*B*) and (*C*) *courtesy of* Steve Beningfield, University of Cape Town, South Africa).

CXR

Effusions are usually accompanied by parenchymal and nodal disease.[17] They may, however, be the only radiographic sign in a minority of primary TB infections. Blunting of the costophrenic angle alone in adults is not considered significant for active disease by the Centers for Disease Control and Prevention (CDC) as a CXR screening criterion. Only larger amounts of pleural fluid are taken into consideration.[21] Pleural apical capping is also not considered to be suggestive of active TB disease and may represent fatty proliferation (**Fig. 17**).[21]

Ultrasound

Ultrasound (US) is a useful and rapid way of detecting pleural fluid and guiding a pleural tap.

CT

Contrast-enhanced scans show thickening of the visceral and parietal pleura ("split-pleura sign").[22]

Fibrosis, Scarring or Destruction

Complete or partial destruction of the lung is not uncommon in the end stage of parenchymal and

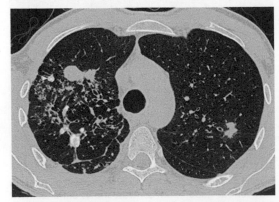

Fig. 13. Tuberculomata. Axial CT scan showing multiple tuberculous granulomas of variable size within the upper lobes. Note central calcification in 1 lesion (*white arrowhead*) and associated thickening of the bronchial walls, thickening of the fissures, and "tree-in-bud" pattern.

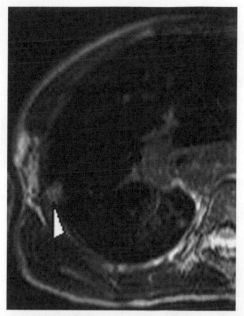

Fig. 14. Tuberculoma. MRI (STIR sequence) shows a peripheral tuberculoma in the right lung (*arrowhead*) with characteristic low signal intensity in keeping with caseous necrosis.

airway involvement. Fibrosis may be stable, progress or regress, but once the lung is destroyed, activity is difficult to assess.

CXR/CT

Cicatrization atelectasis is common after cavitary disease and involves atelectasis of the upper lobe, retraction of the hilum, compensatory hyperinflation of the lower lobe, and mediastinal shift toward the fibrotic lung.[12] Distortion of lung parenchyma with volume loss also results in pleural adhesions (**Fig. 18**) and formation of traction bronchiectasis. Apical pleural thickening is another association of fibrosis and may be caused by proliferation of extrapleural fat and peripheral atelectasis.[12]

IMPORTANT ADDITIONAL CONSIDERATIONS
Drug Resistance (Multidrug-Resistant or Extensive Drug-Resistant TB)

Multidrug-resistant (MDR) TB is resistance to isoniazid and rifampicin. Extensive drug-resistant (XDR) TB is MDR plus resistance to the fluoroquinolones and at least 1 of the second-line injectable

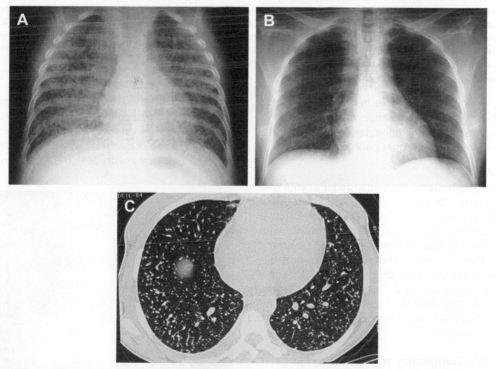

Fig. 15. Miliary tuberculosis. (*A, B*) Plain chest radiographs showing diffuse 2- to 3-mm widespread nodules throughout the lungs. (*From* Andronikou S, Wieselthaler N. Modern imaging of tuberculosis in children: thoracic, central nervous system and abdominal tuberculosis. Pediatr Radiol 2004;34(11):85; with kind permission of Springer Science + Business Media.) (*C*) High-resolution CT showing multiple small nodules in a random distribution. Note subtle subpleural and subfissural nodules.

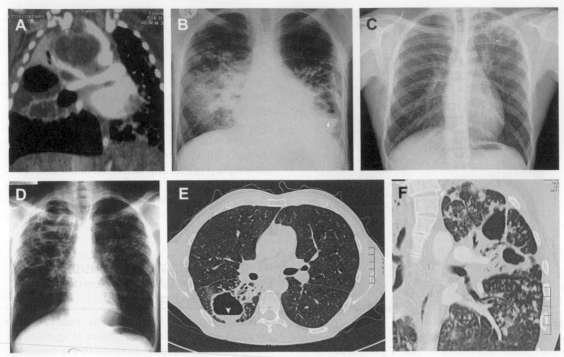

Fig. 16. Cavities. (*A*) Coronal reformatted CT in a child with primary infection showing multiple cavities in the right lung and necrotic mediastinal lymphadenopathy. (*B*) Plain radiograph in an adult showing multiple cavities developing bilaterally within large areas of air-space disease. There are air-fluid levels within some of the cavities (*arrowhead*). (*C*) Plain radiograph of a thick-walled cavity that has developed within an apical tuberculoma (*arrow*). (*D*) Multiple thin-walled cavities within the right upper zone. (*E*) CT image showing an air-fluid level (*arrowhead*) in a cavity within the apex of the right lower lobe. (*F*) Cavities occurring in association with lung distortion and associated endobronchial TB shown on coronal CT scan. There are multiple thick-walled cavities within the left upper lobe, ill defined apicohilar opacities, extensive distortion of the lung parenchyma and hila, and thickening of the apical pleura. Note also traction bronchiectasis and endobronchial spread ("tree-in-bud" sign).

drugs. Imaging plays a role in identifying lesions contributing to drug resistance such as large cavities, which harbor mycobacteria within an area where there is limited drug penetration.

CXR and CT

Two imaging patterns have emerged. Patients with new drug resistance (ie, no previous TB treatment or treatment for ≤1 month) usually show noncavitating disease and pleural effusion. Patients with MDR and a history of previous anti-TB treatment longer than 1 month show cavitating disease. Overall, patients with drug-resistant TB show multiple cavities and bronchiectasis more commonly (**Fig. 19**A, B).[17] Identification and localization of cavities on CT serves as a road map for planning surgery.[17]

AIDS, HIV Coinfection and Immune Reconstitution Inflammatory Syndrome

HIV infection enhances the susceptibility to TB, hastens its progression, and makes it more likely for a patient to be exposed to a case of TB.[15]

Patients infected with HIV can have massive hematogenous dissemination after initial infection, resulting in a higher risk for a fulminant course. TB is a major cause of death in patients with HIV. CXR for TB in patients with HIV may be confusing

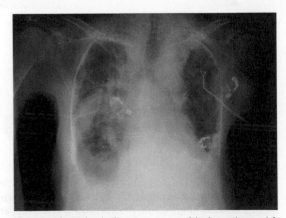

Fig. 17. Pleural calcifications in an elderly patient with a past history of tuberculous pleuritis. Plain radiograph shows extensive calcification of the pleura.

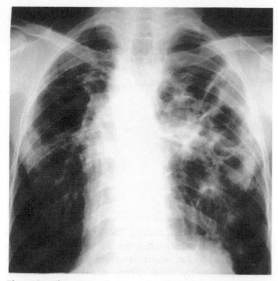

Fig. 18. Fibrosis and scarring. There are long linear densities in the left upper zone with distortion of lung architecture, in addition to multiple cavities. The right and left hila are displaced superiorly by traction from the fibrotic scarring.

because TB and HIV share some imaging features, TB features may be more severe in patients with HIV, there are multiple possible pathologic conditions that may occur simultaneously (Kaposi

sarcoma, lymphocytic interstitial pneumonitis, bacterial pneumonia), and because CXR in patients with TB and HIV coinfection may be normal.[15]

CXR and CT
Appearances depend on the level of immunosuppression.[23]

- Early stage (immunocompetent) CD4 200–500/mm^3: appearances are those of postprimary disease[24]
- Late stage (immunosuppression) CD4 <200/mm^3: up to 20% of CXR may be normal[12,25]; findings are usually those of lymph node TB regardless of previous exposure[24,26]
- Severe and advanced (immunosuppression) CD4 <100/mm^3: nonspecific findings with diffuse coarse pattern[24]
- All stages and degrees of immunosuppression: miliary[23,27]
- Post-HAART initiation (restored immunity): development of immune reconstitution inflammatory syndrome (IRIS) represents a paradoxic clinical and radiological reaction to antigens from TB infection that provokes an inflammatory response. Worsening or new lymphadenopathy, pulmonary disease, and/or effusion are the major chest features.[28]

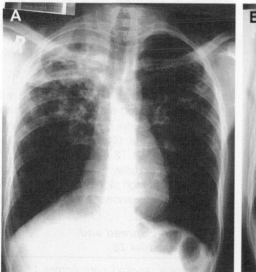
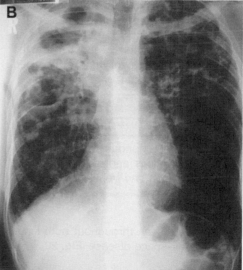

Fig. 19. Multidrug-resistant (MDR) TB with (A) initial, and (B) 5-month follow-up radiographs. (A) The initial radiograph shows that in addition to the bilateral upper zone ring shadows representing traction bronchiectasis and thin-walled cavities, there is a confluent process in the right upper zone containing thick-walled cavities suggestive of active disease. The active cavitating disease indicates a higher risk for relapse of disease. (B) The routine follow-up radiograph (for management decisions in MDR TB) at 5 months shows that the right upper zone process has extended rather than resolved, with further cavitation and fluid levels in the right mid-zone. There was no culture conversion of sputum in this patient requiring revision of therapy and further drug susceptibility testing.

Infection Versus Disease, Active Versus Inactive Disease

Distinguishing TB infection from disease is important as treatment differs (from 1 drug to 3–4 drugs) and because laboratory tests are often unable to make this distinction. This is difficult in children because of the rapid progression from infection to disease. Parenchymal air-space or miliary patterns, lymphadenopathy, and pleural effusion are considered to represent disease. A single non-cavitating, calcified granuloma (Ghon focus) is considered to represent previous infection.

The distinction between active and inactive disease has numerous implications including therapeutic and social (immigration, employment, and health care benefit). Once the lung is destroyed, activity is difficult to assess with radiology studies because fibrosis is known to regress or remain stable. Air-space disease and cavities, with or without lymphadenopathy, are considered active disease. High-resolution CT shows large nodules, "tree-in-bud" densities, lobular consolidation, or mass lesions, and is considered the most accurate imaging method for determining activity.[29] Nodules and scars may contain slowly multiplying TB bacilli and have the potential to progress to active disease.[21] Patients infected with HIV are a greater challenge as even a normal CXR may be associated with active disease.[21] Labeling CXR features as inactive TB should be done with caution. Pulmonary nodules without fibrotic scars and volume loss are considered to represent old healed TB, but it is better to only consider these findings as inactive when smear or culture is negative and the CXR findings are stable over time.[12] Calcified nodular lesions have a low risk of active disease.[21]

COMPLICATIONS
Progressive Primary TB

Children with progressive primary disease tend to have extensive cavitations and are very ill. They often require admission and ventilation. There is a high mortality rate.

CXR and CT
Multiple cavities are seen throughout both lungs with surrounding air-space disease (**Fig. 20**).[30]

Lymphobronchial TB

Lymph node TB may be complicated by perforation of adenopathy into a bronchus with obstructive pneumonia/atelectasis (epituberculosis).

CXR
The lung parenchyma may show air-space disease (consolidation) or obstructive

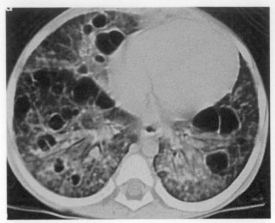

Fig. 20. Progressive primary TB. Axial CT scan shows extensive bilateral air-space disease and multiple cavities in this young child who required ventilation and subsequently died. (*From* Griffith-Richards SB, Goussard P, Andronikou S, et al. Cavitating pulmonary tuberculosis in children: correlating radiology with pathogenesis. Pediatr Radiol 2007;37(8):802; with kind permission of Springer Science + Business Media.)

hyperinflation.[19] This usually affects the right main bronchus or bronchus intermedius (**Fig. 9**).[12,31,32]

CT
A progression from postobstructive air-space disease to bronchial filling by fluid (wet lung), progressive necrosis with loss of vascular markings, lack of lung parenchymal enhancement, bulging fissures, and eventual cavitation is well shown (**Fig. 21**).[30,33]

MRI
Lung necrosis shows nonenhancement within an area of consolidated enhancing lung parenchyma and a range of signal intensity possibilities on T2-weighted imaging. Caseous necrosis is of low signal intensity on T2-weighted images, whereas liquefactive necrosis, which is a precursor to cavitation, is of high signal intensity, and eventual cavitation with air shows signal void (**Fig. 22**).

Bronchogenic Spread and Tracheobronchial TB

Bronchogenic spread complicates 2% to 4% of pulmonary TB disease.[34] This originates when there is perforation of lymphadenopathy into a bronchus.

CXR
Usually the radiograph is normal but parenchymal opacities, seen as ill defined micronodules that tend to coalesce in some parts, are noted

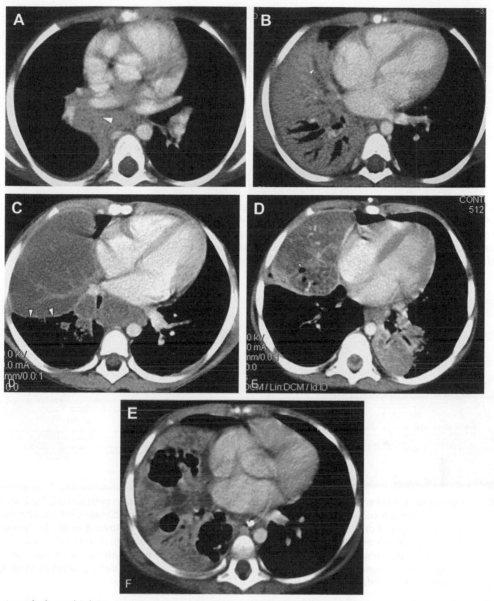

Fig. 21. Lymphobronchial TB. Progressive stages of the effects on the lung shown on contrast-enhanced CT (in different patients) from earliest (*A*) to latest (*E*). (*A*) Lymphadenopathy is seen involving the right hilum (*arrowhead*) and, unlike on the left, the right bronchus is not visible (it is compressed). (*B*) Distal to a right-sided compression, there is air-space disease. Posteriorly in the parenchyma there are air bronchograms and visible vessels. Anteriorly (the right middle lobe) the bronchi are filled with fluid (wet lung) (*arrowhead*). The lung enhances throughout. (*C*) Distal to the bronchus intermedius compression (by hilar and subcarinal lymphadenopathy) the right middle lobe shows nonenhancement, lack of visible bronchi, and a bulging margin (*arrowheads*) indicating a necrotic lung lobe that is expansile. (*D*) The right middle lobe necrosis shows early breakdown with air pockets (*arrowhead*). In contrast, the left lower lobe shows air-space disease with air bronchograms and enhancing parenchyma (in keeping with viability). (*E*) Advanced cavitation (air-filled areas) in multiple locations within the right lung, which also shows some areas of necrosis (low density, nonenhancing) and some areas of viable consolidated lung (enhancing with air bronchograms). (Parts (*C*), (*D*) and (*E*) *from* Andronikou S, Wieselthaler N. Imaging for tuberculosis in children. In: Schaaf HS, Zumla A, editors. Tuberculosis: a comprehensive clinical reference. Philadelphia: Saunders Elsevier; 2009. p. 270; with permission.)

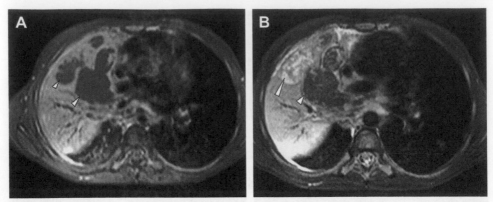

Fig. 22. MRI of lung necrosis. (*A*) Postgadolinium T1-weighted MR image shows right-sided necrosis as geographic areas of nonenhancing low signal (*arrowheads*) compared with the enhancing "solid" air-space disease containing air bronchograms. (*B*) STIR/T2 imaging shows that some areas of necrosis have characteristic low signal (caseous necrosis) (*short arrowhead*), whereas other areas show very high signal (liquefactive necrosis) (*long arrowhead*) easily distinguished from air-space disease, which is generally of high signal with air bronchograms.

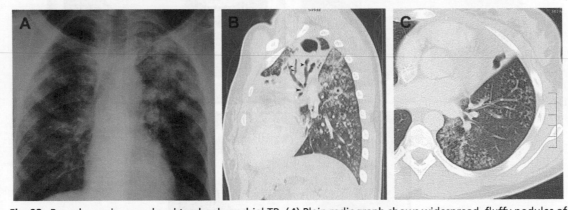

Fig. 23. Bronchogenic spread and tracheobronchial TB. (*A*) Plain radiograph shows widespread, fluffy nodules of various sizes with ill defined edges tending to confluence into areas of air-space disease (*left upper zone*) representing bronchogenic spread of TB. (*B*) Sagittal reformatted CT of the left lung showing multiple stenoses along the course of the left upper bronchi (*arrowheads*), thickening of the bronchial wall, ill defined opacity within the upper lobe, and linear branching opacities within the lower lobe ("tree-in-bud" pattern). Note associated cavitation in the apicoposterior segment of the left upper lobe. (*C*) Axial image in the same patient as in (*B*) showing "tree-in-bud" pattern in the left lower lung.

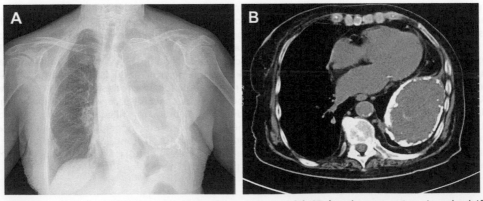

Fig. 24. Extensive pleural calcifications. (*A*) Plain radiographs and (*B*) CT showing extensive pleural calcifications on the left side.

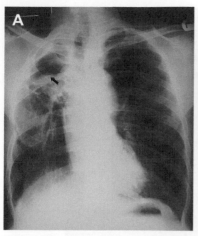

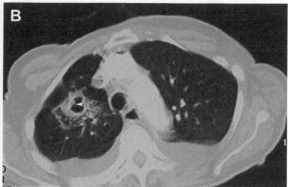

Fig. 25. Aspergilloma. (*A*) Plain radiograph shows a crescent lucency outlining an aspergilloma lying within a right upper zone cavity. Note the elevation of the right hilum caused by apical scarring on the right compared with the left. (*B*) Small aspergilloma (*arrowhead*) in a thick-walled cavitation in the right upper lobe. Note associated pleural effusion bilaterally.

(**Fig. 23**A). This is distinguished from miliary nodules, which have sharp edges and are discreet (ie, separable from each other).

HRCT
Acute tracheobronchial TB is seen as circumferential bronchial narrowing with mural thickening.[35,36] In the late phase the effects on the bronchus are cicatricial bronchiectasis (**Fig. 23**B).[36] Bronchogenic spread of TB is seen earlier and more often on HRCT than plain radiographs and presents as nodular and sharply branching opacities ("tree-in-bud" sign) (**Fig. 23**C).[37]

Empyema, Bronchopleural Fistula, and Fibrothorax

TB pleurisy may become localized causing an empyema. This can also break through the parietal pleura to form a subcutaneous abscess[38] or communicate with the bronchial tree as a bronchopleural fistula.

CXR and CT
Empyema is shown as a focal fluid collection with pleural thickening (with or without calcification) (**Fig. 24**). Fibrothorax is shown as diffuse pleural thickening without pleural effusion and suggests inactivity.[30] Bronchopleural fistula shows air in the pleural space that has a changing air-fluid level on sequential CXR. On CT a direct communication may be seen between the pleural space and bronchial tree or lung parenchyma.[39]

Aspergilloma

A residual TB cavity can be colonized by *Aspergillus* and presents as an aspergilloma with

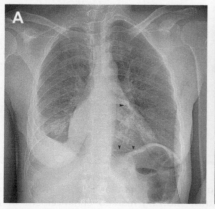

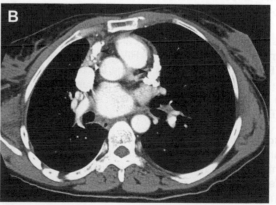

Fig. 26. Tuberculous pleuritis and sequelae of tuberculous pericarditis. (*A*) Plain radiograph showing right pleural effusion and coarse calcification of the pericardium (*arrowheads*). (*B*) Contrast-enhanced CT confirms thickening and coarse calcification of the pericard (*arrowheads*). (*Courtesy of* Dr. A. Snoeckx, Antwerp, Belgium.)

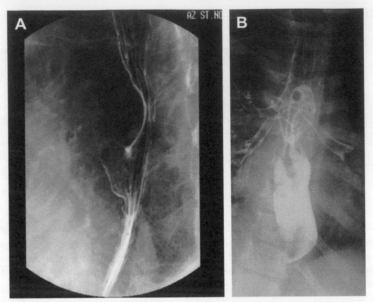

Fig. 27. Esophageal TB and trachea-esophageal fistula. (*A*) Traction diverticulae of the esophagus on a barium study, as a result of longstanding TB. (*B*) Contrast swallow in a child shows contrast entering the trachea and main bronchi in the absence of aspiration indicating a trachea-esophageal fistula. This was repaired using an esophageal stent.

hemoptysis in 60% of cases (and results in death in 5%).

CXR and CT
Early on there is thickening of the walls of a TB cavity and later a spherical nodule is seen with a crescent area of air separating the nodule from the adjacent cavity wall (**Fig. 25**).[40] The nodule is mobile on supine or prone positioning.

TB Pericarditis and Pericardial Effusion

TB pericarditis complicates 1% of TB cases and especially affects immunosuppressed individuals. In sub-Saharan Africa TB is the most common cause of pericardial effusion in adults[41] and effusion is seen in 14% of all TB cases (as high as 22% in those coinfected with HIV).[42] In children with TB, pericardial effusion may be the result of severe malnutrition.[41] Constrictive pericarditis is a late complication affecting 10% of patients with TB pericarditis.[36]

Ultrasound and CT
Pericardial thickening with or without effusion are evident. There may be associated distension of the inferior vena cava, pleural effusions, and deformation of the interventricular septum.[43] Constrictive pericarditis is shown as thickening of the pericardium greater than 3 mm with or without calcification (**Fig. 26**).

Myocardial TB

This is a rare complication of TB usually associated with other foci of TB.

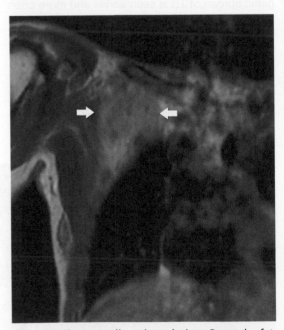

Fig. 28. Chest wall tuberculosis. Coronal fat-suppressed T1-weighted image after gadolinium contrast showing marked enhancement of a large soft tissue lesion at the right thoracic wall. The areas of central nonenhancement reflect caseation and/or liquefaction necrosis.

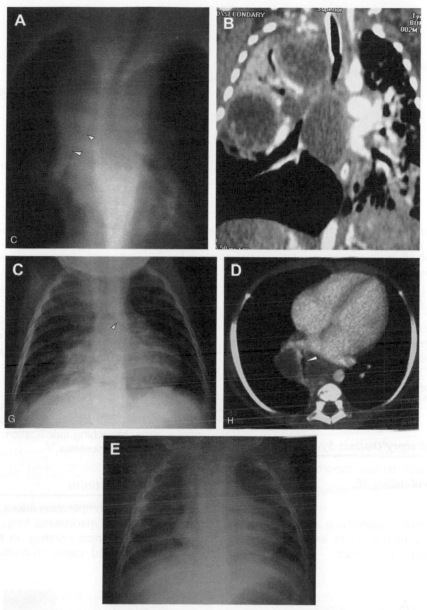

Fig. 29. Airway compression. (*A*) Cropped and contrast manipulated view of the airway in a child showing significant compression of the right main bronchus and bronchus intermedius (*arrowheads*) and less obvious compression of the left main bronchus by TB lymphadenopathy. (*B*) Coronal reformat of a contrast-enhanced CT of the chest in a child showing the significant airway compression of the right main bronchus and bronchus intermedius by massive rim-enhancing TB lymphadenopathy. (*C*) Chest radiograph shows complete obliteration of the right main bronchus and bronchus intermedius with resultant right upper lobe and right middle lobe parenchymal lung disease in addition to partial compression of the left main bronchus (*arrowhead*). (*D*) Corresponding CT of the patient in (*C*) shows the offending lymphadenopathy and the severe compression of the bronchus intermedius (*arrowhead*). (*E*) Follow-up radiograph of the patient in (*C*) after surgical enucleation of the right hilar and subcarinal lymphadenopathy shows reconstitution of the caliber of right- and left-sided airways and resolution of the parenchymal disease. (Parts (*A*), (*C*) and (*D*) *from* Andronikou S, Wieselthaler N. Imaging for tuberculosis in children. In: Schaaf HS, Zumla A, editors. Tuberculosis: a comprehensive clinical reference. Philadelphia: Saunders Elsevier; 2009. p. 272–3; with permission.)

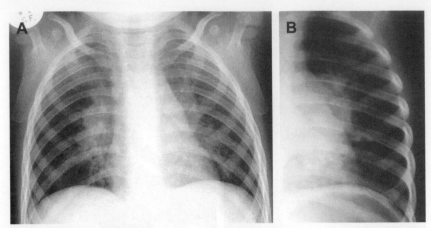

Fig. 30. Lymphadenopathy. (*A*) There is a lobulated mass projecting beyond the cardiac margin on the right at the hilum in keeping with hilar lymphadenopathy. (*B*) A cropped image of the left chest shows a lobulated mass at the left hilum projecting beyond the cardiac margin in keeping with lymphadenopathy. In addition, there is air-space disease posterior to the heart.

CT and MRI

Single or multiple cardiac tuberculomas may be shown as sharply demarcated lesions especially involving the right heart chambers. CT shows calcification more successfully[44] with or without thrombus formation, which may extend into the vena cava.[45]

Acute Respiratory Distress Syndrome

Acute respiratory distress syndrome may result as an evolution of miliary TB.

CXR

A "snow-storm" appearance is characteristic. After recovery, multiple cystic lesions (pneumatocoeles or bullae) may remain.

Broncholithiasis

Broncholithiasis is an uncommon complication occurring after rupture of a calcified peribronchial lymph node into a bronchus.[46]

CT

CT shows the calcified lymph node associated with bronchial obstruction, atelectasis, obstructive pneumonitis, branching calcification, focal hyperinflation, or bronchiectasis.[12]

Fibrosing Mediastinitis

This uncommon complication arises after coalescence of multiple mediastinal lymph nodes and multiple tuberculomas creating an acute inflammatory reaction and reactive fibrosis.

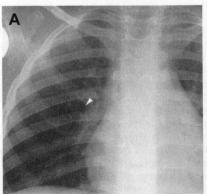
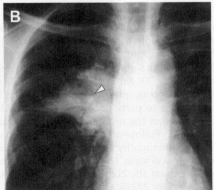

Fig. 31. Hilar point and lymphadenopathy. (*A*) Cropped radiograph of the right chest shows the right hilum where large upper zone and large lower zone vessels meet (*arrowhead*). This normal hilar point is outwardly concave and appears like a horizontally oriented V. (*B*) On the right there is filling in of the horizontal V, which is just visible (*arrowhead*) through the mass of TB lymph nodes.

CT

A mediastinal and hilar mass with calcification, tracheobronchial narrowing, and vascular encasement (and in some cases superior vena cava syndrome) are evident.[47]

Pneumothorax

Pneumothorax may complicate severe cavitary disease and heralds the onset of a bronchopleural fistula.[12]

CXR and CT

A crescent of air (with no discernable lung markings) is seen in the nondependent portion of the chest (erect, apicolateral; supine, inferiorly and medial). There may be mass effect phenomena on the mediastinum when the pneumothorax is large.

Esophageal TB and Tracheo-esophageal Fistula

Esophageal TB is more common in patients infected with HIV.[48] It results from ingestion of

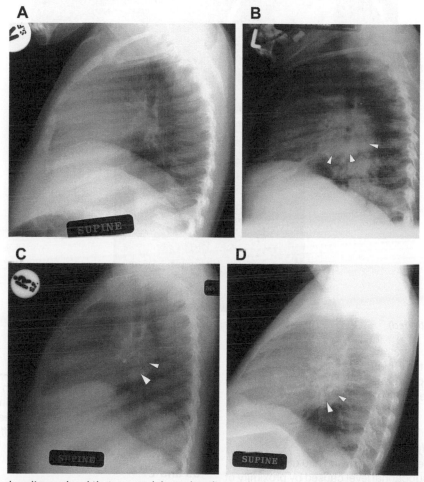

Fig. 32. Lateral radiographs. (*A*) A normal lateral radiograph shows no oval densities behind the trachea/bronchus intermedius or below its apparent termination. The density of the main pulmonary arteries and posterior aspect of the aortic arch are visible. (*B*) Obvious lymphadenopathy on a lateral radiograph is shown as oval densities posterior and inferior to the trachea/bronchus intermedius (*arrowheads*). Associated with the normal dense structures more superiorly, this fits the description known as the "doughnut sign". There is also lower lobe consolidation projected over the distal visible vertebral bodies. (*C*) Oval density representing subcarinal lymphadenopathy is noted posterior and inferior to the trachea/bronchus intermedius (*arrowheads*). (*D*) Another example where oval density representing subcarinal lymphadenopathy is noted posterior and inferior to the trachea/bronchus intermedius (*arrowheads*). (*E*) Multiplanar CT reconstruction with cross-hair cross-referencing used to show the positional projection of subcarinal and hilar lymphadenopathy on a lateral radiograph, by inference from the sagittal reconstruction (*top right corner*). (*F*) Sagittal STIR/T2 MRI shows the hilar mass of low signal TB lymph nodes (*large arrowhead*) which would be shown as a doughnut on a lateral image. On MRI the triad of normal vessels that form the superior aspect of the doughnut show flow void (*small arrowheads*).

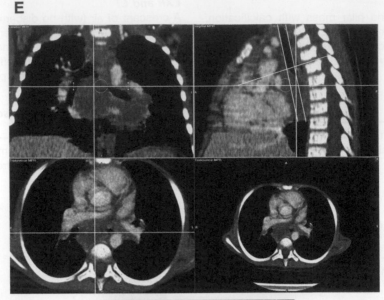

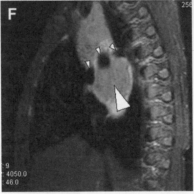

Fig. 32. (*continued*)

infected sputum (intrinsic), spread from an adjacent TB lymph node or pulmonary TB (extrinsic) or may be the result of hematogenous or lymphatic spread.[49]

Barium study

Barium studies show narrowing and displacement, often at the subcarinal level caused by proximity of the esophagus to the lymphadenopathy in this region. Advanced disease results in esophageal ulceration, fistula formation, stricture, and traction diverticula (**Fig. 27**A).[48,49] Tracheo-esophageal fistula may develop and is shown with contrast in the airways (in the absence of aspiration) (**Fig. 27**B).[50]

CT

The extent of disease and the extrinsic causes may be evident.

Chylous Effusion

This is an extremely rare complication described in children caused by infiltration or compression of the thoracic duct by right paratracheal lymphadenopathy. The chylous nature of the effusion is best determined with an aspirate.

US and CT

Large effusions are shown either uni- or bilaterally (10–20 HU). The enlarged lymph nodes in the right paratracheal and other locations may be a clue to TB as the cause.[51]

Phrenic Nerve Palsy

This is a rare complication reported in children. Large lymphadenopathy in the AP window causes compression and infiltration of the phrenic nerve causing diaphragmatic paralysis.[52]

CXR and CT

The elevated hemidiaphragm is always on the left. Usually there is accompanying left-sided consolidation with volume loss. On CT this is shown to be caused by compression of the left main bronchus. This is not only caused by lymphadenopathy but also because the mediastinum is displaced to the right allowing the displaced aorta to contribute to the compression of the bronchus.[52]

Chest Wall TB

The ribs are a frequent location for involvement of tuberculous osteomyelitis. TB granulomatous inflammation and abscesses of the chest wall are most commonly found at the parasternal region,

costovertebral junction, and along the shafts of the ribs. It is thought that lymph node enlargement and subsequent caseation necrosis may burrow through the chest wall.[53]

CXR and CT

CT is more accurate to show subtle rib involvement than CXR. There is usually associated TB pleuritis and intrathoracic lymph node enlargement in contiguity with these chest wall collections. The internal mammary nodes are most commonly involved.

MRI

MRI is the preferred imaging method to assess isolated pyomyositis of the chest wall. The lesion

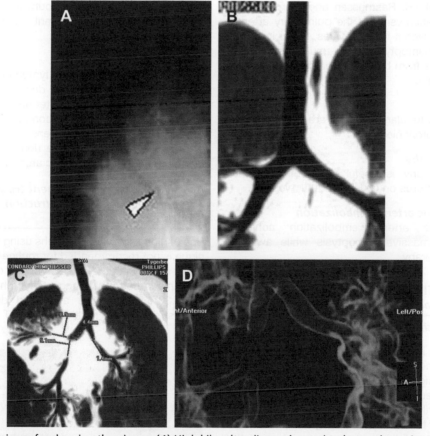

Fig. 33. Techniques for showing the airway. (*A*) High kilovolt radiographs used to better show airway stenosis of the left main bronchus (*arrowhead*). (*From* Andronikou S, Wieselthaler N. Imaging for tuberculosis in children. In: Schaaf HS, Zumla A, editors. Tuberculosis: a comprehensive clinical reference. Philadelphia: Saunders Elsevier; 2009. p. 272; with permission.) (*B*) Thick slab minimum intensity projection CT reconstruction shows a normal airway caliber and outline. (*C*) Thick slab minimum intensity projection CT reconstruction shows how the technique is used to identify stenoses caused by TB and show their length (an advantage over bronchoscopy when the scope cannot pass a compressed area). (*D*) Three-dimensional volume rendered CT reconstruction technique with transparent setting. The bronchus intermedius and right lower lobe bronchus narrowing are well shown. (*From* du Plessis J, Goussard P, Andronikou S, Gie R, George R. Comparing three-dimensional volume-rendered CT images with fibreoptic tracheobronchoscopy in the evaluation of airway compression caused by tuberculous lymphadenopathy in children. Pediatr Radiol 2009;39(7):696; with kind permission of Springer Science + Business Media.)

is of low signal intensity on T1-weighted images and of high signal intensity on T2-weighted images. There is marked contrast enhancement after intravenous administration of gadolinium (**Fig. 28**). Abscess formation is the rule in all cases of advanced pyomyositis. The peripheral wall of the abscess shows a subtle hyperintensity on T1-weighted images and hypointensity on T2-weighted images. On gadolinium-enhanced images, a peripheral enhancing rim corresponding to the abscess wall is observed.

Vascular

Pulmonary arteries and veins in an area of active TB may show vasculitis and thrombosis. Bronchial arteries may be enlarged in TB bronchiectasis or parenchymal TB. Rasmussen aneurysms, which are pseudoaneurysms of the pulmonary arteries occurring adjacent to TB cavities, occur in 5% of patients.[54] Hemoptysis is the usual presentation and it ranges from being minimal to massive and life-threatening.

CXR and CT
Nodular and tubular structures are seen adjacent to areas of bronchiectasis.

CT angiography
CT angiography is useful for confirming that tubular structures on CXR are ectatic vessels.

Angiographic arterial embolization
Angiographic arterial embolization achieves control of massive hemoptysis while awaiting definitive therapy.

IMAGING TIPS AND NOVEL IDEAS
Tips for Reading Chest Radiographs

AP CXR in children

- The most important feature to detect is airway displacement or compression. This may be an indirect sign of lymphadenopathy but is the most objective radiological sign as the airway is the only discernable structure within the density of the mediastinum (**Fig. 29**A).[14] Airways in normal children are compressible and the normal trachea should be positioned to the right of the midline. Normal bronchi should taper distally and should also be of similar size at an equal distance from the carina on both sides. Lymphadenopathy causes compression of the major airways and may displace the trachea to the left (**Fig. 29**B).[10,14,55] Offending lymphadenopathy can be enucleated to relieve the obstruction and allow re-expansion of the lung (**Fig. 29**C–E).

- The lobulated soft tissue masses of lymphadenopathy at the paratracheal region and hilar regions are often hidden behind the thymic shadow or the heart shadow, which is relatively large in children. Noting only the outwardly convex lobulated masses that extend beyond the cardiac margin ensures that only definite lymphadenopathy is recorded (**Fig. 30**).

PA CXR in adults
Lymphadenopathy is represented by a polycyclic, curvilinear or lobulated outline to the mediastinum.[56] Enlarged paratracheal or pretracheal lymph nodes result in widening or obliteration of the right paratracheal stripe within a wide mediastinum.[56] A normal hilar point should show a V on its side, convex outward (**Fig 31**A). Filling of this point, failure to identify it, or an outwardly convex or lobulated margin may represent a mass, including lymphadenopathy (**Fig. 31**B).

Lateral CXR in children
Subcarinal and retrocarinal lymphadenopathy is represented as a lobulated density inferior and posterior to the bronchus intermedius.[56] Lymphadenopathy in this region completes the lower half of a doughnut-shaped density (the upper half of which is made up of the right and left main pulmonary arteries and aortic arch) (**Fig. 32**).[14]

Advanced Airway Assessment (High Kilovolt, Three-dimensional Reconstruction, Virtual Bronchoscopy)

Use of high kilovolt radiographs using a filter technique is not recommended for routine use but can assist in showing the airway, which if compressed or displaced strongly suggests lymphadenopathy (**Fig. 33**A).[55] In more advanced departments, reconstruction of multidetector CT (MDCT) is

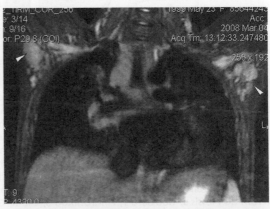

Fig. 34. Axillary lymphadenopathy. STIR/T2 MRI shows the large axillary lymph nodes (*arrowheads*) in this patient with mediastinal and hilar TB lymphadenopathy.

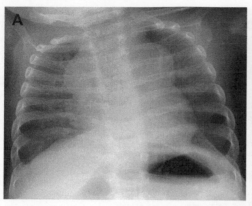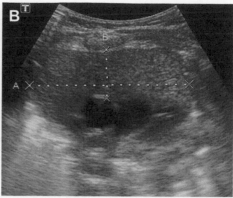

Fig. 35. Thymus. (*A*) Plain radiograph shows how the normal thymus can cause the mediastinum to appear wide and have outwardly convex margins. There is no displacement or compression of mediastinal structures by normal thymic tissue. (*B*) When there is doubt about a mediastinal width, suggesting lymphadenopathy or a mass, ultrasound is useful to show the homogenous texture of the normal thymus seen here (as opposed to the nodular heterogenous appearance of a mass or lymphadenopathy).

possible in many ways including minimum intensity projections (**Fig. 33**B, C), volume rendered three-dimensional (**Fig. 33**D) and virtual bronchoscopy. The three-dimensional volume rendered technique has been assessed against bronchoscopy for detection and characterization of the airway and the causative extrinsic mass. The CT technique was shown to not only match bronchoscopy but also to assess the degree of compression more accurately, and managed to show more distal obstructions of bronchi where the bronchoscope could not navigate because of proximal obstruction.[10] Bronchoscopy can be reserved for when biopsy may be necessary.

Routine Availability of HRCT with MDCT (Combi-scanning)

Current MDCT scanning produces slices thin enough to be useful as high-resolution imaging (after reconstruction with appropriate filters). This means that every time an MDCT is performed with contrast for visualization of mediastinal nodes, effusions, air-space disease, and other complications of TB, the data set is available for reconstruction and review as an HRCT study. This is useful for detecting miliary and other interstitial nodules (and lines), bronchiectasis, tree-in-bud features of bronchogenic spread, and air-filled cysts. This is known to add to the diagnostic confidence in TB assessment and the determination of outcome, and can affect management (eg, detection of cavities and bronchiectasis).[57] The converse is also possible; that is, when clinicians request HRCT for TB, the study should be performed as a postcontrast, thin-slice mediastinal study (combi-scan) and the HRCT component

can be produced in addition to the mediastinal window with a comment on the presence of lymphadenopathy and other information.

Ultrasound for Diagnosis

Ultrasound has been used successfully to detect mediastinal lymphadenopathy via the suprasternal and parasternal approaches in children,[58] Follow-up

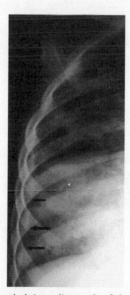

Fig. 36. Cropped plain radiograph of the right chest to show how effusion, termed laminar effusions, in children spares the costophrenic angle and tracks superiorly along the lateral chest wall. A tip for detecting these is to check that the lung reaches the rib margins. In normal children there are no significant companion shadows and when a linear density separates the ribs from the lung an effusion is suspected.

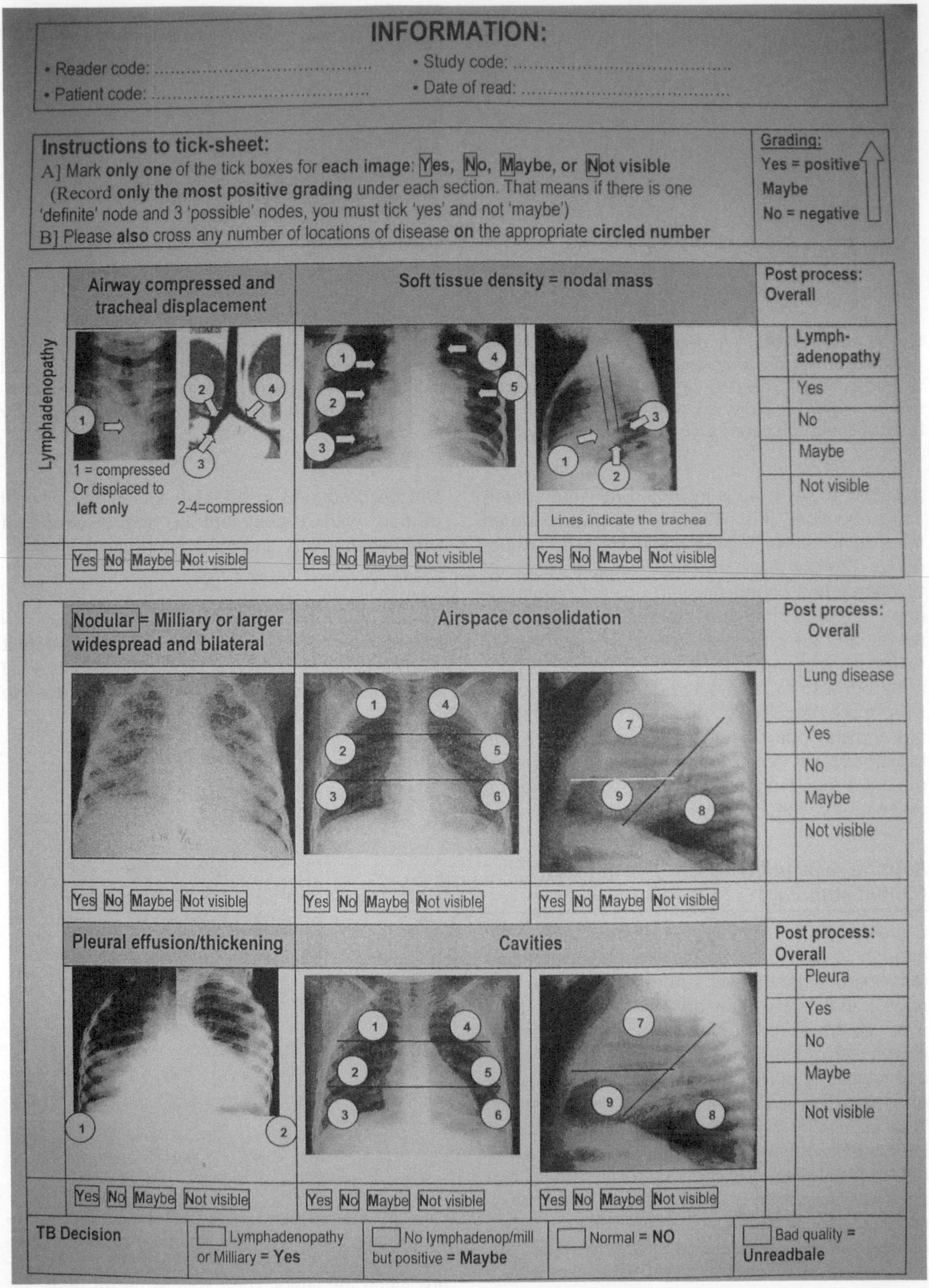

INFORMATION:

- Reader code: ....
- Study code: ....
- Patient code: ....
- Date of read: ....

Instructions to tick-sheet:

A] Mark only one of the tick boxes for **each image**: Yes, No, Maybe, or Not visible
(Record **only the most positive grading** under each section. That means if there is one
'definite' node and 3 'possible' nodes, you must tick 'yes' and not 'maybe')

B] Please **also** cross any number of locations of disease **on** the appropriate **circled number**

Grading:
Yes = positive
Maybe
No = negative

Lymphadenopathy	Airway compressed and tracheal displacement	Soft tissue density = nodal mass		Post process: Overall
				Lymph-adenopathy
	1 = compressed Or displaced to left only 2-4=compression		Lines indicate the trachea	Yes
				No
				Maybe
				Not visible
	Yes No Maybe Not visible	Yes No Maybe Not visible	Yes No Maybe Not visible	

Nodular = Milliary or larger widespread and bilateral	Airspace consolidation		Post process: Overall
			Lung disease
			Yes
			No
			Maybe
			Not visible
Yes No Maybe Not visible	Yes No Maybe Not visible	Yes No Maybe Not visible	

Pleural effusion/thickening	Cavities		Post process: Overall
			Pleura
			Yes
			No
			Maybe
			Not visible
Yes No Maybe Not visible	Yes No Maybe Not visible	Yes No Maybe Not visible	

TB Decision	Lymphadenopathy or Milliary = **Yes**	No lymphadenop/mill but positive = **Maybe**	Normal = **NO**	Bad quality = Unreadbale

Fig. 37. A tick sheet designed for use in children investigated for TB to record information in a retrievable manner and to ensure that the correct aspects of diagnosis are reviewed by the readers in order of priority. (*Courtesy of* S. Moyo, M. Hatherill, and the South African Tuberculosis Vaccine Intitiative, Cape Town, South Africa; with permission.)

ultrasound using the same method has successfully showed response to therapy with decrease in size or disappearance of lymphadenopathy.[59] Using ultrasound to diagnose pulmonary TB by identifying associated abdominal lymphadenopathy has been suggested but shown to be positive in only 25% of patients.[60] The increasing incidence of extrapulmonary TB may make this more important over time especially when used to additionally detect axillary lymphadenopathy (**Fig. 34**) (shown to have a moderate correlation with the presence of intrathoracic lymphadenopathy using CT[61]) and cervical lymphadenopathy. Fine-needle aspiration biopsy can be guided by ultrasound in various locations including the mediastinum.[62]

CONSIDERATIONS IN CHILDREN
Thymus

The mediastinum on CXR in children less than 5 years of age shows a prominent thymus that can be as wide as the thoracic cavity. Even though it may have a variable size, margin, and appearance, the thymus is a soft organ and never displaces or compresses the airways (unless infiltrated and abnormal or replaced by lymphadenopathy) (**Fig. 35**A). Suprasternal ultrasound, CT or MRI can identify normal thymic tissue (**Fig. 35**B) and distinguish it from lymphadenopathy.

Heart

The heart occupies a larger proportion of the chest in a child than in an adult. This masks the hila making it difficult to evaluate the hilar points for lymphadenopathy as described in adults. Instead of considering this a disadvantage, identification of lobulated shadows projecting beyond the cardiac margins should add confidence to the certainty of the presence of lymphadenopathy.

Trachea and Bronchi

Children have soft and compressible airways, which results in the complication of lymphobronchial TB (with compression and distal parenchymal disease) more often than in adults. However, the compressibility of the airways can be used to advantage to infer the presence of lymphadenopathy when noted on CXR.

Effusions

In children, effusions seen on CXR tend to spare the costophrenic angle and extend cranially along the lateral chest wall as they increase in amount. They are termed lamellar effusions and should be checked by looking for a linear density separating the air-filled edge of lung from the lateral chest wall

(**Fig. 36**). Children lack the soft tissue companion shadows noted in adults that would be difficult to distinguish from this imaging pattern.

Radiation

Children are more vulnerable to radiation from medical investigations because of the immature developing organs, the close proximity of sensitive areas (shorter bodies), and the longer life ahead in which to develop malignancies. The lateral CXR is not only an additional view but it imparts approximately twice the radiation dose of the AP CXR. However, the dose is relatively low compared with traditional CT, which is equivalent to approximately 100 CXR. Modern departments have reduced CT doses dramatically by decreasing the tube current setting.[63]

Lymphadenopathy: What Size is Abnormal?

This is a relevant question that has been raised regarding chest CT imaging for TB in children[64] but has also been addressed with regard to abdominal lymphadenopathy in children.[65] Because normal children have been shown to have lymphadenopathy up to 5 mm, the authors recommend noting only lymphadenopathy greater than 1 cm unless there is clear central necrosis on CT, calcification, or low signal intensity on T2-weighted MRI images.

RECORDING SYSTEMS AND TICK SHEETS

Many recording systems have been devised to assist recording of features of TB (**Fig 37**), particularly for the purposes of research, screening, and data collection. These systems not only ensure that a systematic approach is followed but also systematic recording of the findings using a common language. This makes reporting applicable for follow-up especially if this is not always by the same physician or radiologist. These systems are useful for training residents and non-radiologists in identifying and recording the pertinent features of TB in an organized fashion. Testing of 1 such tick sheet has suggested that CXR may be more useful as a screening tool for TB than previously recognized.[66]

SUMMARY

This article reviews the ongoing role of imaging in the diagnosis of TB and its complications. The blurring of differences in the presentation patterns must be absorbed into daily practice. Communication between radiologists and clinicians and improved interpretation skills by clinicians is increasingly important in the field for making management decisions, especially where there are limited resources. Recognition of special imaging, anatomic, and vulnerability differences between children and adults is more important than trying to define patterns of disease exclusive to children. Most importantly, radiologists must continue to push ahead with research into identifying more accurate and cheaper methods of diagnosing TB. Even though some aspects of imaging are being discredited, they persist in practice because laboratory and clinical tests have been disappointing or unaffordable. High-end imaging should be used to confirm the most confident and reliable aspects of diagnosis on cheaper modalities such as plain radiographs. These can then be used with greater confidence in the less fortunate parts of the world that suffer the most from this disease.

ACKNOWLEDGMENT

The authors wish to thank Paul Van den Brande, MD, PhD, for his contribution in the preparation of this manuscript.

REFERENCES

1. Reid MJA, Shah NS. Approaches to tuberculosis screening and diagnosis in people with HIV in resource-limited setting. Lancet Infect Dis 2009;9: 173–84.
2. Zellweger JP, Heinzer R, Touray M, et al. Intra-observer and overall agreement in the radiological assessment of tuberculosis. Int J Tuberc Lung Dis 2006;10:1123–6.
3. Swingler GH, du Toit G, Andronikou S, et al. Diagnostic accuracy of chest radiography in detecting mediastinal lymphadenopathy in suspected pulmonary tuberculosis. Arch Dis Child 2005;90(11): 1153–6.
4. Marais BJ, Parker SK, Verver S, et al. Primary and postprimary or reactivation tuberculosis: time to revise confusion terminology? AJR Am J Roentgenol 2009;192(4):W198 [author reply W199–200].
5. Stead WW. Tuberculosis among elderly persons, as observed among nursing home residents. Int J Tuberc Lung Dis 1998;2:S64–70.
6. Van Rie A, Warren R, Richardson M, et al. Exogenous reinfection as a cause of recurrent tuberculosis after curative treatment. N Engl J Med 1999;341: 1174–9.
7. Verver S, Warren RM, Munch Z, et al. Proportion of tuberculosis transmission that takes place in households in a high-incidence area. Lancet 2004;363: 212–4.
8. Verver S, Warren RM, Beyers N, et al. Rate of reinfection tuberculosis after successful treatment

is higher than rate of new tuberculosis. Am J Respir Crit Care Med 2005;171:1430–5.
9. Hamilton CD, Stout JE, Goodman PC, et al. The value of the end-of-treatment chest radiograph in predicting pulmonary TB relapse. Int J Tuberc Lung Dis 2008;12:1059–64.
10. du Plessis J, Goussard P, Andronikou S, et al. Comparing three-dimensional volume-rendered CT images with fibreoptic tracheobronchoscopy in the evaluation of airway compression caused by tuberculous lymphadenopathy in children. Pediatr Radiol 2009;39(7):694–702.
11. De Backer AI, Vanhoenacker FM, Van den Brande P. Computed tomography, magnetic resonance imaging and PET in tuberculosis. In: Schaaf HS, Zumla A, editors. Tuberculosis: a comprehensive clinical reference. Philadelphia: Saunders Elsevier; 2009. p. 296–314.
12. Van Dyck P, Vanhoenacker FM, Van den Brande P, et al. Imaging of pulmonary tuberculosis. Eur Radiol 2003;13(8):1771–85.
13. Woodring JH, Vandiviere HM, Lee C. Intrathoracic lymphadenopathy in post primary TB. South Med J 1988;81:992–7.
14. Andronikou S, Wieselthaler N. Modern imaging of tuberculosis in children: thoracic, central nervous system and abdominal tuberculosis. Pediatr Radiol 2004;34(11):861–75 [Epub 2004 Sep 15].
15. Lighter J, Rigaud. Diagnosing childhood TB: traditional and innovative modalities. Curr Probl Pediatr Adolesc Health Care 2009;39:61–88.
16. Kim WS, Moon WK, Kim IO, et al. Pulmonary tuberculosis in children: CT evaluation. AJR Am J Roentgenol 1997;168:1005–9.
17. Jeong YJ, Lees KS. Pulmonary tuberculosis: up-to-date imaging and management. Am J Roentgenol 2008;191:834–44.
18. Hartman TE, Primack SL, Muller NL, et al. Diagnosis of thoracic complications in AIDS: accuracy of CT. Am J Roentgenol 1994;162:547–53.
19. Leung AN, Muller NL, Pineda PR, et al. Primary tuberculosis in childhood: radiographic manifestations. Radiology 1992;182:87–91.
20. Hopewell PC. A clinical view of tuberculosis. Radiol Clin North Am 1995;33:641–53.
21. Available at: http://www.lumrix.net/medical/radiology/ tuberculosis_radiology.html. Accessed July 4, 2009.
22. Yilmaz MU, Kumcuoglu Z, Utkaner G, et al. CT findings of tuberculous pleurisy. Int J Tuberc Lung Dis 1998;2:164–7.
23. Goodman PC. Pulmonary tuberculosis in patients with acquired immunodeficiency syndrome. J Thorac Imaging 1990;5:38–45.
24. Wall SD, Edinburgh KJ. Invited commentary. Abdominal findings in AIDS-related pulmonary tuberculosis correlated with associated CD4 levels. Abdom Imaging 1998;23:578–9.

25. Perlman DC, el-Sadr WM, Nelson ET, et al. Variation of chest radiographic patterns in pulmonary tuberculosis by degree of HIV-related immunosuppression. The Terry Beirn Community Programs for Clinical Research on AIDS (CPCRA). The AIDS Clinical Trials Group (ACTG). Clin Infect Dis 1997;25:242–56.

26. Haramati LB, Jenny-Avital ER, Alterman DD. Effect of HIV status on chest radiographic and CT findings in patients with tuberculosis. Clin Radiol 1997;52:31–5.

27. Raviglione MC, Narain JP, Kochi A. HIV-associated tuberculosis in developing countries: clinical features, diagnosis and treatment. Bull World Health Organ 1992;70:515–26.

28. Buckingham SJ, Haddow LJ, Shaw PJ, et al. Immune reconstitution inflammatory syndrome in HIV-infected patients with mycobacterial infections starting highly active anti-retroviral therapy. Clin Radiol 2004;59(6):505–13.

29. Nakanishi M, Demura Y, Ameshima S, et al. Utility of high-resolution computed tomography for predicting risk of sputum smear-negative pulmonary tuberculosis. Eur J Radiol 2009. Jan 22 [Epub ahead of print].

30. Griffith-Richards SB, Goussard P, Andronikou S, et al. Cavitating pulmonary tuberculosis in children: correlating radiology with pathogenesis. Pediatr Radiol 2007;37(8):798–804 [quiz 848–9. Epub 2007 May 26].

31. Andronikou S, Joseph E, Lucas S, et al. CT scanning for the detection of tuberculous mediastinal and hilar lymphadenopathy in children. Pediatr Radiol 2004; 34(3):232–6.

32. Maydell AT, Goussard P, Andronikou P. Radiological changes post lymph node enucleation for airway obstruction in children with pulmonary TB. Pediatr Radiol 2009;39(Suppl 3):517.

33. Andronikou S, Wieslthaler N. Imaging for tuberculosis in children. In: Schaaf HS, Zumla A, editors. Tuberculosis: a comprehensive clinical reference. Philadelphia: Saunders Elsevier; 2009. p. 261–95.

34. Lee KS, Kim YH, Kim WS, et al. Endobronchial tuberculosis: CT features. J Comput Assist Tomogr 1991; 15:424–8.

35. Moon WK, Im JG, Yeon KM, et al. Tuberculosis of central airways: CT findings of active and fibrotic disease. Am J Roentgenol 1997;169:649–53.

36. Kim Y, Song KS, Goo JM, et al. Thoracic sequelae and complications of tuberculosis. Radiographics 2001;21:839–58.

37. Im JG, Itoh H, Han MC. CT of pulmonary tuberculosis. Semin Ultrasound CT MR 1995;16:420–34.

38. Glicklich M, Mendelson DS, Gendal ES, et al. Tuberculous empyema necessitatis: CT findings. Clin Imaging 1990;14:23–5.

39. Westcott JL, Volpe JP. Peripheral bronchopleural fistula: CT evaluation in 20 patients with pneumonia, empyema or postoperative air leak. Radiology 1995; 196:175–81.

40. Fraser RS. Pulmonary aspergillosis: pathologic and pathogenetic features. Pathol Annu 1993;28:231–77.

41. Ahmad A, Ellis J, Nesbill A, et al. Pericardial effusions in children with severe protein energy malnutrition resolve with therapeutic feeding: a prospective cohort study. Arch Dis Child 2008;93:1033–6.

42. Casas E, Blanco JR, Ibara V, et al. Incidence of pericardial effusion in pulmonary tuberculosis. Int J Tuberc Lung Dis 2000;4:1172–5.

43. Burrill J, Williams CJ, Bain G, et al. Tuberculosis: a radiologic review. Radiographics 2007;27(5): 1255–73.

44. Rodriguez E, Soler R, Juffé A, et al. CT and MR findings in a calcified myocardial tuberculoma of the left ventricle. J Comput Assist Tomogr 2001;25:577–9.

45. Al-Nasser I, Anwar AM, Nosir YF, et al. Bicaval obstruction complicating right atrial tuberculoma: the diagnostic value of cardiovascular MR. J Cardiovasc Magn Reson 2008;10(1):60.

46. Conces DJ Jr, Tarver RD, Vix VA. Broncholithiasis: CT features in 15 patients. Am J Roentgenol 1991; 157:249–53.

47. Lee JY, Kim Y, Lee KS, et al. Tuberculous fibrosing mediastinitis: radiological findings. Am J Roentgenol 1996;167:1598–9.

48. Vanhoenacker FM, De Backer AI, Op de Beeck B, et al. Imaging of gastrointestinal and abdominal tuberculosis. Eur Radiol 2004;14:E103–15.

49. De Backer AI, Mortelé KJ, De Keulenaer BL, et al. CT and MRI of gastrointestinal tuberculosis. JBR-BTR 2006;89:190–4.

50. Erlank A, Goussard P, Andronikou S, et al. Oesophageal perforation as a complication of primary pulmonary tuberculous lymphadenopathy in children. Pediatr Radiol 2007;37(7):636–9.

51. Grobbelaar M, Andronikou S, Goussard P, et al. Chylothorax as a complication of pulmonary tuberculosis in children. Pediatr Radiol 2008;38(2): 224–6.

52. Goussard P, Gie RP, Kling S, et al. Phrenic nerve palsy in children associated with confirmed intrathoracic tuberculosis: diagnosis and clinical course. Pediatr Pulmonol 2009;44(4):345–50.

53. Morris BS, Maheshwari M, Chalwa A. Chest wall tuberculosis: a review of CT appearances. Br J Radiol 2004;77:449–57.

54. Santelli ED, Katz DS, Goldschmidt AM, et al. Embolization of multiple Rasmussen aneurysms as a treatment of hemoptysis. Radiology 1994;193:396–8.

55. De Villiers RV, Andronikou S, Van de Westhuizen S. Specificity and sensitivity of chest radiographs in the diagnosis of paediatric pulmonary tuberculosis and the value of additional high-kilovolt radiographs. Australas Radiol 2004;48(2):148–53.

56. Neufang KFR, Beyer D, Peters PE. Conventional Roentgen diagnosis of mediastinal lymphadenopathy. Review article (Part 1). Lymphology 1982;4:132–42.

57. Erlank A, Andronikou S, Ackermann C, et al. Does the routine availability of a high-resolution CT (multidetector CT) on the chest in children add significant information? An African setting. 31 Postgraduate Course and 45th Annual meeting of European Society of Paediatric Radiology (EPR), Edinburgh. Pediatr Radiol 2008;38(Suppl 2):S533.

58. Bosch-Marcet J, Serres-Creixams X, Zuasnahar-Cono A, et al. Comparison of ultrasound with plain radiography and CT for the detection of mediastinal lymphadenopathy in children with tuberculosis. Pediatr Radiol 2004;4:895–900.

59. Bosch-Marcet J, Serres-Creixams X, Borras-Perez V, et al. Value of sonography for follow-up of mediastinal lymphadenopathy in children with tuberculosis. J Clin Ultrasound 2007;35:118–24.

60. Scheepers S, Andronikou S, Mapukata A, et al. Abdominal lymphadenopathy in children with tuberculosis presenting with respiratory symptoms. Pediatr Radiol 2009;39(Suppl 3):S513.

61. Theron S, Andronikou S. Comparing axillary and mediastinal lymphadenopathy on CT in children with suspected pulmonary tuberculosis. Pediatr Radiol 2005;35(9):854–8.

62. Gulati M, Venkataramu NK, Gupta S, et al. Ultrasound guided fine needle aspiration biopsy in mediastinal tuberculosis. Int J Tuberc Lung Dis 2000;4:1164–8.

63. Andronikou S, Fink AM. Radiation risk in paediatric CT. S Afr Med J 2002;92(7):516.

64. Andronikou S. Pathological correlation of CT-detected mediastinal lymphadenopathy in children: the lack of size threshold criteria for abnormality. Pediatr Radiol 2002;32(12):912.

65. Karmazyn, Werner EA, Rejaie B, et al. Mesenteric lymph nodes in children: what is normal. Pediatr Radiol 35: 774–7.

66. den Boon S, Bateman ED, Enarson DA, et al. Development and evaluation of a new chest radiograph reading and recording system for epidemiological surveys of tuberculosis and lung disease. Int J Tuberc Lung Dis 2005;9:1088–96.

Update on Tuberculosis of the Central Nervous System: Pathogenesis, Diagnosis, and Treatment

Guy E. Thwaites, MA, MBBS, MRCP, FRCPath, PhD[a],*,
Johan F. Schoeman, MMed Paed, FCPaed(SA), MD[b]

KEYWORDS

• Tuberculous meningitis • Diagnosis • Hydrocephalus
• Treatment • Pathophysiology • Pathology

Central nervous system (CNS) tuberculosis accounts for approximately 1% of all of disease caused by *Mycobacterium tuberculosis* but kills and disables more sufferers than any other form of tuberculosis.[1] Tuberculous meningitis is the most common form of CNS tuberculosis and is characterized by a slowly progressive granulomatous inflammation of the basal meninges that results in hydrocephalus, brain infarction, and death if left untreated. Several general reviews of the pathogenesis, diagnosis, and treatment of tuberculous meningitis have been recently published.[2–6] Instead of writing another review of these topics, the authors focus upon three important and controversial topics that are often neglected in the literature. First, how does *M tuberculosis* reach the brain? Second, what is the best way of identifying patients who require early empiric antituberculosis therapy? Third, what is the best way of managing tuberculous hydrocephalus?

THE PATHOGENESIS OF CENTRAL NERVOUS SYTEM TUBERCULOSIS: HOW DOES *M TUBERCULOSIS* REACH THE BRAIN?

The investigations of Arnold Rich and Howard McCordock, published more than 75 years ago,[7] remain central to our current understanding of CNS tuberculosis pathogenesis. They began with the simple clinical observation that not all patients with miliary tuberculosis (hematogenously disseminated disease of multiple organs) developed tuberculous meningitis. At the time, most authorities believed that tuberculous meningitis occurred as a consequence of the direct and simultaneous invasion of the meninges by mycobacteria from the blood. The frequent occurrence of miliary tuberculosis with meningitis lent support to this view, but the observation that this association was not invariable led Rich and McCordock to investigate its accuracy. First, they showed that the intravenous injection of virulent *M tuberculosis* into numerous rabbits and guinea pigs did not result in immediate meningitis in any of the animals. Second, by meticulous postmortem examinations they found small foci of infection (or granulomas) in communication with the subarachnoid space in 77 of 82 people with fatal tuberculous meningitis (not all the brain could be examined in the five without these lesions). These foci, now called Rich foci, were found predominantly within the brain parenchyma, rather than the meninges, and were believed to develop during a preceding

The authors declare that they have no conflicts of interest. Dr. Thwaites is funded by the Wellcome Trust, London, UK
[a] Department of Microbiology, Imperial College, South Kensington, London, SW7 2AZ UK
[b] Department of Paediatrics and Child Health, Faculty of Health Sciences, University of Stellenbosch, Francie van Zijlrylaan, Tygerberg 7500, South Africa
* Corresponding author.
E-mail address: guy.thwaites@btinternet.com (G.E. Thwaites).

Clin Chest Med 30 (2009) 745–754
doi:10.1016/j.ccm.2009.08.018
0272-5231/09/$ – see front matter © 2009 Elsevier Inc. All rights reserved.

bacteremia. Meningitis occurred once mycobacteria contained within these lesions were released into the subarachnoid space, an event that might happen months or years after the initial bacteremia. Thus, the two-step model of CNS tuberculosis pathogenesis was born and it has remained largely unchallenged ever since.

Attempts to further understand the pathogenesis of CNS tuberculosis have generally depended upon the development of disease models. Cynomolgus monkeys[8] and pigs[9] developed tuberculous meningitis with similar pathologic appearances to humans following intratracheal or intravenous inoculation of mycobacteria, but these models have not been used to investigate how mycobacteria enter the brain. Efforts to develop a mouse model of CNS tuberculosis have been frustrated by the poor clinical and pathologic correlation between mouse and human CNS tuberculosis.[10,11] Intracerebral inoculation of mice with *M tuberculosis* does not produce the pathologic hallmarks of human tuberculous meningitis. However, *M tuberculosis* has been found within the brain following intravenous challenge, a finding recently used by one group to investigate how mycobacteria invade the brain during the initial bacteraemia.[12] These investigators compared the cerebral invasion of a clinical *M tuberculosis* strain with 28 transposon mutants of the same strain following pooled intravenous inoculation.[12] Their aim was to identify mycobacterial genes responsible for the passage of bacteria across the blood-brain barrier. Five of the mutants were found in far lower concentrations in the brain than the lung, suggesting the affected genes might be important for mycobacterial cerebral invasion. The function of these genes is currently unclear, although some are believed to be involved in cellular adhesion and entry. In an earlier study, the same investigators used a human brain microvascular endothelial cell model of the blood-brain barrier to identify bacterial genes responsible for CNS invasion.[13] In common with their findings in mice, they found mycobacteria with a mutation in a gene probably responsible for cellular adhesion and virulence failed to invade the cells of the model as efficiently as wild-type bacteria.

The ability of *M tuberculosis* to disseminate within blood appears to be a key component of tuberculosis pathogenesis. Even pulmonary tuberculosis may require bacteremia to seed lobes of the lung unaffected by the primary infection.[14,15] However, how mycobacteria leave the lungs and enter the blood is poorly understood. Bacteria must breach the alveolar epithelium, and there is evidence that *M tuberculosis* can invade and survive within type II alveolar epithelial cells.[16] Investigations using a bilayer of epithelial and endothelial cells as a model of the alveolar wall have suggested mycobacteria might gain access to deeper tissues by translocation across epithelial cells and by travelling within monocytes.[17] In addition, Pethe and colleagues[18] demonstrated that disruption of the *M tuberculosis* gene encoding the heparin binding hemagglutinin adhesin affected mycobacterial interaction with epithelial cells in vitro and resulted in impaired dissemination to the spleen in mice. Despite these findings, the pulmonary alveolar macrophage represents the most plausible vehicle of *M tuberculosis* transport from alveolar lumen to blood. A fascinating insight into this process was recently provided by Davis and Ramakrishnan working with *Mycobacterium marinum* in embryonic zebra fish.[19] By infecting the hindbrain ventricle of the transparent embryonic fish with virulent and attenuated mycobacteria they were able to observe the dynamic interactions between bacteria, macrophages, and developing granulomas. They found that virulent mycobacteria initiated rapid granuloma formation through the attraction and aggregation of uninfected macrophages to infected macrophages. Once macrophages were infected they were capable of leaving the granulomas and migrating through blood and tissue to form distant secondary foci of infection. Also, in an earlier publication they demonstrated that super-infecting mycobacteria hone to preexisting granulomas.[20] These investigations provide compelling evidence for the dynamic role of macrophages and granulomas in early mycobacterial dissemination and challenges Rich and McCordock's model of CNS tuberculosis pathogenesis. Their model depends upon the traditional notion of a static, protective granuloma (the Rich focus) forming a physical and temporal barrier between bacteria in blood and infection of the subarachnoid space. Davis and Ramakrishnan's findings suggest the interactions between bacteria in blood, the Rich focus, and the subarachnoid space may be more dynamic than previously thought. Indeed, recent MRI studies from children who had miliary tuberculosis with meningitis revealed the majority had numerous concurrent leptomeningeal granulomas, suggesting Rich and McCordock may have over-exaggerated the dissociation between miliary tuberculosis and cerebral disease with meningitis.[21] Much uncertainty remains, but novel disease models and improved imaging of the brains of patients who have CNS tuberculosis promises a welcome re-appraisal of the pathogenesis of CNS tuberculosis.

WHAT IS THE BEST WAY OF IDENTIFYING PATIENTS WHO REQUIRE EARLY EMPIRIC ANTITUBERCULOSIS THERAPY?

An early diagnosis, before the onset of coma and focal neurologic deficit, is the greatest contribution a physician can make toward improving outcome from tuberculous meningitis.[4] Yet the diagnosis is often elusive, obscured by nonspecific symptoms and signs and insensitive laboratory tests. Many less experienced physicians believe the slow onset of tuberculous meningitis means they can safely delay treatment for a few days while they review the results of investigations and consider the diagnosis. This delay is a dangerous practice; disease progression is not linear and patients can progress to deep coma over hours following days of mild symptoms.[22,23] As with pyogenic bacterial meningitis, tuberculous meningitis should be considered a medical emergency that requires rapid assessment and treatment.

Despite the critical importance of early treatment to outcome, few studies have addressed the common reasons for treatment delay or examined the consequences of reducing treatment threshold. A detailed analysis of five subjects who had tuberculous meningitis in the Netherlands revealed diagnostic delay was most strongly associated with a lack of epidemiologic risk factors for tuberculosis infection and a failure to perform a timely lumbar puncture.[24] However, reducing the threshold for starting antituberculosis treatment may result in large numbers of patients receiving unnecessary and potentially toxic drugs. Investigators from Ecuador modeled the effect of lowering the treatment threshold for tuberculous meningitis and found it produced only a modest increase in the numbers treated.[25] Whether the same will apply to settings with much lower disease incidence is uncertain and merits further investigation.

One of the critical steps in the timely treatment of tuberculous meningitis is identifying those at high risk of the disease in whom the diagnosis should be initially suspected, regardless of the presenting clinical features. There are two components to this risk assessment: first, to identify those at risk of M tuberculosis exposure and infection; and second, to identify those at risk of M tuberculosis disease. Immigrants from high tuberculosis-incidence regions constitute the major risk group for tuberculous meningitis in settings of low

tuberculosis incidence.[26] A history of recent household exposure or previous tuberculosis treatment is important to elicit in all suspected cases, but especially from children and their parents in tuberculosis-endemic regions.[27] Immune suppression is the primary determinant of risk of active tuberculosis disease and patients who have HIV infection, or those at the extremes of age, should be considered at the highest risk.[27–29]

Once the possibility of tuberculous meningitis has been raised, how does a physician decide which patients should receive early empiric antituberculosis therapy? A rapid bacteriologic diagnosis can be made by finding acid-fast bacilli or M tuberculosis DNA within the cerebrospinal fluid (CSF), but even in ideal circumstances these tests fail to detect approximately 50% of patients who have tuberculous meningitis.[4,30] Therefore, early diagnosis is usually dependent upon presenting clinical features. Several recent studies have highlighted the clinical features most predictive of tuberculous meningitis. A recent Iranian study of older children and adults identified four variables independently associated with tuberculous meningitis: duration of symptoms greater than 4 days, age greater than 30 years, CSF white cells less than or equal to 1000 cells/mm,[3] and greater than or equal to 70% lymphocytes in the CSF.[31] The strongest predictor was the duration of symptoms, adjusted odds ratio of 21.9, which is a simple but potentially powerful clinical finding. Indeed, one of the most striking features of the results of the study is their similarity to those previously published (**Table 1**). Investigators in India,[32] Vietnam,[33] and Egypt[34] all found a similar set of variables predict the diagnosis of tuberculous meningitis, with duration of symptoms and the percentage of CSF lymphocytes as the strongest diagnostic predictors in all the studies. The different cutoffs used to dichotomize these variables should not detract from their potential clinical utility. The message is simple: strongly suspect tuberculous meningitis in patients who have meningitis with more than 5 days of symptoms, and less than 1000 × 10^3/ml white cells in the CSF of which lymphocytes form the majority. The only important caveat to this rule is for patients who are HIV-infected, in whom cryptococcal meningitis can cause indistinguishable clinical features.[35] These simple clinical predictors do not represent a universal panacea to the problems of diagnosing tuberculous meningitis, but if they serve to rapidly highlight the possibility of tuberculous meningitis, and the urgent need

Table 1
Comparison of the presenting clinical variables independently predictive of tuberculous meningitis in four published studies

Study	Kumar et al, 1999[32]	Youssef et al, 2006[34]	Thwaites et al, 2002[33]	Moghtaderi et al, 2009[31]
Setting	India	Egypt	Vietnam	Iran
Age group	Children (1 month –12 years)	Children and adults (5 months –56 years)	Adults (16–70 years)	Older children and adults (9–80 years)
Variables predictive of tuberculous meningitis	History of illness >6 days CSF lymphocytes >50% total white cells Optic atrophy Abnormal movements Focal neurological deficit	History of illness >5 days CSF lymphocytes >30% total white cells CSF white cell count <1000 $\times 10^3$/ml Clear CSF CSF protein >100 mg/dL	History of illness $\geq$6 days CSF lymphocytes >10% CSF white cell count <750 $\times 10^3$/ml Age <36 years Blood white cell count (103/ml) <15,000 $\times 10^3$/ml	History of illness >5days CSF lymphocytes >70% total white cells CSF white cell count $\leq$1000 $\times 10^3$/ml Age >30 years

to consider empiric treatment, they will save lives.

WHAT IS THE BEST WAY OF MANAGING TUBERCULOUS HYDROCEPHALUS?

It is generally agreed that hydrocephalus is the most common, treatable complication of tuberculous meningitis. As early as 1768 Whytt described the clinical course of patients who died after a prolonged febrile illness and who had hydrocephalus at autopsy.[36] This report most likely represents the first description of tuberculous hydrocephalus although the author did not recognize it as such. Cairns described one of the first attempts at neurosurgical intervention by advocating intermittent ventricular drainage through frontal burr holes.[37]

Several pathologic processes including mass lesions (tuberculoma and tuberculous abscess), cerebral ischemia, and diffuse demyelination (tuberculous encephalopathy) can contribute to raised intracranial pressure (ICP) in the acute stage of tuberculous meningitis.[38] However, modern neuroimaging, such as CT and MRI, has clearly shown that obstructive hydrocephalus plays the most important role in this regard. A recent report on a large cohort of children who had tuberculous meningitis demonstrated hydrocephalus in 70% of cases.[27] Most were of the communicating type caused by obstruction of CSF in the cisterna interpeduncularis and ambiens causing a bottleneck at the level of the tentorium.[39] Obstruction of the

fourth ventricular outlet foramina results in noncommunicating hydrocephalus, which occurs much less commonly (about 20% of cases).[27] Proximal CSF obstruction (at the level of foramen of Munro or aqueduct of Sylvius) is a rare cause of noncommunicating hydrocephalus in tuberculous meningitis.[40]

Diagnosis

All the signs of acute and chronic raised ICP have been described in tuberculous meningitis, but they correlate poorly with monitored CSF pressure.[41] In addition, clinical signs of raised ICP are a poor predictor of underlying hydrocephalus. In a large cohort of children who had tuberculous meningitis of whom 70% showed hydrocephalus on CT, only 22% had any clinical evidence of raised ICP.[27] This discrepancy probably relates to the fact that the tuberculous infection itself can mimic many of the signs of raised ICP, including depressed level of consciousness, cranial nerve palsies, absent brainstem responses and decerebration.

Because tuberculous hydrocephalus is mostly communicating, lumbar CSF pressure will accurately reflect ICP in most cases. The continuous fluctuation of baseline pressure is best demonstrated by continuous CSF pressure monitoring, which also portrays other dynamic aspects of CSF pressure, such as pulse pressure and pressure waves (B waves and plateau waves).[42] A normal baseline pressure and absence of high-amplitude B waves after the first month of treatment also correlate well with CT evidence of compensated hydrocephalus. As a research tool, continuous ICP monitoring is invaluable in elucidating the complex pressure/volume dynamics of tuberculous hydrocephalus. However, because of time and cost constraints neuroimaging has remained the cornerstone in diagnosis and management.

The classical CT and MRI appearance of tuberculous hydrocephalus is that of pan-ventricular dilatation, decrease of the subarachnoid space over the convexities, and obliteration of the basal cisterns with enhancement after contrast.[38,43] Communicating and noncommunicating hydrocephalus have an identical appearance on CT and cannot be differentiated by routine imaging.[44] Because cerebral herniation is a possible complication of noncommunicating tuberculous hydrocephalus, determining the site of CSF block is important.[37,45] Lowering of the CSF pressure after lumbar puncture in this condition may result in downward displacement of the brain because of lack of communication between the ventricular and extra-ventricular CSF spaces. In contrast, lumbar puncture is generally regarded as safe in communicating tuberculous hydrocephalus because of free communication between these CSF spaces and has even been advocated as a treatment option in this condition.[46] Limited air-encephalography, based on the work of Lorber,[47] is an inexpensive and safe method in differentiating communicating from noncommunicating hydrocephalus. The procedure entails injection of 5 to 8 cc of air during lumbar puncture immediately followed by a lateral radiograph of the skull. Whenever air is shown in the ventricular system (usually lateral ventricles) the hydrocephalus is regarded as being communicating. Air demonstrated at the base of the brain (eg, prepontine cistern) without any air visible in the lateral ventricles is regarded as indicative of noncommunicating hydrocephalus.[48] More sophisticated ways of differentiation (MRI, contrast and isotope studies) are not freely available in resource-poor countries where tuberculous meningitis is common. Even air-encephalography, which identifies patients in need of an urgent ventriculo-peritoneal shunt, has limited value in situations where neurosurgical treatment is not available. Medical treatment of hydrocephalus (diuretics) is probably the best option under these circumstances.

Management of Hydrocephalus

There is no consensus in the literature regarding the most appropriate treatment for tuberculous hydrocephalus, mainly because of lack of well-designed,

prospective controlled trials. Cairns observed that only one third of 125 children who had tuberculous meningitis needed any neurosurgical intervention to relieve ICP; all the others developed arrested hydrocephalus.[37] This tendency of hydrocephalus to resolve on antituberculosis therapy only, is often not taken into account by the protagonists of early ventriculo-peritoneal shunting.[49,50] In addition, response to surgical treatment is mostly assessed clinically without the backup of intracranial pressure monitoring and neuroimaging. Although CT and MRI are equally sensitive in the diagnosis of tuberculous hydrocephalus, MRI is significantly superior to CT in demonstrating infarcts, basal enhancement, and possibly tuberculomas.[51] The varying clinical response to shunt surgery is most likely related to the presence and degree of underlying ischemic disease.[49,52]

The spectrum of surgical treatment proposed for tuberculous hydrocephalus ranges from early ventriculo-peritoneal shunting in all patients who have signs of raised ICP and early disease, to selective shunting according to type of CSF block, results of ICP monitoring, neuroimaging findings, and clinical response to medical treatment.[49,52,53] Palur advised early shunting for all subjects who had grade 1 and 2 tuberculous meningitis but only for those with grade 3 and 4 disease that showed some degree of improvement after external ventricular drainage.[49] In this study, tuberculous meningitis was graded as follows: grade 1, normal sensorium and no neurologic deficit; grade 2, normal sensorium with neurologic deficit; grade 3, altered sensorium with/without dense neurologic deficit; and grade 4, deeply comatose with/without decerebrate or decorticate posturing. These authors found that subjects who had grade 1 and 2 disease benefited most from shunt surgery, but that all subjects who were deeply comatose or had decerebrate/decorticate posturing (stage 4 disease) at the time of surgery died. This approach, however, does not take into account that most cases of hydrocephalus will compensate on medical treatment only, therefore unnecessarily subjecting many patients to the complications of shunt surgery.[54] It is now generally accepted that many cases of advanced tuberculous meningitis and severe brain damage will not benefit from shunt surgery.[55]

Another approach to the management of acute hydrocephalus and raised ICP in tuberculous meningitis is that of selective shunting. Noncommunicating hydrocephalus, which carries the risk of herniation, is treated by immediate ventriculo-peritoneal shunt, whereas communicating hydrocephalus, which carries no immediate risk, is first given a trial of medical treatment.[48] Medical and surgical treatment was compared in children who had stage 2 and 3 tuberculous meningitis by means of a controlled clinical trial. Subjects who had noncommunicating hydrocephalus who received a ventriculo-peritoneal shunt, constituted the surgical treatment group. All subjects who had communicating hydrocephalus were randomized to a month of antituberculosis treatment only (control group) or intrathecal hyaluronidase or daily diuretics (acetazolamide and furosemide). Groups were compared with regard to CSF pressure, ventricular size, and clinical outcome after the first month of treatment. More children who received acetazolamide and furosemide had normalization of intracranial pressure than those treated with antituberculosis medication only (78% versus 41%; P = .072). Excellent correlation was found between normalization of CSF pressure and compensated hydrocephalus as demonstrated by CT (**Fig. 1**). In contrast, subjects whose lumbar CSF pressure failed to normalize on medical treatment showed progressive hydrocephalus on follow-up CT and were shunted (**Fig. 2**). The medical and surgical treatment groups did not differ in clinical outcome or resolution of hydrocephalus (ventricular size on CT) after completing 6 months of antituberculosis therapy. A large follow-up study recently confirmed that

approximately 70% of cases of communicating hydrocephalus will respond to medical therapy (antituberculosis treatment and diuretics), which reduces the need for shunt surgery significantly.[27] The benefits of this, especially in resource limited countries where tuberculous meningitis occurs most commonly, are many. The risk of shunt dysfunction (obstruction or infection) in tuberculous meningitis has been reported to be as high as 30%. This percentage has been attributed to the high CSF protein content and also the high incidence of shunt infection resulting from shunts being performed mostly in general emergency theaters by junior staff.[46,52,56,57] Late shunt dysfunction in a patient who has become shunt-dependent may have serious consequences if left undiagnosed or untreated because of unavailability of neurosurgical services. Endoscopic third ventriculostomy reduces these complications, but carries the risk of damage to the basilar artery in cases where the floor of the third ventricle is clouded by a thick basal exudate.[58,59]

The effect of HIV-coinfection on the course of tuberculous hydrocephalus has not been well documented. One study reported a lower incidence of obstructive hydrocephalus and basal enhancement on CT in children who were coinfected with HIV.[60] Limited personal experience

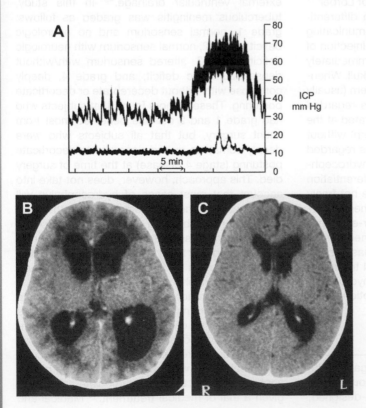

Fig. 1. Successful medical treatment of hydrocephalus. (*A*) Continuous lumbar CSF pressure recordings in a child before and after 1 month of medical treatment of hydrocephalus with acetazolamide and furosemide. The initial recording (*top*) shows a markedly raised baseline CSF pressure and a plateau wave and repeated high-amplitude B waves. These findings are indicative of acutely raised ICP. The follow-up recording (*bottom*) shows normal baseline CSF pressure (<15 mmHg) and only a few high-pressure B waves at the start of the recording. (*B*) Cranial CT of the above child before treatment. Note the degree of dilatation of the lateral ventricles and periventricular lucency indicative of acute hydrocephalus. (*C*) Cranial CT 1 month after successful medical treatment. Note the decrease in the size of the lateral ventricles and the absence of periventricular edema in comparison with the pretreatment tomogram (*B*). The subarachnoid space absent on the previous CT scan is now visible. All these findings indicate that the hydrocephalus has become compensated and that medical treatment was successful.[65]

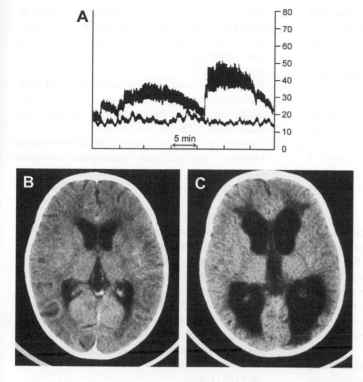

Fig. 2. Unsuccessful medical treatment of hydrocephalus. (*A*) Continuous lumbar CSF pressure recordings before and after 1 month of medical treatment (furosemide and acetazolamide) of tuberculous hydrocephalus. The initial recording (*top*) shows a markedly raised baseline CSF pressure and two pressure waves (plateau waves). The mean baseline pressure after 1 month (*bottom*) is significantly lower than before treatment. However, the baseline pressure (>15 mmHg) and the presence of many high-amplitude B waves are both indicative that the hydrocephalus has not become compensated. (*B*) Cranial CT before medical treatment. (*C*) Cranial CT after 1 month of treatment with diuretics (acetazolamide and furosemide) shows that the hydrocephalus has deteriorated (ventricles larger and periventricular lucency has increased). The patient received a ventriculo-peritoneal shunt.[65]

suggests that endoscopic third ventriculostomy may be the preferred surgical procedure in this cohort because of the increased risk for shunt infection and the decreased basal exudate, which allows permeability of the floor of the third ventricle.

Prognosis

Hydrocephalus has been identified as one of the poor prognostic factors in tuberculous meningitis.[38,60-62] This finding is not unexpected as its presence and degree closely relate to disease progression and stage of disease.[48] A retrospective, controlled study showed that children who had tuberculous hydrocephalus who were referred for surgery did clinically better than those who were not.[63] Despite lack of other controlled trials, there is general agreement in the literature that active treatment of raised ICP and hydrocephalus in tuberculous meningitis improves clinical outcome. The exception seems to be cases with clinical and radiological evidence of irreversible brain damage at the time of presentation. The large number of handicapped survivors after tuberculous meningitis underlines the importance of other mechanisms of brain damage, especially vasculitis and stroke, in the outcome of the disease.[64]

REFERENCES

1. Iserman MD. A clinician's guide to tuberculosis. Philadelphia: Lippincott Williams and Wilkins; 2000. p. 173–81.
2. Be NA, Kim KS, Bishai WR, et al. Pathogenesis of central nervous system tuberculosis. Curr Mol Med 2009;9(2):94–9.
3. Rock RB, Olin M, Baker CA, et al. Central nervous system tuberculosis: pathogenesis and clinical aspects. Clin Microbiol Rev 2008;21(2): 243–61.
4. Thwaites GE, Tran TH. Tuberculous meningitis: many questions, too few answers. Lancet Neurol. 2005; 4(3):160–70.
5. Woodfield J, Argent A. Evidence behind the WHO guidelines: hospital care for children: what is the most appropriate anti-microbial treatment for tuberculous meningitis? J Trop Pediatr 2008;54(4):220–4.
6. Rowe JS, Shah SS, Marais BJ, et al. Diagnosis and management of tuberculous meningitis in HIV-infected pediatric patients. Pediatr Infect Dis J 2009; 28(2):147–8.
7. Rich AR, McCordock HA. The pathogenesis of tuberculous meningitis. Not Found In Database 1933;52:5–37.
8. Walsh GP, Tan EV, dela Cruz EC, et al. The Philippine cynomolgus monkey (*Macaca fasicularis*) provides a new nonhuman primate model of tuberculosis that resembles human disease. Nat Med 1996;2(4):430–6.

9. Bolin CA, Whipple DL, Khanna KV, et al. Infection of swine with *Mycobacterium bovis* as a model of human tuberculosis. J Infect Dis 1997;176(6): 1559–66.

10. Mazzolla R, Puliti M, Barluzzi R, et al. Differential microbial clearance and immunoresponse of Balb/c (Nramp1 susceptible) and DBA2 (Nramp1 resistant) mice intracerebrally infected with *Mycobacterium bovis* BCG (BCG). FEMS Immunol Med Microbiol 2002;32(2):149–58.

11. van Well GT, Wieland CW, Florquin S, et al. A new murine model to study the pathogenesis of tuberculous meningitis. J Infect Dis 2007;195(5): 694–7.

12. Be NA, Lamichhane G, Grosset J, et al. Murine model to study the invasion and survival of Mycobacterium tuberculosis in the central nervous system. J Infect Dis 2008;198(10):1520–8.

13. Jain SK, Paul-Satyaseela M, Lamichhane G, et al. Mycobacterium tuberculosis invasion and traversal across an in vitro human blood-brain barrier as a pathogenic mechanism for central nervous system tuberculosis. J Infect Dis 2006;193(9): 1287–95.

14. McMurray DN. Hematogenous reseeding of the lung in low-dose, aerosol-infected guinea pigs: unique features of the host-pathogen interface in secondary tubercles. Tuberculosis (Edinb). 2003;83(1–3):131–4.

15. Balasubramanian V, Wiegeshaus EH, Taylor BT, et al. Pathogenesis of tuberculosis: pathway to apical localization. Tuber Lung Dis 1994;75(3): 168–78.

16. Mehta PK, King CH, White EH, et al. Comparison of in vitro models for the study of Mycobacterium tuberculosis invasion and intracellular replication. Infect Immun 1996;64(7):2673–9.

17. Bermudez LE, Sangari FJ, Kolonoski P, et al. The efficiency of the translocation of Mycobacterium tuberculosis across a bilayer of epithelial and endothelial cells as a model of the alveolar wall is a consequence of transport within mononuclear phagocytes and invasion of alveolar epithelial cells. Infect Immun 2002;70(1):140–6.

18. Pethe K, Alonso S, Biet F, et al. The heparin-binding haemagglutinin of M tuberculosis is required for extrapulmonary dissemination. Nature 2001; 412(6843):190–4.

19. Davis JM, Ramakrishnan L. The role of the granuloma in expansion and dissemination of early tuberculous infection. Cellule 2009;136(1):37–49.

20. Cosma CL, Humbert O, Sherman DR, et al. Trafficking of superinfecting Mycobacterium organisms into established granulomas occurs in mammals and is independent of the Erp and ESX-1 mycobacterial virulence loci. J Infect Dis 2008;198(12): 1851–5.

21. Janse van Rensburg P, Andronikou S, van Toorn R, et al. Magnetic resonance imaging of miliary tuberculosis of the central nervous system in children with tuberculous meningitis. Pediatr Radiol 2008; 38(12):1306–13.

22. Thwaites GE, Simmons CP, Than Ha Quyen N, et al. Pathophysiology and prognosis in vietnamese adults with tuberculous meningitis. J Infect Dis 2003;188(8):1105–15.

23. Thwaites G, Caws M, Chau TT, et al. Relationship between *Mycobacterium tuberculosis* genotype and the clinical phenotype of pulmonary and meningeal tuberculosis. J Clin Microbiol 2008;46(4): 1363–8.

24. Joosten AA, van der Valk PD, Geelen JA, et al. *Tuberculous meningitis*: pitfalls in diagnosis. Acta Neurol Scand 2000;102(6):388–94.

25. Moreira J, Alarcon F, Bisoffi Z, et al. Tuberculous meningitis: does lowering the treatment threshold result in many more treated patients? Trop Med Int Health 2008;13(1):68–75.

26. Bidstrup C, Andersen PH, Skinhoj P, et al. Tuberculous meningitis in a country with a low incidence of tuberculosis: still a serious disease and a diagnostic challenge. Scand J Infect Dis 2002; 34(11):811–4.

27. van Well GT, Paes BF, Terwee CB, et al. Twenty years of pediatric tuberculous meningitis: a retrospective cohort study in the western cape of South Africa. Pediatrics 2009;123(1):e1–8.

28. Berenguer J, Moreno S, Laguna F, et al. Tuberculous meningitis in patients infected with the human immunodeficiency virus. N Engl J Med 1992;326(10): 668–72.

29. Forssbohm M, Zwahlen M, Loddenkemper R, et al. Demographic characteristics of patients with extrapulmonary tuberculosis in Germany. Eur Respir J 2008;31(1):99–105.

30. Pai M, Flores LL, Pai N, et al. Diagnostic accuracy of nucleic acid amplification tests for tuberculous meningitis: a systematic review and meta-analysis. Lancet Infect Dis 2003;3(10): 633–43.

31. Moghtaderi A, Alavi-Naini R, Izadi S, et al. Diagnostic risk factors to differentiate tuberculous and acute bacterial meningitis. Scand J Infect Dis 2009;41(3):188–94.

32. Kumar R, Singh SN, Kohli N. A diagnostic rule for tuberculous meningitis. Arch Dis Child 1999;81(3): 221–4.

33. Thwaites GE, Chau TT, Stepniewska K, et al. Diagnosis of adult tuberculous meningitis by use of clinical and laboratory features. Lancet 2002;360(9342): 1287–92.

34. Youssef FG, Afifi SA, Azab AM, et al. Differentiation of tuberculous meningitis from acute bacterial

meningitis using simple clinical and laboratory parameters. Diagn Microbiol Infect Dis 2006;55(4): 275–8.

35. Checkley AM, Njalale Y, Scarborough M. Sensitivity and specificity of an index for the diagnosis of TB meningitis in patients in an urban teaching hospital in Malawi. Trop Med Int Health Jul 8 2008.

36. Whytt R. Observations on the dropsy in the brain. Edinburgh: Aulde and Smelle 1768. p. 24–34.

37. Cairns H. Neurosurgical methods in the treatment of tuberculous meningitis with a note on some unusual manifestations of the disease. Arch Dis Child 1951; 26(129):373–86.

38. Schoeman JF, Van Zyl LE, Laubscher JA, et al. Serial CT scanning in childhood tuberculous meningitis: prognostic features in 198 cases. J Child Neurol 1995;10(4):320–9.

39. Dastur DK, Manghani DK, Udani PM. Pathology and pathogenetic mechanisms in neurotuberculosis. Radiol Clin North Am 1995;33(4): 733–52.

40. Ravenscroft A, Schoeman JF, Donald PR. Tuberculous granulomas in childhood tuberculous meningitis: radiological features and course. J Trop Pediatr 2001;47(1):5–12.

41. Schoeman JF, le Roux D, Bezuidenhout PB, Donald PR. Intracranial pressure monitoring in tuberculous meningitis: clinical and computerized tomographic correlation. Dev Med Child Neurol 1985, 27(5):644–54.

42. Schoeman JF, Laubscher JA, Donald PR. Serial lumbar CSF pressure measurements and cranial computed tomographic findings in childhood tuberculous meningitis. Childs Nerv Syst 2000;16(4): 203–8.

43. Andronikou S, Smith B, Hatherhill M, et al. Definitive neuroradiological diagnostic features of tuberculous meningitis in children. Pediatr Radiol 2004;34(11): 876–85.

44. Bruwer GE, Van der Westhuizen S, Lombard CJ, et al. Can CT predict the level of CSF block in tuberculous hydrocephalus? Childs Nerv Syst 2004;20(3): 183–7.

45. Bharucha PE, Iyer CG, Bharucha EP, et al. Tuberculous meningitis in children: a clinico-pathological evaluation of 24 cases. Indian Pediatr 1969;6(5): 282–90.

46. Visudhiphan P, Chiemchanya S. Hydrocephalus in tuberculous meningitis in children: treatment with acetazolamide and repeated lumbar puncture. J Pediatr 1979;95(4):657–60.

47. Lorber J. Studies of the cerebrospinal fluid circulation in tuberculous meningitis in children. Part II. A review of 100 pneumoencephalograms. Arch Dis Child 1951;26(125):28–44.

48. Schoeman J, Donald P, van Zyl L, et al. Tuberculous hydrocephalus: comparison of different treatments with regard to ICP, ventricular size and clinical outcome. Dev Med Child Neurol 1991;33(5): 396–405.

49. Palur R, Rajshekhar V, Chandy MJ, et al. Shunt surgery for hydrocephalus in tuberculous meningitis: a long-term follow-up study. J Neurosurg 1991;74(1):64–9.

50. Agrawal D, Gupta A, Mehta VS. Role of shunt surgery in pediatric tubercular meningitis with hydrocephalus. Indian Pediatr 2005;42(3):245–50.

51. Pienaar M, Andronikou S, van Toorn R. MRI to demonstrate diagnostic features and complications of TBM not seen on CT. Childs Nerv Syst 2009;25: 941–7.

52. Lamprecht D, Schoeman J, Donald P, et al. Ventriculoperitoneal shunting in childhood tuberculous meningitis. Br J Neurosurg 2001;15(2):119–25.

53. Bullock MR, Welchman JM. Diagnostic and prognostic features of tuberculous meningitis on CT scanning. J Neurol Neurosurg Psychiatr 1982; 45(12):1098–101.

54. Kumar R. Role of shunt surgery in pediatric tubercular meningitis with hydrocephalus. Indian Pediatr 2005;42(7):735–6.

55. Mathew JM, Rajshekhar V, Chandy MJ. Shunt surgery in poor grade patients with tuberculous meningitis and hydrocephalus: effects of response to external ventricular drainage and other variables on long term outcome. J Neurol Neurosurg Psychiatr 1998;65(1):115–8.

56. de Villiers JC, Cluver PF, Handler L. Complications following shunt operations for post-meningitic hydrocephalus. Adv Tech Stand Neurosurg 1978; 6:23–7.

57. Gourie-Devi M, Satish P. Hyaluronidase as an adjuvant in the treatment of cranial arachnoiditis (hydrocephalus and optochiasmatic arachnoiditis) complicating tuberculous meningitis. Acta Neurol Scand 1980;62(6):368–81.

58. Figaji AA, Fieggen AG, Peter JC. Endoscopy for tuberculous hydrocephalus. Childs Nerv Syst 2007; 23(1):79–84.

59. Jha DK, Mishra V, Choudhary A, et al. Factors affecting the outcome of neuroendoscopy in patients with tuberculous meningitis hydrocephalus: a preliminary study. Surg Neurol 2007;68(1):35–41.

60. van der Weert EM, Hartgers NM, Schaaf HS, et al. Comparison of diagnostic criteria of tuberculous meningitis in human immunodeficiency virus-infected and uninfected children. Pediatr Infect Dis J 2006;25(1):65–9.

61. Mahadevan B, Mahadevan S, Serane VT. Prognostic factors in childhood tuberculous meningitis. J Trop Pediatr 2002;48(6):362–5.

62. Karande S, Gupta V, Kulkarni M, et al. Prognostic clinical variables in childhood tuberculous meningitis: an experience from Mumbai, India. Neurol India 2005;53(2):191–5.

63. Peacock WJ, Deeny JE. Improving the outcome of tuberculous meningitis in childhood. S Afr Med J 1984;66(16):597–8.

64. Sil K, Chatterjee S. Shunting in tuberculous meningitis: a neurosurgeon's nightmare. Childs Nerv Syst 2008;24(9):1029–32.

65. Donald PR, Schoeman JF. Central nervous system tuberculosis in children. In: Schaaf SH, Zumla A, editors. Tuberculosis: a comprehensive clinical reference. London: Saunders, Elsevier; 2009. p. 413–23.

Toward an Optimized Therapy for Tuberculosis? Drugs in Clinical Trials and in Preclinical Development

Zhenkun Ma, PhD[a],*, Christian Lienhardt, MD, PhD[b]

KEYWORDS

- Tuberculosis • Chemotherapy • Novel mechanism of action
- Drug combination • Drug resistance
- Drug persistence • MDR-TB • XDR-TB

After decades of neglect, tuberculosis (TB) drug research and development is attracting renewed interest, with the discovery of several promising new drug candidates over the past 10 years that spark hope for the possibility to improve the treatment and control of this terrible scourge. The situation is indeed critical: According to the World Health Organization (WHO), there were an estimated 9.27 million new cases of TB in the world in 2007, of which about 4 million were sputum smear–positive, the most infectious form of the disease.[1] About 1.7 million people died of TB in 2007, Including 456,000 patients who were coinfected with HIV. About 9% of the new TB cases in the world today are attributable to human immunodeficiency virus (HIV), and this amounts to 31% in sub-Saharan Africa, where nearly 40% of TB deaths are attributable to HIV/AIDS. Multidrug-resistant TB (MDR-TB) is becoming prevalent in many parts of the world, with 0.5 million estimated new cases in 2007, and extensively drug-resistant TB (XDR-TB) is emerging rapidly. An improved therapy that can shorten and simplify the treatment of both drug-susceptible and drug-resistant TB, be effective against MDR-TB and XDR-TB, and be compatible with antiretroviral therapy (ART) for the treatment of TB and HIV coinfections will clearly have significant impact on the prevention, treatment, and control of this devastating disease.

HISTORY OF TUBERCULOSIS DRUG DISCOVERY AND DEVELOPMENT

The discovery of streptomycin the first effective antituberculosis agent, in 1943, brought much excitement and hope to the world: a cure against this ancient disease was finally in sight.[2] However, this hope was short lived. It was soon observed that *Mycobacterium tuberculosis*, the causative pathogen, developed resistance to this drug rapidly and a stable cure was clearly unattainable with streptomycin monotherapy. To prevent the development of resistance and produce a stable cure, a combination therapy was needed.[3] Since that time the search for better TB therapy has been driven by two intertwining activities: the search for new drugs and the development of efficacious regimens (**Fig. 1**).

Since the discovery of streptomycin, huge progress has been made in the development of an efficacious treatment of TB, with the aim of obtaining rapid sterilization of lesions and avoiding patients' failure to comply with long-lasting treatments.[3] In the first-ever conducted randomized controlled TB trial, streptomycin (S) was found to be very

[a] Global Alliance for TB Drug Development, 40 Wall Street, New York, NY 10005, USA
[b] Stop TB Partnership & Stop TB Department, World Health Organization, 20 Avenue Appia, CH - 1211 Geneva 27, Switzerland
* Corresponding author.
E-mail address: zhenkun.ma@tballiance.org (Z. Ma).

Clin Chest Med 30 (2009) 755–768
doi:10.1016/j.ccm.2009.08.011

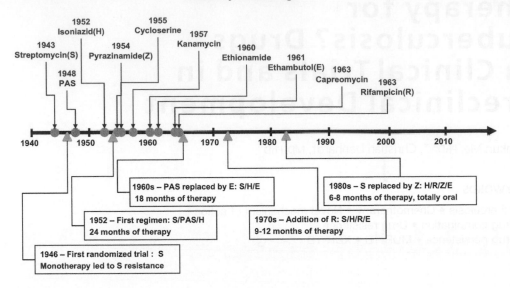

Development of Regimens

Fig. 1. History of TB drug discovery and regimen development.

efficacious compared with bed rest alone. The occurrence of high rates of resistance to this drug in the 5 years following treatment, however, led to the joint introduction of *para*-aminosalicylic acid (PAS) and isoniazid (H) in addition to streptomycin. This first combination therapy, given for 24 months, became the basis for treatment of TB in the developed world for about a decade. In the mid 1960s, PAS was replaced by ethambutol (E), a better-tolerated drug, and the treatment duration was reduced from 24 to 18 months. The discovery of rifampicin in the late 1960s was a major advance that allowed the development of a more powerful therapeutic combination when added to the isoniazid, ethambutol, and streptomycin regimen. This rifampicin-containing regimen offered a predictable cure in more than 95% of patients with 9- to 12-month duration of therapy. Another significant improvement was realized in the early 1980s with the discovery of the effect of adding pyrazinamide (Z) in the intensive phase of treatment, thus accelerating time to culture conversion and decreasing the duration of a fully orally administered treatment to 6 to 8 months. Studies conducted in East Africa showed that the relapse rate after a 6-month regimen was reduced from 22% to 8% by the addition of pyrazinamide, and to 3% by the addition of rifampicin.[4]

Since the 1980s the 6- to 8-month regimen, using a 4-drug combination (HRZE) in the initial phase followed by a 2-drug combination (HR or HE) in the continuation phase, has been widely accepted for the treatment of drug-susceptible TB.[5] This treatment norm was challenged, however, in 2004 with the results of a multicenter randomized clinical trial (Study A), showing higher efficacy of the 6-month regimen (2 months of HRZE plus 4 months of HR: 2HRZE/4HR) compared with the 8-month therapy (2HRZE/6HE).[6] Subsequent to this and recent meta-analyses, the current WHO treatment guidelines are being revised.

CURRENT THERAPIES

Drug-Susceptible Tuberculosis

The accepted standard regimen for the treatment of drug-susceptible TB at present is the 6-month, 4-drug combination therapy (2HRZE/4HR). A classic model established by Mitchison[7] suggests that there are at least 4 different populations of TB bacilli present in lung lesions: (1) bacteria that are actively growing, killed primarily by isoniazid; (2) bacteria that have spurts of metabolism, mainly killed by rifampicin; (3) bacteria that are characterized by low metabolism and reside in an acidic environment, killed by pyrazinamide; and (4) bacteria that are "dormant" or "persistent" that are not killed by current drugs. The 4 drugs used in the 2-month initial phase of therapy have been selected to kill actively metabolizing bacilli in the lung cavities, to destroy less actively replicating bacilli in acidic and anoxic closed lesions, and to kill near-dormant bacilli that may cause relapse.

During the 4-month continuation phase, rifampicin and isoniazid are given to kill any residual dormant bacilli and the rifampicin-resistant mutants that may replicate.[8] Most of the currently available TB drugs are able to kill *M tuberculosis* in the actively replicating stage of growth. However, the sterilizing activity of these agents, characterized by their ability to eliminate "dormant" or "persistent" bacteria, is relatively weak, which explains the remaining risk of relapse after successful cure, due to the persistence of "dormant" bacteria not killed by either rifampicin or pyrazinamide.[9] For this reason, patients who receive inadequate or incomplete treatment are more likely to fail or relapse, contributing to the continuous spread of TB infection in communities and increasing the risk of drug resistance. In the context of severely overstretched and resource-limited National TB Control Programs, new drug combinations with a shorter duration of therapy would be a significant step forward in reducing the global burden and spread of TB, including in those areas with rising multidrug resistance. To do so, new TB drugs with a mechanism of action effective against the "dormant" or "persistent" *M tuberculosis* populations are in great demand.

Fixed-dose combination (FDC) drugs have been advocated both by the International Union Against Tuberculosis and Lung Disease (IUATLD) and the WHO as a useful tool for the treatment of TB by National TB Control Programs.[10] Advantages of FDCs include preventing the emergence of drug resistance due to inappropriate drug intake, reducing the risk of incorrect dosage, simplifying drug procurement and prescribing practices, aiding adherence, and facilitating directly observed treatment. Procurement aspects are, however, important to consider, because the bioavailability of various preparations may vary and only preparations produced by WHO-approved laboratories should be used.[11]

Multidrug-Resistant Tuberculosis

Treatment of MDR-TB is based on the use of any of the first-line drugs to which the strains are still susceptible together with alternative "second-line drugs."[12] The second-line drugs include aminoglycosides (amikacin and kanamycin), fluoroquinolones (ofloxacin, levofloxacin, gatifloxacin, and moxifloxacin), ethionamide or prothionamide, cycloserine or terizidone, capreomycin, and PAS. Treating MDR-TB is difficult, expensive, and lengthy, and requires the availability of appropriate clinical and laboratory infrastructures. According to the WHO guidelines, treatment of MDR-TB should include at least 4 drugs with almost certain effectiveness based on drug-susceptibility testing or the history of the patient's drug use.[13] The injectable agents (amikacin, kanamycin, and capreomycin) must be given for a minimum duration of 6 months. In some cases, more than 4 drugs may be started, for instance when susceptibility patterns are unknown, when the effectiveness of an agent is questionable, or in clinically serious cases such as those with extensive, bilateral pulmonary disease. The drugs should be administered 6 days a week using directly observed therapy throughout treatment, which should last at least 18 months beyond culture conversion (usually 24 months).[13] Most second-line drugs are costly or associated with a high frequency of adverse effects, making the treatment of MDR-TB extremely difficult to implement under routine program conditions. Adverse effects and long duration of treatment may also be conducive to the patient abandoning treatment prematurely against medical advice.[14] This abandonment can lead to further failure or relapse, with serious consequences both at the individual and community levels in terms of the patient's survival and the spread of resistance. Lastly, little is known about potential drug-drug interactions with other drugs and antiretroviral agents, as this area has not been studied sufficiently. For all these reasons, the search for new drugs with a novel mechanism of action and new drug combinations that are effective against MDR-TB is of high priority.[15] This search includes conducting clinical trials to determine the best combinations, and clarifying the role of new drugs within the armamentarium for the treatment of MDR-TB.[16]

Tuberculosis and Human Immunodeficiency Virus Coinfection

The early introduction of ART has been reported to reduce the incidence of HIV-associated TB.[17] Although the precise timing of when to start ART in HIV-infected TB patients has yet to be determined, current guidelines recommend starting ART before the completion of treatment in all TB patients with CD4 lymphocyte counts of less than 200 cells per microliter. The main difficulty in combining these drugs derives from the fact that rifampicin is a potent inducer of certain cytochrome P450 enzymes, which reduces the bioavailability of coadministered ART drugs metabolized through this pathway. ART drugs that can be affected by rifampicin include the nonnucleoside reverse transcriptase inhibitors (such as nevirapine and efavirenz), as well as the protease inhibitors (such as boosted lopinavir [LPV/r]).[18] In addition, the initiation of ART during treatment of TB can lead to the emergence of the immune reconstitution inflammatory syndrome (IRIS), which is characterized by a worsening of signs and symptoms or the appearance of new TB lesions.[19] This problem arises most frequently when ART is started early in the course of TB treatment (ie, in the first 2 months) and when the patient has a low CD4 lymphocyte count (<100 cells/μL). Lastly, the combined toxicities of anti-TB and ART medications may reduce patients' adherence to treatment and therefore, the effectiveness of both HIV and TB treatment components. Developing new TB drugs that could be safely taken with ART is a priority for countries with high burdens of TB and HIV.

Latent Tuberculosis Infection

The objective of treating latent TB infection (LTBI) is to avoid development of active disease, and is usually geared toward contacts of infectious TB cases or HIV-infected persons. It is essential to ensure full adherence with the prophylaxis regimen.[20] Because individuals with LTBI do not usually feel sick, the treatment of LTBI needs to have both low toxicity and high efficacy. Isoniazid has long been the drug of choice for the treatment of LTBI. A large clinical trial of isoniazid for treatment of LTBI indicates the 12-month regimen has better efficacy (93%) than the 6-month regimen (69%).[21] However, reanalysis of the early isoniazid prophylaxis trials among Alaskan Eskimos (the Bethel isoniazid studies) showed an optimal effect of the 9-month regimen.[22] A Cochrane review of randomized controlled trials for treatment of LTBI among HIV-negative persons showed that daily dosing of isoniazid during a period of 6 to 12 months substantially reduced the risk of developing active TB by 40% over 2 years or longer, but no significant difference between 6- and 12-month courses was observed.[23]

Rifampicin-containing regimens have also been proposed for the treatment of LTBI. The advantage is that these regimens are shorter and have fewer adverse events. The British Thoracic Society has recommended a 3-month regimen of rifampicin and isoniazid combination therapy,[24] whereas the American Thoracic Society recommends 4 months of rifampicin therapy without isoniazid.[25] In children, isoniazid monotherapy is usually given for 6 months, but a 9-month therapy has been judged by some to have optimal effectiveness.[25] A combination of isoniazid and rifampicin for 3 months has been shown to be a promising alternative, as it is effective and increases adherence to treatment.[26]

The spread of HIV has changed the natural history of infection with *M tuberculosis*. Whereas persons who are infected with *M tuberculosis* alone have a lifetime risk of 10% to 20% of developing the disease, persons living with HIV have a 10% annual risk of developing active TB.[27] Preventive treatment of TB has thus been proposed to reduce the burden of TB in people infected with HIV. A Cochrane review of 11 trials showed that the administration of preventive therapy with isoniazid reduced the risk of TB by 60% (95% confidence interval 51%–81%) in HIV-infected individuals. This benefit was more pronounced in individuals with a positive tuberculin skin test (62%) than in those who had a negative test (17%).[28] Efficacy was similar for all drug regimens, although isoniazid monotherapy was associated with better adherence than multidrug regimens (rifampicin and pyrazinamide with or without isoniazid in various combinations). In HIV-infected children, isoniazid prophylaxis reduced TB incidence and death. However, data are insufficient to guide the duration of prophylaxis and to support its use in children who take ART.[29] Further studies are needed to address the efficacy and cost-effectiveness of TB preventive therapy in HIV-infected adults and children, the optimal duration of preventive therapy, and the potential long-term adverse events, irrespective of the use of ART.

GLOBAL TUBERCULOSIS DRUG PIPELINE

There have been some promising developments in TB drug research and development since the turn of the century. Based on information compiled by the Stop TB Partnership Working Group on New Drugs, the global TB drug pipeline has increased steadily over the past few years. There are about 15 compounds and 28 projects currently in the global portfolio, including 9 compounds in different stages of clinical development, 6 compounds in preclinical development, and 28 projects at various stages of discovery (**Fig. 2**).[30]

Among the 9 compounds in clinical development, 6 of them, including 2 fluoroquinolones, 1 rifamycin, 1 diarylquinoline, and 2 nitroimidazoles, have passed proof-of-concept and are currently in Phase 2 and 3 clinical trials. The 3 remaining compounds, including 1 ethylenediamine and 2 oxazolidinones, are in phase 1 trials (**Table 1**).

Fluoroquinolones: Gatifloxacin and Moxifloxacin

Fluoroquinolones belong to a well-known class of broad-spectrum antimicrobial agents that exert their antibacterial activity by targeting bacterial DNA gyrase, an essential enzyme associated

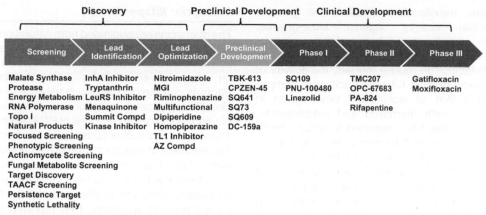

Fig. 2. Current global TB drug research and development portfolio, based on information compiled by the Stop TB Partnership Working Group on New Drugs.

with DNA replication, transcription, and repair. Members of the drug class have been used as second-line therapy for the treatment of MDR-TB. Current clinical trials are focused on fluoroquinolone-containing regimens that have potential to shorten duration of therapy. Gatifloxacin and moxifloxacin are the 2 most advanced compounds currently in clinical development. Both gatifloxacin and moxifloxacin have demonstrated potent activity against *M tuberculosis* in vitro, and seem to be more active than the older fluoroquinolones, ofloxacin and ciprofloxacin.[31–34] Both compounds are currently being investigated as first-line drugs in regimens that have the potential to shorten the duration of TB therapy to 4 months.

Gatifloxacin has been found to have in vitro and in vivo bactericidal activity against *M tuberculosis*, comparable with the bactericidal activity of rifampicin.[35] When tested in mice in combination with ethionamide and pyrazinamide (150 mg/kg, 5 days per week), the combination was able to clear the lungs of infected animals after 2 months of treatment.[36] In an early bactericidal activity (EBA) study, the bactericidal activity exhibited by gatifloxacin (as well as moxifloxacin and levofloxacin) from days 0 to 2 was slightly inferior to that of isoniazid, but extended bactericidal activity from days 2 to 7 was greater.[37] In a Phase 2 controlled trial in which patients were randomized to receive 8 weeks of therapy with either standard treatment or the combination of isoniazid, pyrazinamide, rifampin, and with either ofloxacin, moxifloxacin, or gatifloxacin, the rates of elimination of *M tuberculosis* from serial sputum cultures were more rapid in the gatifloxacin- and moxifloxacin-containing regimens than in the ofloxacin-containing or the standard regimen.[38]

Table 1
TB drugs and regimens currently under clinical development

Drug Class	Drug Target/MoA	Compound	Regimen	Indication	Stage
Fluoroquinolone	DNA gyrase	Gatifloxacin (G)	RHZG/RHG	DS	Phase 3
		Moxifloxacin (M)	RMZE/RM	DS	Phase 3
			RHZM/RHM	DS	Phase 3
Rifamycin	RNA polymerase	Rifapentine (P)	PHZE/PH	DS	Phase 2b
Diarylquinoline	ATP synthase	TMC-207 (J)	BR + J	MDR-TB	Phase 2b
Nitroimidazole	Bioreduction	OPC-67683 (O)	BR + O	MDR-TB	Phase 2b
		PA-824 (Pa)			Phase 2a
Ethylenediamine	Cell wall Synthesis	SQ109			Phase 1
Oxazolidinone	Ribosome	Linezolid			Phase 1
		PNU-100480			Phase 1

Abbreviations: BR, background regimen; DS, drug-susceptible TB; E, ethambutol; H, isoniazid; MDR, multidrug-resistant; MoA, mode of action; R, rifampicin; Z, pyrazinamide.

In vitro, moxifloxacin exhibited the greatest bactericidal activity against slow-growing tubercle bacilli and best activity against persisters, when compared with ciprofloxacin and ofloxacin.[31] In mouse models, the activity of moxifloxacin against tubercle bacilli was comparable with that of isoniazid.[39] When given in combination with rifampicin and pyrazinamide, moxifloxacin has been reported to reduce treatment time by up to 2 months compared with an isoniazid, rifampicin, and pyrazinamide combination.[40] In a Phase 2a EBA study conducted in Tanzania, moxifloxacin (400 mg daily) was as efficacious as isoniazid (300 mg daily) and more efficacious than rifampicin (600 mg daily).[41] In a smaller EBA study performed in Germany, the bactericidal activity of moxifloxacin over 5 days of monotherapy was similar to that of isoniazid.[42] In a Phase 2b clinical trial conducted in the United States in which moxifloxacin was substituted for ethambutol during the 2-month intensive Phase, the moxifloxacin-containing regimen was no better in achieving culture conversion at 2 months than the ethambutol-containing regimen.[43] In a similar but more recent Phase 2b trial conducted in Brazil, however, the moxifloxacin-containing regimen achieved a higher rate of culture conversion at 2 months compared with the standard ethambutol-containing regimen.[44]

Two Phase 3 randomized controlled trials are presently underway which investigate the safety and efficacy of 4-month treatment regimens including those that replace ethambutol or isoniazid with gatifloxacin or moxifloxacin.[45] The safety and efficacy of a 4-month regimen including gatifloxacin substituted for ethambutol is presently being evaluated in a pivotal open-label, noninferiority, multicenter, Phase 3 randomized controlled trial, conducted in Africa under the supervision of the European Commission–funded OFLOTUB Consortium and WHO/ Tropical Disease Research. Enrollment is presently complete and patients are being followed for combined failure/relapse over a period of 18 months post randomization. Moxifloxacin is presently being evaluated in a Phase 3 multicenter double-blind randomized controlled trial (REMox TB) under the umbrella of a Bayer Healthcare and Global Alliance for TB Drug Development (TB Alliance) partnership. This trial evaluates the ability of 2 moxifloxacin-based regimens (one substituting moxifloxacin for ethambutol and another substituting moxifloxacin for isoniazid) to shorten treatment from 6 months to 4 months for active, drug-susceptible pulmonary TB. The trial is presently enrolling patients.

Rifamycin: Rifapentine (P)

The rifamycins are originated from natural products first isolated in 1957.[46] Rifamycins are potent and selective inhibitors of bacterial RNA polymerase, an essential enzyme for DNA transcription. Bacteria can rapidly develop resistance to rifamycins through point mutations in the rifamycin-binding region of the β-subunit of RNA polymerase. There are 3 rifamycins currently on the market for the treatment of various microbial infections: rifampicin, rifapentine, and rifabutin. These compounds are all semisynthetic, and have improved potency and pharmacokinetic profiles compared with their natural product ancestors. First reported in 1963 and introduced into the clinic in 1968, rifampicin has become the cornerstone of the current 6-month, 4-drug combination, short-course therapy. Rifabutin received regulatory approval in 1992 for the prevention of disseminated *Mycobacterium avium* complex disease in patients with advanced HIV infection.[47] As compared with other rifamycins, rifabutin is a relatively poor inducer of cytochrome P450 enzymes and therefore has potential use in the treatment of the TB and HIV coinfected patient population. However, TB and HIV coinfected patients—the group most likely to benefit from rifabutin use—have been underrepresented in clinical trials to date, and further trials with these patients are needed.[48] Rifapentine was discovered in 1965, soon after the discovery of rifampicin, but this agent was not introduced to the clinic until 1998.[49] Rifapentine is structurally a close analogue to rifampicin and therefore is not active against rifampicin-resistant mutants. However, unlike rifampicin, rifapentine has an extended terminal half-life and therefore can be used as intermittent therapy.[50]

Rifapentine is indicated for the treatment of pulmonary TB. During clinical studies conducted by Aventis in the 1990s, rifapentine was given twice weekly in the initial 2-month intensive Phase of treatment in combination with daily doses of isoniazid, pyrazinamide, and ethambutol. In the 4-month continuation Phase, rifapentine was given together with isoniazid once weekly. The rifapentine-treated group was compared with the standard rifampicin-containing therapy. During the 6-month follow-up after therapy, there was a 10% relapse rate in the rifapentine group compared with a 5% relapse rate in the rifampicin group.[51] Despite the higher relapse rate, the US Food and Drug Administration approved the drug, based on the assumption that an intermittent therapy would improve patient compliance and reduce the development of resistance.

A preclinical study in a mouse TB infection model recently conducted by a group at Johns Hopkins University suggested that substituting rifapentine for rifampicin in the standard regimen could dramatically shorten the duration of treatment.[52] Daily regimens comprising rifapentine, isoniazid, and pyrazinamide produced a stable cure in mice after 10 weeks of therapy, whereas mice receiving standard RHZ regimen relapsed after 12 weeks of treatment. Another preclinical study by the same group showed that a novel combination containing rifapentine, moxifloxacin, and pyrazinamide in daily or thrice-weekly therapy allowed shortening of treatment from 6 to 3 months or less in mice.[53]

These preclinical findings have stimulated interest to reevaluate the role of rifapentine in shortening the duration of therapy for drug-susceptible TB. Several Phase 1 and 2 clinical trials have been planned to explore the potential utility of this promising agent.

Diarylquinoline: TMC-207

Among the newly discovered novel drugs, TMC-207 (formerly R207910, Tibotec BVBA) is the most advanced compound presently in clinical development. TMC-207 belongs to the diarylquinoline class discovered through a random high-throughput screening against *Mycobacterium smegmatis*. The target of TMC-207 was later identified as adenosine triphosphate synthase, the "powerhouse" of the tubercle bacillus. Because of its novel mechanism of action, TMC-207 has been shown to be highly potent against both drug-susceptible and drug-resistant strains of *M tuberculosis*.[54] The minimum inhibitory concentration (MIC) against *M tuberculosis* H37Rv strain is 0.06 µg/mL. TMC-207 has also been shown to have potent activity against other *Mycobacterium* species, such as *M avium, M marinum, M fortuitum, M abscessus,* and *M smegmatis.* In a mouse model of "nonestablished" infection, TMC-207 (50 mg/kg) was more efficacious than isoniazid (25 mg/kg). The minimal effective dose and the bactericidal doses are very similar, suggesting that killing is time dependent but not concentration dependent. More importantly, TMC-207 has potent late bactericidal activity in a mouse model of "established infection." Substitution of rifampicin, isoniazid, or pyrazinamide with TMC-207 accelerated bactericidal activity, leading to complete culture conversion after 2 months of treatment in some combinations. In particular, the TMC-207/HZ and TMC-207/RZ combinations cleared the infections in the lungs of all mice after 2 months of therapy. TMC-207 has been also tested in various combinations with amikacin,

ethionamide, moxifloxacin, and pyrazinamide in mice infected with the drug-susceptible virulent *M tuberculosis* strain H37Rv. All TMC-207–containing regimens were significantly more active than the amikacin/ethionamide/moxifloxacin/pyrazinamide combination used in the treatment of MDR-TB. Culture negativity of the lungs and spleens was reached after 2 months of treatment in almost every animal.[55] The superior sterilizing activity of TMC-207 was further confirmed using a guinea pig TB infection model. Compared with the standard combination RHZ, TMC-207 at 5, 10, and 15 mg/kg exhibited better bactericidal activity than the 3-drug combination after 6 weeks of therapy.[56]

Pharmacokinetic and pharmacodynamic studies in mice demonstrated long plasma and tissue half-life and high tissue penetration, which are valuable characteristics for the development of simpler dosing regimens. In a mouse model of established infection, the triple combination TMC-207/PZ given once weekly for 2 months was significantly more active than TMC-207 monotherapy or in other combinations, and was more active than the current standard regimen RHZ given 5 times per week.[57]

TMC-207 has demonstrated a good safety and tolerability profile so far, with linear pharmacokinetics in humans. Absorption is dependent on food, with a twofold increase in serum concentration when delivered in the fed versus the fasted state. The drug is metabolized by the cytochrome P450 3A4 enzyme, which may create an unfavorable interaction with rifampicin. TMC-207 exhibited a minimal EBA for at least the first 4 days compared with either isoniazid or rifampicin. However, from days 5 to 7, TMC-207 at 400 mg per day demonstrated an EBA similar to that of either isoniazid or rifampin during the same time period.[58]

The safety and efficacy of TMC-207 is presently being evaluated in a Phase 2b placebo-controlled, double-blind, randomized trial in newly diagnosed MDR-TB patients, in which the drug is given in addition to the individualized background drug-resistant therapy. Treatment is given for 2 months in a first stage and then for 6 months. Preliminary results of the 2-month treatment Phase showed that the combination of the background MDR-TB treatment with TMC-207 provided a higher sputum culture conversion (48%) in patients than the background regimen combined with placebo (9%). The second stage of the study is presently underway.[59]

Nitroimidazoles: PA-824 and OPC-67683

Nitroimidazoles constitute another novel class of antituberculosis agents currently in late-stage clinical development. There are 2 subclasses in the family, the nitroimidazo-oxazines and the nitroimidazo-oxazoles. Compounds in the nitroimidazole class show equal activity against drug-susceptible and drug-resistant organisms, indicating a novel mechanism of action. However, the mechanism of action is not fully understood. It seems that nitroimidazoles exert their antimycobacterial action through bioreduction of the nitroimidazole pharmacophore mediated by 2 deazaflavin-dependent enzymes in a cascade fashion.[60] Reactive chemical species generated through this bioreduction process is presumed responsible for the killing effect. It is worth pointing out that nitroimidazoles are active under both aerobic and anaerobic conditions, and the mechanism of action of these agents could differ under these 2 conditions. Two compounds in the class, PA-824, a nitroimidazo-oxazine developed by the TB Alliance,[61] and OPC-67683, a nitroimidazo-oxazole developed by Otsuka,[62] are presently in Phase 2 clinical trials.

PA-824 exhibits potent in vitro activity against a variety of drug-susceptible and MDR-TB clinical isolates, with MICs in the range of 0.015 to 0.25 μg/mL. The activity is highly specific, with potent activity only against bacillus Calmette-Guérin and M tuberculosis among mycobacterial species tested, and without significant activity against a broad range of gram-positive and gram-negative bacteria (with the exception of Helicobacter pylori and some anaerobes). More importantly, PA-824 has activity against nonreplicating bacilli, indicating its potential for activity against persisting organisms and shortening duration of treatment. In vivo studies using a mouse infection model with PA-824 at 50 mg/kg/d demonstrated reductions of the bacterial burden in lungs similar to those treated by isoniazid at 25 mg/kg/d, with all mice treated with PA-824 surviving and all untreated control animals dying by day 35. In a guinea pig aerosol TB infection model, daily oral administration of PA-824 at 37 mg/kg/d for 35 days produced reductions of M tuberculosis burden in lungs and spleens comparable with those produced by isoniazid.[61] Another in vivo mouse study indicates that the minimal effective dose (MED) for PA-824 was 12.5 mg/kg/d and the minimal bactericidal dose (MBD) was 100 mg/kg/d. PA-824 exhibited promising bactericidal activity in mice during the initial intensive Phase of therapy, similar to that of the equipotent dose of isoniazid in humans. PA-824 has also demonstrated potent activity during the continuation Phase of therapy in mice, during which it targeted bacilli that had persisted through an initial 2-month intensive Phase of treatment with RHZ.[63]

PA-824 seems to be nonmutagenic based on a battery of in vitro and in vivo assays. When tested in the Ames assay, both with and without S9 activation, PA-824 showed no evidence of mutagenicity. Furthermore, chromosomal aberration, mouse micronucleus, and mouse lymphoma tests have all been negative, confirming no evidence of genotoxic potential for the compound. PA-824 does not seem to have significant interactions with cytochrome P450 enzymes in vitro. Pharmacokinetic studies of PA-824 in mice and rats indicate excellent tissue penetration. Total exposure in various tissues as measured by area under the concentration-time curve (AUC) is 3- to 8-fold higher than that in plasma. PA-824 is orally bioavailable and has pharmacokinetic profiles consistent with once daily or less frequent dosing.

The TB Alliance has completed a series of PA-824 Phase 1 trials to study its safety and pharmacokinetic profiles. Based on the findings from Phase 1, an EBA study in drug-susceptible, smear-positive, adult pulmonary TB patients was conducted in South Africa. This study demonstrated clinically significant bactericidal activity for this drug over a 14-day dosing period when administered orally at 200 to 1200 mg per day.[64]

The nitroimidazo-oxazole OPC-67683 has potent in vitro antimicrobial activity against M tuberculosis. MICs against a large number of M tuberculosis clinical isolates range from 0.006 to 0.024 μg/mL. Similar to PA-824, OPC-67683 shows no cross-resistance with any of the currently used first-line TB drugs. There is no sign of mutagenicity or potential for P450 enzyme mediated drug-drug interactions. In a mouse model of established infection, the efficacy of OPC-67683 is superior to that of currently used TB drugs. The plasma concentration required to achieve an efficacy equivalent to that of rifampicin at a human equipotent dose was only 0.100 μg/mL, which was achieved with an oral dose of 0.625 mg/kg. The combination of OPC-67683 with rifampicin and pyrazinamide resulted in a quicker eradication of viable TB bacilli in the lung of mice in comparison with the standard regimen consisting of RHZE.[62] Otsuka has completed a series of Phase 1 and EBA studies with OPC-67683, and the compound is currently in a Phase 2b trial for the treatment of MDR-TB.

Ethylenediamine: SQ109

SQ109 is a derivative of ethambutol identified from a synthetic compound library based on the same ethylenediamine scaffold. This compound seems to have a different mode of action from that of ethambutol, and is believed to have synergistic interactions with both isoniazid and rifampicin.[65] The oral bioavailability of SQ109 in dogs, rats, and mice are 2.4% to 5%, 12%, and 3.8%, respectively. SQ109 is metabolized by rat, mouse, dog, and human liver microsomes, resulting in 22.8%, 48.4%, 50.8%, or 58.3%, respectively, of SQ109 remaining after a 10-minute incubation at 37°C.[66] In a mouse model of established infection, substituting SQ109 for ethambutol in the standard regimen demonstrated an improved efficacy.[67] A Phase 1 single-dose, dose-escalation study has been completed and a Phase 1 multiple-dose study has been planned.

Oxazolidinones: Linezolid and PNU-100480

Oxazolidinones are a relatively new class of antimicrobial agents, exerting their antimicrobial activity by inhibiting protein synthesis through binding to the 70S ribosomal initiation complex. Compounds in the oxazolidinone class have a relatively broad spectrum of activity, including activity against anaerobic and Gram-positive aerobic bacteria as well as mycobacteria.[68,69] Linezolid, the only approved drug in the class, has modest in vitro activity against M tuberculosis, and has been used off-label in combination regimens to treat MDR-TB. However, the precise contribution of linezolid to the efficacy of such combinations is unclear. In a recent EBA study, linezolid showed modest EBA against rapidly dividing tubercle bacilli in patients with cavitary pulmonary TB during the first 2 days of administration, but little extended EBA between days 2 and 7.[70] In the meantime, there are emerging reports of accumulative toxicity with the use of this drug in conditions such as peripheral and optic neuropathy, and long-term use of linezolid has become a significant concern.[71]

PNU-100480 is a close analogue of linezolid developed by Pfizer. This compound has demonstrated slightly better in vitro activity against M tuberculosis than linezolid, and has significantly improved bactericidal activity in mouse infection models.[72] In addition, incorporation of PNU-100480 dramatically improved the bactericidal activity of regimens containing current first-line TB drugs and moxifloxacin. A regimen combining PNU-100480, moxifloxacin, and pyrazinamide, which contains neither rifampicin nor isoniazid, was more active than the RHZ combination. These findings suggest that PNU-100480 may have the potential to significantly shorten the duration of therapy for both drug-susceptible and drug-resistant TB.[73] Pfizer has recently filed an Investigational New Drug application and has initiated a Phase 1 clinical trial for PNU-100480.

Preclinical Discovery Pipeline

Due to the lack of market incentives in TB drug research and development, the TB drug pipeline was almost empty at the turn of the century. There are some encouraging developments recently with a large number of new projects introduced into the global portfolio, largely through an innovative Private-Public Product Development Partnership (PDP) mechanism. Based on a recent survey conducted by the Stop TB Partnership Working Group on New TB Drugs,[30] there are about 43 compounds and projects in the global pipeline. The majority of them (34) are in preclinical and discovery stage, including 6 compounds in preclinical development, 8 projects in lead optimization, 6 projects in lead identification, and 14 projects in screening stage (**Fig. 2**).

At present, TB drug discovery efforts are focused on addressing two of the most fundamental issues associated with the current TB therapy: drug resistance and drug persistence. Drug resistance is a man-made phenomenon, requiring integrated approaches to alleviate. The first approach is to discover new drugs with novel mechanisms of action, which by virtue should be active against M tuberculosis strains that are resistant to the currently available drugs and therefore effective against MDR-TB and XDR-TB. The second approach is to develop strategies that could prevent future drug resistance development. In this regard, compounds that have a low propensity to develop resistance and that can help to improve adherence to treatment (eg, high tolerability and short treatment duration) should be considered a high priority for development. Drug persistence is a noninheritable phenomenon due to bacteria adopting a highly drug-tolerant state of growth within certain microenvironments, which is believed to be responsible for the long duration of the current therapy. The ability of a drug or drug combination to eradicate these drug-persistent populations determines the duration of the therapy. It seems that the ability of a given drug to kill the drug-persistent population is directly associated with its mechanism of action. Therefore, identifying drug targets that are associated with persistence is one of the top priorities of current TB drug discovery efforts.

The ultimate solution to address the problems associated with current TB therapy is to develop novel drug combinations that consist of at least 3 new drugs, each with a novel mechanism of action. Such combinations should be equally effective against both drug-susceptible and drug-resistant TB, including MDR and XDR-TB. Drugs in the combination ideally should have potent and complementary activities against various *M tuberculosis* subpopulations, which should lead to a faster cure for patients. In addition, drugs in the combination should have no or minimal interactions with P450 enzymes to allow for coadministration with ART. To achieve this goal, a large number of new drugs with novel mechanisms of action and activity against drug-persistent *M tuberculosis* need to be discovered and developed in the coming years, to create a critical mass of new drugs that will enable the rational selection of novel drug combinations.

Drugs in the discovery and development pipeline to treat TB, as with any other therapeutic area, will suffer a high attrition rate. Based on industry experience, the success rates to advance a project from a given stage to the next, and ultimately to successful registration, are summarized in **Table 2**. Based on these success rates, the number of compounds or projects that will be required in each stage to bring one compound to successful registration could also be estimated.[74] For the purpose of comparison, the number of projects in the global TB drug pipeline is also summarized in the last row of **Table 2**. Assuming the same success rates, the current TB drug pipeline will only be able to produce a very small number of new drugs in the coming years. The current TB drug pipeline, without significant enhancement, will not be able to deliver a critical mass of new drugs to allow for a rational selection and development of novel drug combinations.

CHALLENGES IN TUBERCULOSIS DRUG CLINICAL DEVELOPMENT

Clinical development of new TB drugs faces several unique challenges. The first challenge is the long timeline for clinical trials due to the long periods of time required for patient recruitment and treatment, and the lack of predictive surrogate markers that could replace the measurement of relapse rate as a primary efficacy end point. Phase III trials are presently a very lengthy and complicated undertaking. As the 6-month standard regimen is 95% efficacious under trial conditions, the only appropriate design is one of noninferiority. Such a trial design requires the recruitment of a large number of patients, who have to be followed up closely for a long period of time (usually 12 to 24 months post treatment) to assess the occurrence of relapses and avoid the loss to follow-up that may bias or dilute the results.

A second challenge in TB drug development is the need for combination therapy to prevent the development of drug resistance. New drugs are currently added to, or substituted into, the current regimen one at a time, requiring 6 to 8 years to evaluate each new drug in sequence, and potentially 2 to 3 decades to develop a new regimen

Table 2
Drug discovery and development stages, success rates, and number of projects required in each stage for a successful registration compared with global pipeline

Stage	Discovery			Preclinical Development	Clinical Development			
	HTS	Lead ID	Lead OP		Phase 1	Phase 2	Phase 3	Registration
Success rate to the following stage[a]	63	60	63	57	58	45	58	85
Accumulative success rate for registration[b]	1.7	2.7	4.6	7.3	13	22	49	85
No. of projects needed for one registration	57	36	22	14	8	4.5	2	1.2
No. of projects in global portfolio[c]	14	6	8	6	3	4	2	0

Abbreviations: HTS, high-throughput screening; Lead ID, lead identification; Lead OP, lead optimization.
[a] Success rate: represents the probability of a given project or compound to be advanced into the next stage.
[b] Accumulative success rate: represents the probability of a given project or compound to reach final regulatory approval.
[c] Based on survey conducted by Stop TB Partnership Working Group on New TB Drugs.

that contains 3 or 4 new drugs.[45] New regimens that take full advantage of the existing and future TB drug pipeline and dramatically shorten the treatment duration will surely require more than one new drug. To bring such a regimen to patients quickly, a new paradigm for TB drug development is needed, one that requires drastic updating and revision of the current steps of clinical development. Once a new agent is discovered, appropriate tools are needed to define its role within multidrug regimens. In this regard, animal models that reliably predict human treatment duration would be an important asset. EBA studies are presently limited to 2 weeks, as it is not possible to subject a patient to monotherapy for a longer period of time under present conditions. Therefore, it is necessary to develop innovative approaches to test potential new drug combinations in Phase 2 trials to select reliably optimal combinations of treatments that would then go on to Phase 3 trials.

A third challenge in TB drug development is the lack of global clinical trial capacity to conduct late-stage controlled trials to support the registration of compounds currently in clinical development. This lack of clinical trial capacity will likely become more severe and restricting in the coming years as more drug candidates enter clinical trials as a result of intensified TB drug discovery activities. This necessitates wide investment in knowledge transfer, structure upgrading, and capacity building to expand the number of sites capable of running trials in accordance with Good Clinical and Good Laboratory Practice standards.[75]

Lastly, there is a large funding gap to meet the needs for the discovery of new drugs with novel modes of action, and the development of novel drug combinations that can drastically shorten the duration of therapy and improve the treatment of MDR-TB. It is a major challenge to access increased and sustainable funding to ensure that new optimized regimens are ultimately made accessible to those who need them most.

SUMMARY

TB continues to be one of the greatest challenges in the global public health arena. Current therapeutic agents against TB are old and inadequate, particularly in the face of many new challenges. MDR-TB has become prevalent in many parts of the world, and XDR-TB is emerging rapidly. There are few safe and effective drugs available to treat these drug-resistant forms of TB. TB and HIV coinfections have become another major problem in areas with a high HIV infection prevalence.

Simultaneous treatment of TB and HIV is difficult due to the drug-drug interactions between the first-line rifamycin-containing TB therapy and ART. There have been some encouraging developments in TB drug research and development during the past decade. At present there are 6 compounds—2 fluoroquinolones, a diarylquinoline, 2 nitroimidazoles, and a rifamycin—in late stages of clinical development. The fluoroquinolones (gatifloxacin and moxifloxacin) and the rifamycin (rifapentine) belong to known classes of antibiotics, and are currently being studied for their potential to shorten duration of therapy against drug-susceptible TB. The diarylquinoline TMC-207, and the nitroimidazoles PA-824 and OPC-67683 are new molecular entities that have a novel mechanism of action. These 3 novel agents are currently being studied for their potential in the treatment of both drug-susceptible and drug-resistant diseases. There is an even larger TB drug pipeline in the discovery stage and in the early Phases of development. The primary goal for these early-stage projects is to discover new drugs that can play a role in treatment shortening and overcoming drug resistance. Despite these encouraging advances, the current TB drug pipeline is not strong enough to produce an adequate number of new drugs to allow for the rational selection of novel TB drug combinations. A stronger TB drug pipeline and a new paradigm for the development of novel TB drug combinations are needed.

REFERENCES

1. World Health Organization. Global tuberculosis control—epidemiology, strategy, financing. Geneva: World Health Organization; 2009. WHO/HTM/TB/2009.411.

2. Jones D, Metzger HJ, Schatz A, et al. Control of gram-negative bacteria in experimental animals by streptomycin. Science 1944;100(2588):103–5.

3. Fox W. Whither short-course chemotherapy? Br J Dis Chest 1981;75:331–57.

4. Fox W, Ellard GA, Mitchison DA. Studies on the treatment of tuberculosis undertaken by the British Medical Research Council Tuberculosis Units, 1946–1986. Int J Tuberc Lung Dis 1999;3(10):S231–79.

5. World Health Organization. Treatment of tuberculosis: guidelines for national programmes. Geneva: World Health Organization; 2003. WHO/CDS/TB/2003.313.

6. Jindani A, Nunn AJ, Enarson DA. Two 8-month regimens of chemotherapy for treatment of newly diagnosed pulmonary tuberculosis: international

multicentre randomised trial. Lancet 2004;364: 1244–51.

7. Mitchison DA. Basic mechanisms of chemotherapy. Chest 1979;76:771–81.

8. Mitchison DA. Treatment of tuberculosis. The Mitchell lecture 1979. J R Coll Physicians Lond 1980;14: 91–5 and 98–99.

9. McCune RM Jr, Tompsett R. Fate of *Mycobacterium tuberculosis* in mouse tissues as determined by the microbial enumeration technique. I. The persistence of drug-susceptible tubercle bacilli in the tissues despite prolonged antimicrobial therapy. J Exp Med 1956;104:737–62.

10. International Union Against Tuberculosis and Lung Disease. The promise and reality of fixed-dose combinations with rifampicin. A joint statement of the International Union Against Tuberculosis and Lung Disease and the Tuberculosis Programme of the World Health Organization. Tuber Lung Dis 1994;75(3):180–1.

11. Quality assurance of fixed-dose combinations of anti-tuberculosis medications. Proceedings of an IUATLD/WHO workshop, 29th IUATLD World Conference. Int J Tuberc Lung Dis 1999;3(11): S281–388.

12. Mukherjee JS, Rich ML, Socci AR, et al. Programmes and principles in treatment of multidrug resistant tuberculosis. Lancet 2004;363(9407): 474–81.

13. World Health Organization. Guidelines for the programmatic management of drug-resistant tuberculosis. Geneva: World Health Organization; 2006. WHO/HTM/TB/2006.361.

14. Nathanson E, Gupta R, Huamani P, et al. Adverse events in the treatment of multidrug-resistant tuberculosis: Results from the DOTS-Plus initiative. Int J Tuberc Lung Dis 2004;8:1382–4.

15. Cobelens FG, Heldal E, Kimerling ME, et al. Scaling up programmatic management of drug-resistant tuberculosis: a prioritized research agenda. PLoS Med 2008;5(7):e150.

16. Espinal M, Farmer P. The Cambridge declaration: towards clinical trials for drug-resistant tuberculosis. Int J Tuberc Lung Dis 2009;13:1–2.

17. Lawn SD, Badri M, Wood R. Risk factors for tuberculosis among HIV-infected patients receiving antiretroviral treatment. Am J Respir Crit Care Med 2005;172(10):1348.

18. Niemi M, Backman JT, Fromm MF, et al. Pharmacokinetic interactions with rifampicin: clinical relevance. Clin Pharm 2003;42:819–50.

19. Lawn SD, Gail-Bekker L, Miller R. Immune reconstitution disease associated with mycobacterial infections in HIV-infected individuals receiving antiretrovirals. Lancet Infect Dis 2005;5:361–73.

20. Jereb J, Etkind SC, Joglar OT, et al. Tuberculosis contact investigations: outcomes in selected areas of the United States, 1999. Int J Tuberc Lung Dis 2003;7(Suppl 3):S384–90.

21. IUAT. Efficacy of various durations of isoniazid preventive therapy for tuberculosis: five years of follow-up in the IUAT trial. International Union Against Tuberculosis Committee on Prophylaxis. Bull World Health Organ 1982;60:555–64.

22. Comstock GW, Baum C, Snider DE Jr. Isoniazid prophylaxis among Alaskan Eskimos: a final report of the Bethel isoniazid studies. Am Rev Respir Dis 1979;119:827–30.

23. Smieja MJ, Marchetti CA, Cook DJ, et al. Isoniazid for preventing tuberculosis in non-HIV infected persons. Cochrane Database Syst Rev 1999;(1):CD001363.

24. British Thoracic Society. Control and prevention of tuberculosis in the United Kingdom: code of practice 2000. Joint Tuberculosis Committee of the British Thoracic Society. Thorax 2000;55: 887–901.

25. American Thoracic Society. Targeted tuberculin testing and treatment of latent tuberculosis infection. Am J Respir Crit Care Med 2000;161:S221–47.

26. Spyridis NP, Spyridis PG, Gelesme A, et al. The effectiveness of a 9-month regimen of isoniazid alone versus 3- and 4-month regimens of isoniazid plus rifampin for treatment of latent tuberculosis infection in children: results of an 11-year randomized study. Clin Infect Dis 2007;45(6):715–22.

27. Corbett EL, Watt CJ, Walker N, et al. The growing burden of tuberculosis: Global trends and interactions with the HIV epidemic. Arch Intern Med 2003; 163:1009–21.

28. Woldehanna S, Volmink J. Treatment of latent tuberculosis infection in HIV infected persons. Cochrane Database Syst Rev 2006;(3):CD000171.

29. Gray DM, Zar H, Cotton M. Impact of tuberculosis preventive therapy on tuberculosis and mortality in HIV-infected children. Cochrane Database Syst Rev 2009;(1):CD006418.

30. Stop T.B. Partnership working group on new drugs. Working group TB drug R&D portfolio. Web publication. Available at: http://www.stoptb.org/wg/new_drugs/projects.asp.

31. Hu Y, Coates AR, Mitchison DA. Sterilizing activities of fluoroquinolones against rifampin-tolerant populations of *Mycobacterium tuberculosis*. Antimicrobial Agents Chemother 2003;47:653–7.

32. Paramasivan CN, Sulochana S, Kubendiran G, et al. Bactericidal action of gatifloxacin, rifampin, and isoniazid on logarithmic- and stationary-phase cultures of *Mycobacterium tuberculosis*. Antimicrobial Agents Chemother 2005;49:627–31.

33. Rodriguez JC, Ruiz M, Climent A, et al. In vitro activity of four fluoroquinolones against *Mycobacterium tuberculosis*. Int J Antimicrob Agents 2001;17: 229–31.

34. Sulochana S, Rahman F, Paramasivan CN. In vitro activity of fluoroquinolones against *Mycobacterium tuberculosis*. J Chemother 2005;17:169–73.

35. Alvirez-Freites EJ, Carter JL, Cynamon MH. In vitro and in vivo activities of gatifloxacin against *Mycobacterium tuberculosis*. Antimicrobial Agents Chemother 2002;46:1022–5.

36. Cynamon MH, Sklaney M. Gatifloxacin and ethionamide as the foundation for therapy of tuberculosis. Antimicrobial Agents Chemother 2003;47:2442–4.

37. Johnson JL, Hadad DJ, Boom WH, et al. Early and extended early bactericidal activity of levofloxacin, gatifloxacin and moxifloxacin in pulmonary tuberculosis. Int J Tuberc Lung Dis 2006;10(6):605–12.

38. Rustomjee R, Lienhardt C, Kanyok T, et al. A Phase II study of the sterilizing activities of ofloxacin, gatifloxacin and moxifloxacin in pulmonary tuberculosis. Int J Tuberc Lung Dis 2008;12(2):128–38.

39. Miyazaki E, Miyazaki M, Chen JM, et al. Moxifloxacin (BAY12-8039), a new 8-methoxyquinolone, is active in a mouse model of tuberculosis. Antimicrobial Agents Chemother 1999;43:85–9.

40. Nuermberger EL, Yoshimatsu T, Tyagi S, et al. Moxifloxacin-containing regimen greatly reduces time to culture conversion in murine tuberculosis. Am J Respir Crit Care Med 2004;169:421–6.

41. Gosling RD, Uiso LO, Sam NE, et al. The bactericidal activity of moxifloxacin in patients with pulmonary tuberculosis. Am J Respir Crit Care Med 2003;168:1342–5.

42. Pletz MWR, De Roux A, Roth A, et al. Early bactericidal activity of moxifloxacin in treatment of pulmonary tuberculosis: a prospective, randomized study. Antimicrobial Agents Chemother 2004;48(3):780–2.

43. Burman WJ, Goldberg S, Johnson JL, et al. Moxifloxacin versus ethambutol in the first 2 months of treatment for pulmonary tuberculosis. Am J Respir Crit Care Med 2006;174:331–8.

44. Conde MB, Efron A, Loredo C, et al. Moxifloxacin versus ethambutol in the initial treatment of tuberculosis: a double-blind, randomised, controlled Phase II trial. Lancet 2009;373:1183–9.

45. Ginsberg AM, Spigelman M. Challenges in tuberculosis drug research and development. Nat Med 2007;13(3):290–4.

46. Ma Z, Ginsberg AM, Spigelman M. In: Taylor JB, Triggle D, editors. Comprehensive medicinal chemistry II, Antibacterial: anti-mycobial agents, vol 7. Oxford: Elsevier; 2007. p. 699–730.

47. Maddix DS, Tallian KB, Mead PS. Rifabutin: a review with emphasis on its role in the prevention of disseminated *Mycobacterium avium* complex infection. Ann Pharmacother 1994;28(11):1250–4.

48. Davies G, Cerri S, Richeldi L. Rifabutin for treating pulmonary tuberculosis. Cochrane Database Syst Rev 2007;(4):CD005159.

49. Munsiff SS, Kambili C, Ahuja SD. Rifapentine for the treatment of pulmonary tuberculosis. Clin Infect Dis 2006;43(11):1468–75.

50. Temple ME, Nahata MC. Rifapentine: its role in the treatment of tuberculosis. Ann Pharmacother 1999;33(11):1203–10.

51. The Tuberculosis Trials Consortium. Rifapentine and isoniazid once a week versus rifampicin and isoniazid twice a week for treatment of drug-susceptible pulmonary tuberculosis in HIV-negative patients: a randomized clinical trial. Lancet 2002;360(9332):528–34.

52. Rosenthal IM, Williams K, Tyagi S, et al. Potent twice-weekly rifapentine-containing regimens in murine tuberculosis. Am J Respir Crit Care Med 2008;178(9):989–93.

53. Rosenthal IM, Zhang M, Williams KN, et al. Daily dosing of rifapentine cures tuberculosis in three months or less in the murine model. PLoS Med 2007;4(12):e344.

54. Andries K, Verhasselt P, Guillemont J, et al. A diarylquinoline drug active on the ATP synthase of *Mycobacterium tuberculosis*. Science 2005;307:223–7.

55. Lounis N, Veziris N, Chauffour A, et al. Combinations of R207910 with drugs used to treat multidrug-resistant tuberculosis have the potential to shorten treatment duration. Antimicrobial Agents Chemother 2006;50:3543–7.

56. Lenaerts AJ, Hoff D, Aly S, et al. Location of persisting mycobacteria in a guinea pig model of tuberculosis revealed by R207910. Antimicrobial Agents Chemother 2007;51(9):3338–45.

57. Veziris N, Ibrahim M, Lounis N, et al. A once-weekly R207910-containing regimen exceeds activity of the standard daily regimen in murine tuberculosis. Am J Respir Crit Care Med 2009;179(1):75–9.

58. Rustomjee R, Diacon AH, Allen J, et al. Early bactericidal activity and pharmacokinetics of the diarylquinoline TMC-207 in treatment of pulmonary tuberculosis. Antimicrobial Agents Chemother 2008;52(8):2831–5.

59. Diacon AH, Pym A, Grobusch M, et al. The diarylquinoline TMC207 for multidrug-resistant tuberculosis. N Engl J Med 2009;360:2397–405.

60. Singh R, Manjunatha U, Boshoff HI, et al. PA-824 kills nonreplicating *Mycobacterium tuberculosis* by intracellular NO release. Science 2008;322(5906):1392–5.

61. Stover CK, Warrener P, VanDevanter DR, et al. A small-molecule nitroimidazopyran drug candidate for the treatment of tuberculosis. Nature 2000;405(6789):962–6.

62. Matsumoto M, Hashizume H, Tomishige T, et al. OPC-67683, a nitro-dihydro-imidazooxazole derivative with promising action against tuberculosis in vitro and in mice. PLoS Med 2006;3(11):e466.

63. Tyagi S, Nuermberger E, Yoshimatsu T, et al. Bactericidal activity of the nitroimidazopyran PA-824 in

a murine model of tuberculosis. Antimicrobial Agents Chemother 2005;49(6):2289–93.

64. Ginsberg AM, Diacon A. Update on PA-824. Symposium 12: Recent Advances in TB Drug Development, 39th Union World Conference on Lung Health 2008; Paris.

65. Protopopova M, Hanrahan C, Nikonenko B, et al. Identification of a new antitubercular drug candidate, SQ109, from a combinatorial library of 1,2-ethylenediamines. Antimicrobial Agents Chemother 2005;56:968–74.

66. Jia L, Noker PE, Coward L, et al. Interspecies pharmacokinetics and in vitro metabolism of SQ109. Br J Pharmacol 2006;147(5):476–85.

67. Nikonenko BV, Protopopova M, Samala R, et al. Drug therapy of experimental tuberculosis (TB): improved outcome by combining SQ109, a new diamine antibiotic, with existing TB drugs. Antimicrobial Agents Chemother 2007;51(4):1563–5.

68. Diekema DJ, Jones RN. Oxazolidinone antibiotics. Lancet 2001;358(9297):1975–82.

69. Sood R, Bhadauriya T, Rao M, et al. Antimycobacterial activities of oxazolidinones: a review. Infect Disord Drug Targets 2006;6(4):343–54.

70. Dietze R, Hadad DJ, McGee B, et al. Early and extended early bactericidal activity of linezolid in pulmonary tuberculosis. Am J Respir Crit Care Med 2008;178(11):1180–5.

71. Ntziora F, Falagas ME. Linezolid for the treatment of patients with mycobacterial infections: a systematic review. Int J Tuberc Lung Dis 2007;11(6): 606–11.

72. Cynamon MH, Klemens SP, Sharpe CA, et al. Activities of several novel oxazolidinones against *Mycobacterium tuberculosis* in a murine model. Antimicrobial Agents Chemother 1999;43(5): 1189–91.

73. Williams 2008 Williams KN, Stover CK, Zhu T, et al. Promising antituberculosis activity of the oxazolidinone PNU-100480 relative to that of linezolid in a murine model. Antimicrobial Agents Chemother 2009;53(4):1314–9.

74. Brown D, Super-Furga G. Rediscovering the sweet spot in drug discovery. Drug Discov Today 2003;8:1067–77.

75. Schluger N, Karunakara U, Lienhardt C, et al. Building clinical trials capacity for tuberculosis drugs in high-burden countries. PLoS Med 2007; 4(11):e302.

Advances in Immunotherapy for Tuberculosis Treatment

Gavin J. Churchyard, MD[a,b,c,*], Gilla Kaplan, PhD[d],
Dorothy Fallows, PhD[d], Robert S. Wallis, MD, FIDSA[e],
Philip Onyebujoh, MD[f], Graham A. Rook, MD[g]

KEYWORDS

- Tuberculosis • Immunotherapeutics • Antituberculous
- Chemotherapy • Pulmonary infection
- Immunopathology • TB treatment

Globally, tuberculosis (TB) rates have started to decline, including in sub-Saharan Africa, apart from South Africa and Lesotho. In high human immunodeficiency virus (HIV)-prevalent countries, the risk of TB in HIV-infected persons is more than 20-fold higher than that of HIV-uninfected persons, and the African region accounted for most of the HIV-infected TB cases (79%) in 2007.[1] An estimated 511,000 multidrug-resistant (MDR) TB cases occurred in 2007, with the greatest numbers reported from India, China, the Russian Federation, South Africa, and Bangladesh.[1] The outbreak of extensively drug-resistant (XDR) TB in HIV-infected adults in the Tugela Ferry district of Kwa-Zulu Natal, South Africa, which was associated with an extremely high mortality rate, drew attention to the threat that XDR-TB poses to TB and HIV control programs.[2] By the end of 2008, XDR-TB had been reported by 55 countries.[1]

Antituberculous chemotherapy remains the cornerstone of TB control. TB treatment, however, is complex, requiring at least 6 months of treatment, and is associated with drug toxicities and drug-interactions. Current anti-TB drugs are not able to fully eradicate *Mycobacterium tuberculosis* at all sites of infection because of their relative inactivity against semidormant or persisting organisms, particularly those in lung granulomas. Treatment of MDR-TB and XDR-TB is even more complex and requires use of toxic, expensive, and less effective second-line drugs for longer duration. Advances in the understanding of the immunopathogenesis of TB allow the possible application of adjunctive immunotherapy for the treatment of TB. Adjunctive immunotherapy, together with chemotherapy, has the potential to shorten TB treatment and improve treatment outcomes of drug-resistant TB.

This article updates a previous review of immunotherapy for TB[3] and highlights the potential usefulness of immunotherapy in optimizing and augmenting current TB chemotherapeutic regimens.

WHAT ROLE MAY IMMUNOTHERAPY PLAY IN TREATING TUBERCULOSIS?

Immunotherapy may have multiple roles to play in TB: improving success rates in the treatment of

a Aurum Institute for Health Research, Suite 300, Private Bag X 30500, Houghton 2041, Johannesburg, South Africa
b Nelson R Mandela School of Medicine, University of Kwa-Zulu Natal, Durban, 4041, South Africa
c Faculty of Health Sciences, University of Cape Town, Cape Town, 7935, South Africa
d The Public Health Research Institute, University of Medicine and Dentistry of New Jersey, Newark, NJ 07103, USA
e Pfizer Global Research & Development, MS 6025 B3149, 50 Pequot Avenue, New London, CT 06320, USA
f Tropical Disease Research, World Health Organization, 1211 Genève 27, Switzerland
g Centre for Infectious Diseases & International Health, Windeyer Institute of Medical Sciences, Royal Free and University College Medical School, London, W1P 7PP, UK
* Corresponding author. Aurum Institute for Health Research, Suite 300, Private Bag X 30500, Houghton 2041, Johannesburg, South Africa.
E-mail address: gchurchyard@auruminstitute.org (G.J. Churchyard).

MDR-TB and XDR-TB; shortening the duration of treatment of drug-susceptible TB; improving immunity; and reducing the pathology in individuals cured by chemotherapy, thereby preventing recurrent disease (whether due to true relapse or to reinfection).

Current candidate TB immunotherapies are at different stages of clinical development. There are immunotherapy approaches that are active in mouse TB models (with or without chemotherapy), which have been produced to good manufacturing practice (GMP) standards. These have not yet been tested in humans. Several immunotherapies have been evaluated in human clinical trials, although not all have been studied in patients with TB.

Immune Protection and Immunopathology

The nature of the immune response to TB infection determines whether protective immunity or active disease will be the result. A mechanistic model of immunity has been proposed to explain the immune responses leading to either protection or disease.[4] The authors suggest that the immune response to M tuberculosis infection may lend itself to manipulation by immunotherapies or vaccines.

Protective immunity is comprised of bacteriostatic and bacteriocidal components. These may be expressed within a single infected host, at different times, or in different parts of affected organs. Although a bacteriostatic response may transiently protect the host from an invasive pathogen, it does so at the cost of creating dormancy, a source of recurrent infection that can be difficult to eradicate. The challenge for immunotherapy is to convert a predominantly bacteriostatic immune response into a bacteriocidal response, or, alternatively, to modify the bacteriostatic response so that it no longer interferes with chemotherapy.

When granulomas are formed around recently TB-infected alveolar macrophages, through the sequential recruitment of peripheral blood leukocytes to the site, a physical barrier that contains infection is created. The microenvironment within the granuloma is hostile to the bacilli because of reduced oxygen tension, lower pH, and limited micronutrient levels. Under these conditions, mycobacteria enter into a latent state, characterized by profoundly altered metabolism and lack of replication. However, in addition to their protective role, granulomas can have a detrimental effect on the infected host because, as granulomas enlarge and differentiate, they can obstruct the airways and cause irreversible damage to lung tissue. Central necrosis of the granuloma (caseation), destruction of lung tissue, and rupture of cavities

into the bronchi leading to spread of TB via coughing, have been reported to be more likely to occur when TB infection involves a mixed Th1/Th2 response.[5] Furthermore, in contrast with macrophages located in the cellular area of the granuloma, macrophages migrating into the luminal aspect of the cavity are permissive and support the growth of M tuberculosis.[6]

Immune protection results from phagocytosis and killing of, or controlling the growth of, mycobacteria by activated macrophages. This cellular response is regulated by antigen-specific T cells that produce interferon γ (IFN-γ). IFN-γ, together with tumor necrosis factor α (TNF-α) and interleukin (IL)-15 (referred to as a type 1 cellular response), are essential for activation of macrophages and immune protection.[7,8] However, M tuberculosis can subvert classic Th1-mediated macrophage activation by blocking or reducing phagosome maturation,[9] lysosome fusion,[7] antigen presentation via major histocompatibility complex (MHC) class I,[10] activation of the inflammasome,[11] and signaling via the IFN-γ receptor.[12] Other immune-mediated mechanisms that may compensate for disabled macrophage and phagosome function and can lead to bactericidal activity include autophagy, apoptosis, and killing by cytotoxic T lymphocytes (CTL).[13,14] CTL contribute to protective immunity by driving apoptosis and by granule-mediated lysis of infected macrophages, which has been shown to result in death of the intracellular organisms. Thus optimal bacteriocidal immunity is probably achieved by a combination of the classic type 1 IFN-γ–mediated response plus CTL.

Significantly, all of these compensatory mechanisms (autophagy, apoptosis and CTL) are susceptible to downregulation by a combination of Th2 cytokines and transforming growth factor β (TGF-β).[13,15,16] That Th2 cytokines dampen the immune response to TB is clearly demonstrated in animal models in which high-dose challenge is used.[17] In these models, after a brief plateau in colony-forming units (CFU) at about 3 weeks when the Th1 response peaks, the CFU increase again. This second period of bacterial growth is accompanied by, and dependent on, expression of IL-4, and is not seen in models of low-dose infection in specific pathogen free (SPF) mice, in which IL-4 is not involved and the CFU plateau is maintained.[18–20] Progressive TB, most frequently seen in developing countries, is often accompanied by high levels of IL-4, and occurs in individuals with suboptimal immunity who experience frequent exposure to infectious bacilli from untreated cases in crowded living conditions.[17]

The shift toward a more Th2-dominated immune response to TB is also partly attributable to a greater risk of exposure to environmental myco-bacteria.[21] The presence of underlying helminth infections, which are more common in low-income environments, can further promote a Th2 response.[22] IL-4 can stimulate macrophages to produce TGF-β, and IL-4 and TGF-β would be expected to downregulate the CTL response. Thus, an immune response that is characterized by an excessive proportion of antigen-specific IL-4–producing T cells, and skewed toward a Th2-type cellular response, is expected to result in increased immunopathology rather than protection.

In conclusion, immunotherapeutic strategies for use in developing countries will need to enhance protective responses while inhibiting Th2 responses. Several immune modifying agents have been shown to have these properties (**Fig. 1**).

OVERVIEW OF IMMUNOTHERAPY AGENTS

The aim of immunotherapy is to "realign" or improve the immune response by either promoting protective T helper 1 (Th1) immunity or blocking harmful immune (Th2) responses. Inducing more protective immunity is not necessarily better as many TB patients already have a robust Th1 response in their lungs. Furthermore, boosting Th1 responses may induce systemic release of Th1-associated cytokines, resulting in necrosis of TB lesions (Koch phenomenon). A better approach may be to optimize the balance between the Th1/Th2 immune response by downregulating the Th2 response.

The three categories of immunotherapeutic agents

1. Immunoregulatory approaches that seek to alter the nature of the immune response. Immunoregulatory agents can be divided into those:
   - For which GMP manufacturing capacity exists
     - High-dose intravenous immunoglobulin (IVIg)
     - HE2000 (16α-bromoepiandrosterone)
     - Multidose heat-killed *Mycobacterium vaccae*
     - Anti-IL-4
   - For which GMP manufacturing capacity can be established
     - DNA vaccine (HSP65)
   - Others
     - Dzherelo
     - SCV-07 SciCLone
     - RUTI
2. Immunosuppressive therapy, to increase access of antibacterial drugs, or susceptibility to them

   - Thalidomide analogs (lower TNF-α levels)
   - Etanercept (blocks TNF-α)
   - Prednisolone (reduces TNF-α levels)
3. Supplement effector cytokines, to assist anti-microbicidal activity
   - Recombinant human (rh) IFN-γ and rh-IFN-α
   - rh-IL-2
   - rh-Granulocyte-macrophage colony-stimulating factor (rh-GM-CSF)
   - IL-12

IMMUNOREGULATORY APPROACHES TO ALTERING THE IMMUNE RESPONSE
Immunotherapeutics for which GMP Manufacture Capacity Exists

High-dose IVIg
High-dose intravenous immunoglobulin (IVIg) is administered routinely as a treatment of a variety of human inflammatory disorders. Because anti-TNF-α, also used in some of the same inflammatory disorders, has been shown to cause reactivation of TB, high-dose IVIg was tested in a mouse model of TB to check its safety. Rather than activating TB, it was found to exert a marked therapeutic effect whether administered early or during infection.[23] Because this material has an excellent safety record, it is an attractive potential immunotherapeutic for human TB, particularly in view of the recent discovery of its mode of action. The effect of high-dose IVIg is pharmacologic because of the subset of immunoglobulin G (IgG) with fully sialylated fragment crystallizable (Fc) oligosaccharides.[24,25] In TB, the Fc oligosaccharides are agalactosyl (also lacking sialic acid).[26] Agalactosyl IgG, in contrast with fully sialylated IgG, is proinflammatory (**Fig. 2**).[27] It could be worthwhile to test this material in patients with XDR-TB, who fail to respond to conventional drug treatment, especially in those with markedly raised agalactosyl IgG.

HE2000 (16α-BROMOEPIANDROSTERONE)
The major steroid produced by the human adrenals is dehydroepiandrosterone (DHEA). HE2000 is a modified form of DHEA that cannot go into the sex steroid pathways (which excess DHEA can do, causing masculinizing side effects). HE2000 was therapeutic in a mouse model of pulmonary TB, even when given late in the infection, without any chemotherapy. The molecule also showed synergy with antibacterial drugs, leading to accelerated bacillary clearance.[28] The mode of action and the receptor used are unknown. HE2000 was well tolerated and safe in patients infected with HIV. No significant change in CD4+ T cell numbers were noted, although

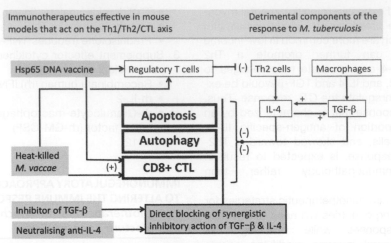

Fig. 1. Probable mode of action of immunotherapeutics that downregulate IL-4 and drive CTL. The major mechanisms that kill *M tuberculosis* are apoptosis, autophagy, and cytotoxic T cells. These are all inhibited by Th2 cytokines. TGF-β is released from macrophages exposed to *M tuberculosis*. TGF-β and IL-4 each enhance production of the other, and work together to inhibit development and function of CTL. Agents that downregulate IL-4, or block its function, are able to exert therapeutic effects in mouse models induced by high-dose challenge, in which the late phase of progressive increase in CFU is IL-4–dependent. If these models parallel the TB seen in developing countries where high-dose challenge of partially immune individuals is common and IL-4 levels are often high, then these strategies should also be therapeutic in human TB.

patients receiving 50 mg doses had a significant decrease in viral load (−0.6 log; P<.01).[29] Moreover, HE2000 was shown to reduce the incidence of TB coinfection by 42.2% (P<.05) in a cohort of antiretroviral therapy-naive HIV-infected subjects with advanced HIV disease.[30]

Multidose heat-killed *M vaccae*

Heat-killed *M vaccae* is a preparation of an environmental saprophyte with unusual immunologic properties. Previous studies in mice have shown that *M vaccae* induces regulatory T cells that inhibit Th2 responses,[31] while simultaneously driving a Th1 response that results in activation of cytotoxic T cells that kill *M tuberculosis*-infected

macrophages.[32] *M vaccae* is therapeutic in a mouse model of pulmonary TB[33] and has shown activity against eczema in a trial in dogs.[34]

M vaccae can induce activation of human monocyte-derived dendritic cells (DCs) via toll-like receptor (TLR)2, but not via other TLRs. *M vaccae* caused maturation of human DC in a dose-dependent manner and induced activation and translocation to the nucleus of the transcription factor NF-κB. In cocultures with naive allogeneic CD4+ T cells, *M vaccae*-primed DC enhanced T cell activation and induced a population of CD25+ FoxP3high cells. Moreover, these DC attenuated maturation of Th2 cells without altering maturation of Th1 cells. New microarray

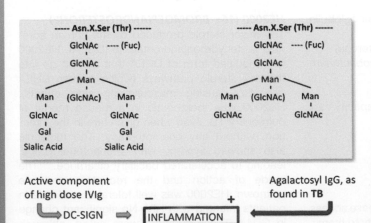

Fig. 2. Mechanisms of action of IVIg. The structures of the N-linked biantennary oligosaccharides situated on the Fc of the active component of high-dose IVIg, and the equivalent oligosaccharide from IgG isolated from the serum of TB patients. The agalactosyl IgG of TB patients is proinflammatory, though the precise mechanism is not known. The fully sialylated fraction of normal IgG exerts complex anti-inflammatory effects, involving DC-SIGN and inhibitory Fc receptors. IVIg, rich in the fully sialylated form, is therapeutic in a mouse model of TB, and could be tested in the human disease.

data have revealed some of the pathways involved when human DC are exposed to *M vaccae*. Bioinformatic comparisons with data derived from DC stimulated with other innate immune stimuli have led to the identification of a transcription factor that is a key component of *M vaccae*-specific effects on DC (Witt N, Rook GAW, and Noursadeghi M, personal communication, 2009).

A single intradermal dose of *M vaccae* given to patients with fully drug-susceptible TB during the first week of treatment does not have a clinically useful effect, although borderline acceleration of sputum culture conversion was reported after 1 month of treatment in a cohort of patients in Uganda ($P = .01$)[35] and after 2 months of treatment in patients in Zambia and Malawi ($P = .06$).[36] The emphasis has now turned to multidose schedules. One fully published non-Good Clinical Practice pilot study of multiple doses of *M vaccae* given during treatment of drug-susceptible TB claimed enhanced clearance of sputum, and normalization of serum IL-4 and TNF-α.[37] In China, multiple injections of *M vaccae* have been given to patients with recurrent or drug-resistant TB. Significant improvements in sputum conversion rates were claimed,[38,39] although the unacceptably poor results in the control group have led to doubts about the trial. Nevertheless, *M vaccae* is now commercially available and licensed as a therapy for TB in China, and a recent meta-analysis of 11 trials of multidose *M vaccae* undertaken in China concluded that it is effective as an adjunctive treatment in MDR-TB.[40]

The need for a full GCP trial of this *M vaccae* in MDR/XDR-TB in the West is highlighted by the recent DARDAR study in which 5 doses of *M vaccae* were given to more than 2000 Tanzanians infected with HIV, which resulted in a significant decrease in definite TB in the *M vaccae* recipients ($P = .027$).[41] This prophylactic study has some overlap with immunotherapy, to the extent that most patients were already TB-infected, even if their disease was latent. The Aeras Global TB Vaccine Foundation, in collaboration with Immodulon, is now attempting to manufacture a new GMP batch for further trials.

Neutralizing antibodies to IL-4, leading to reduced IL-4 and TGF-β

Neutralizing antibodies to IL-4 have a therapeutic effect in the high-dose challenge mouse model.[17,19] Reducing IL-4 in the mouse model caused a secondary decrease in TGF-β.[18] Because TGF-β is known to be detrimental in TB, this suggested that blocking TGF-β might also be a therapeutic alternative to blocking IL-4. When TGF-β was blocked in vivo by administering recombinant soluble type III TGF-β receptor, a therapeutic effect was observed, but there was increased pulmonary inflammation, suggesting that this strategy is not a clinical option.[42] Nevertheless the modest decrease in TGF-β caused by blocking IL-4 might be a part of the therapeutic effect. There is a synergistic downregulation of CD8+ CTL activity by IL-4 and TGF–β (see **Fig. 1**). A humanized antibody to human IL-4 (pascolizumab) has been developed (by Glaxo Smith Kline) that is likely to be a safe strategy and to be effective in patients with high IL-4.

Immunotherapeutics for which GMP Manufacture Capacity can be Established

DNA vaccine encoding a mycobacterial protein (HSP65)

Mycobacterial heat shock protein (HSP) 65 is a major target of the immune response to mycobacteria but also a molecule with profound immunoregulatory properties. In mouse models of TB, the HSP65 DNA vaccine is effective alone[43] and enhances cytotoxic T cells, while inhibiting the IL-4 response. The vaccine also shows synergy with antibacterials,[44] including moxifloxacin.[45] Recent microarray work confirms downregulation of the Th2 response.[46] A single article, using different constructs (some not encoding HSP65), claimed that DNA vaccines caused immunopathology in TB lung lesions in guinea pigs.[47] This has led to concern about safety. However, constructs encoding HSP65 are now known to be safe in humans with cancer,[48] and a similar construct created by Japanese researchers that also encodes IL-12 was safe and therapeutic in TB in cynomolgus monkeys.[49] Phase 1 trials of DNA vaccines encoding HSP65 are planned.

Another group is at an earlier stage in the development of a DNA vaccine encoding 3 other antigens of *M tuberculosis*: Ag85B, MPT-64, and MPT-83. Used together with antibacterial drugs, this vaccine significantly reduced CFU 3 to 5 months after treatment of infected mice ($P<.001$).[50]

Other Immunotherapies for which Little is Known

Dzherelo

There are several publications describing clinical studies using plant extracts (Dzherelo [Immunoxel], Lizorm, and Svitanok). Dzherelo has been marketed for some years by Ekomed LLC (a Ukrainian company) as a nonregulated health supplement. The products are widely used in the Ukraine, and seem to be safe. The new studies describe their use as adjunct immunotherapy against MDR-TB and XDR-TB, and in patients with concomitant HIV and TB.[51–53] The claims are striking and cannot be ignored. There is a need for definitive GCP studies.

SCV-07 SciClone (γ-glutamyl-tryptophan)

γ-Glutamyl-tryptophan is an immunostimulatory peptide with an unknown mechanism of action. One study in a mouse TB model has been reported in a Russian immunology journal,[54] and a small human TB study was reported as a news item in The Lancet Infectious Diseases.[55] The study is doubtful because the results in the group receiving chemotherapy only are poor, and there have been no further announcements.

RUTI

RUTI is a liposome preparation of M tuberculosis cell wall skeleton. RUTI was designed as adjunctive treatment of latent TB infection, and is intended to accelerate treatment after drugs have killed the bulk of the M tuberculosis. It is not intended as an immunotherapeutic for use in cases of drug-resistant disease. In a mouse model, RUTI accelerates bacterial clearance when given late in treatment as an adjunct to conventional chemotherapy.[56,57] The results of a Phase I study of RUTI as an adjunct to conventional therapy in drug-susceptible infection are awaited.

Immunosuppressive Therapy

Immunotherapy that increases chemotherapy access

The difficulty in curing TB is partly attributed to the fact that current antibiotics were selected to kill actively growing M tuberculosis, and do not efficiently kill nonreplicating bacilli. Following infection, M tuberculosis adapts to conditions within granulomas by adopting a dormancy phenotype with reduced replication and aerobic metabolism, and altered biosynthetic pathways, against which most current TB drugs have reduced bactericidal activity. Recent preliminary studies suggest that modulation of the host immune response to alleviate the environmental pressure within the macrophage may render existing antibiotics more effective at killing M tuberculosis. The strategies described later in this article seek to restore these drugs to full effectiveness by modulation of immunity, which would increase drug access or bacillary responsiveness. However, 2 potential concerns must be considered: (1) in the absence of adequate therapeutic regimens (eg, for XDR-TB), reduced immunity may have a detrimental effect on bacillary growth; and (2) there is a risk that generalized immunosuppression may result in opportunistic infections.

Thalidomide analogs

TNF-α is essential for granuloma formation, and also contributes to activation of macrophages, leading to control of growth of M tuberculosis.[58,59] If TNF-α is inhibited, the environment in which the bacilli reside is modified, likely affecting the physiologic state of the organisms. It is hypothesized that, when TNF-α is inhibited and macrophage activation is suboptimal, the bacilli would be more likely to remain in an actively growing state, rather than shifting into latency, rendering them more responsive to the bactericidal action of antibiotics.

Thalidomide (α-N-phthalimidiglutarimide) has been shown to have anti-inflammatory and immunomodulatory effects in various experimental and clinical settings. Thalidomide partially inhibits TNF-α production by monocytes, but not T cells.[60] It has been shown that treatment with thalidomide reduces TNF-α production in patients with pulmonary TB and improves treatment outcome.[61] Thalidomide, when used adjunctively in the treatment of adults infected with HIV with or without TB, was associated with lower TNF-α and HIV viral loads and increased weight gain compared with placebo recipients.[62] Initial studies of adjunctive thalidomide used in the treatment of rabbits and in limited studies in children with TB meningitis showed promise.[63,64] However, a randomized controlled trial of high-dose thalidomide in the treatment of severe TB meningitis, in HIV-uninfected children, showed no benefit and was stopped early due to excess adverse events and all deaths occurring in the thalidomide treatment group.[65] Based on the results of this trial, high-dose thalidomide is not recommended for TB meningitis.

To overcome the side effects of thalidomide, including teratogenicity and peripheral neuropathy, thalidomide analogs have been synthesized (Celgene Corporation, Warren, NJ, USA). These analogs are potent inhibitors of TNF-α, with up to 50,000-fold more activity in in vitro assays compared with the parent drug.[66] One class of these analogs, termed selective cytokine inhibitory drugs (SelCiDs), has been shown to act via inhibition of phosphodiesterase 4 (PDE4), a monocyte/macrophage enzyme involved in regulating intracellular levels of cAMP.[60] Most importantly, the PDE4 inhibitors are nonteratogenic and well tolerated by humans, as shown in Phase 1 clinical studies.[67]

To evaluate the role of TNF-α–induced immune pressure on the response of M tuberculosis to antibiotic treatment, a monocyte/macrophage TNF-α PDE4 inhibitor (thalidomide analog CC-3052) has been used to treat M tuberculosis-infected mice. Preliminary data indicated that co-treatment of infected mice with CC-3052 and isoniazid (INH) resulted in improved M tuberculosis killing and clearance of bacilli from the lungs (Gilla Kaplan, PhD, personal communication, 2009). In contrast, mice treated with INH alone showed reduced bacillary loads at a steady state and less efficient bacillary control. Treatment with CC-3052 alone was associated with control of M tuberculosis growth in the lungs during infection similar to that seen in the untreated control mice, indicating that the drug was not generally immune suppressive.

In contrast, the anti-TNF-α monoclonal antibody TN3-19.12 was highly immune suppressive (Gilla Kaplan, PhD, personal communication, 2009).[68] Control mice treated with IgG1 starting at 14 days postinfection showed a steady-state infection at about 6 $\log_{10}$ from 28 days to the end of the experiment. In animals treated with TN3-19.12 initiated at 14 days postinfection, bacterial growth in the lungs from 28 days was uncontrolled, reaching 9 $\log_{10}$, at which time the mice either died or were moribund. Treatment with INH initiated at 14 days, together with TN3-19.12 or IgG1, resulted in decreased bacillary loads, similar to the results seen with INH alone, showing that TN3-19.12 did not enhance the efficacy of INH.

These observations suggest that CC-3052 acts to enhance M tuberculosis killing through its selective effect on macrophage PDE4, without inhibiting the host immune response required to control M tuberculosis infection. A recent report showed that increased cAMP levels in macrophages can disrupt actin assembly, resulting in reduced phagosome acidification and enhanced mycobacterial growth.[69] Because CC-3052–mediated inhibition of PDE4 leads to elevated cAMP levels, it is possible that CC-3052 may enhance antibiotic killing of M tuberculosis by targeting a second host mechanism involving prevention of phagosome acidification via disruption of actin assembly.

When similar preliminary experiments were performed in rabbits infected with M tuberculosis, improved clearance of the bacilli was again seen in the cotreated animals. In addition, a striking effect of CC-3052 administration to rabbits during INH treatment was the improvement in lung pathology, whereby the drug facilitated accelerated lesion clearance and reduced inflammation. These observations are consistent with previous studies in the rabbit TB meningitis model, in which the extent of pathology was associated with increased levels of TNF-α in the central nervous system, and tissue destruction could be limited by adjunctive treatment with a class I thalidomide analog that reduces TNF-α production.[70] The results of these studies are particularly interesting in light of many published observations suggesting that TB can cause chronic lung

function impairment, involving varying degrees of fibrosis, bronchovascular distortion, emphysema, and bronchiectasis, all known to be associated with inflammation in the lungs. Pulmonary damage associated with chronic impairment and excess mortality in TB patients, despite successful microbiologic cure, has been described in several reports.[71–73]

Etanercept (soluble TNF-α receptor)

The hypothesis that a strong host immune response may interfere with the ability of TB chemotherapy to achieve sterilization is also supported by the results of a clinical trial evaluating the use of adjunctive etanercept (soluble TNF-α receptor) in the treatment of HIV-infected patients with TB.[74] The primary goal of this controlled trial was to evaluate the role of TNF-α in accelerating the progression of HIV disease due to TB coinfection, and microbiologic and clinical data were prospectively collected during the study. The study was performed with HIV-1 infected patients who had relatively intact TB immune responses, based on levels of CD4+ T cells (>200 cells/mm^3) and the presence of cavitary TB disease. Sixteen HIV-infected patients were treated with etanercept (25 mg), administered subcutaneously twice weekly for 8 doses, beginning on day 4 of standard TB antibiotic treatment, and 42 CD4-frequency–matched controls receiving TB chemotherapy alone were included. The median time to sputum culture conversion was significantly reduced ($P = .04$) in the etanercept-treated patients (56 days) compared with the control patients (63 days). In addition, the etanercept-treated subjects tended to show superior change from baseline to month 6 in the number of involved lung zones, closure of cavities, weight gain, and Karnofsky performance score, although these results did not reach statistical significance. Although this is a small study, these results suggest that adjunctive treatment with etanercept, together with conventional TB chemotherapy, can accelerate the microbiologic response and improve outcome in patients with HIV/TB coinfection. Adjunctive etanercept treatment resulted in a trend toward increased CD4+ T cell counts, but there was no effect on plasma HIV RNA levels. Etanercept was well tolerated, showing that this drug can be safely administered during initial TB treatment even in HIV-infected patients.

High-dose prednisolone

A substantially greater microbiologic benefit was observed in a Phase 2 clinical trial performed to evaluate the use of high-dose prednisolone in the treatment of HIV-1 infected patients with TB.[75] In this study, 187 HIV-infected TB patients (CD4+ T cell counts > 200 cells/mm^3) were treated with either prednisolone (at 2.75 mg/kg/d) or placebo during the first month of standard TB chemotherapy. Sputum culture conversion rates after 1 month of treatment were 62% and 37% in subjects treated with prednisolone versus placebo, respectively ($P = .001$), and is the greatest effect on sputum culture conversion observed in any trial of adjunctive therapy in TB, whether chemotherapy or immunotherapy. No previous studies have examined the microbiologic effects of corticosteroid doses of this magnitude in TB patients. The high dose of prednisolone was selected based on a pilot pharmacokinetic study indicating this as a sufficient dose to reduce TNF-α levels by 50%. However, although there were no significant increases in other opportunistic infections in this study, prednisolone treatment led to increased risk of other serious adverse events, including edema, hyperglycemia, electrolyte disturbances, and severe hypertension. In addition, high-dose prednisolone therapy also led to a transient increase in plasma HIV RNA levels, which receded after the end of prednisolone treatment. Two other prospective clinical trials of adjunctive corticosteroids administered at much lower doses in TB patients have shown acceleration of sputum culture conversion,[76,77] providing further support for the hypothesis of an association between release of immune pressure and improved antibiotic-mediated bacillary clearance. Future studies may consider reducing these adverse events by delivering steroid therapy directly to the lung by inhalation, or by using a targeted anti-TNF-α therapy with greater antigranuloma activity, such as infliximab (anti-TNF-α monoclonal antibody).

SUPPLEMENTING EFFECTOR CYTOKINES, TO ASSIST ANTIMICROBICIDAL ACTIVITY

The cytokine therapies have had modest effects. As they are reviewed elsewhere,[3,78–80] only a brief update is provided.

Recombinant Human IFN-γ

IFN-γ is essential for antimycobacterial host defenses. There have been 5 small trials of aerosolized, subcutaneous, or intramuscular recombinant human (rh) IFN-γ or α among patients with multi- or drug-resistant TB. The studies showed minimal to moderate benefit that was not sustained.[81–84] The first placebo-controlled study of inhaled adjunctive IFN-γ in

MDR-TB patients was stopped early because of a lack of effect, and the results have never been published. Preliminary results from another controlled trial of aerosolized or subcutaneous IFN-γ used adjunctively in the treatment of drug-susceptible cavitary pulmonary TB showed a trend toward earlier sputum smear conversion, but the final results of this trial have also not been published. The results of these studies suggest that adjunctive IFN-γ is not able to significantly augment Th1 responses in TB patients who already have upregulated IFN-γ–induced genes, such as IP-10 and iNOS.[85]

rh-IL-2

IL-2 promotes T cell proliferation, differentiation, and activation, and is essential for cellular immune function and granuloma formation. Several studies have shown rh-IL-2 to be safe and well tolerated.[86–89] In 1997, a small, unblinded study in MDR-TB patients of 2 low-dose IL-2 regimens (daily or in 5-day "pulses") found that the daily regimen appeared to decrease sputum acid-fast bacilli (AFB) counts.[88] Based on this preliminary observation, a randomized, double-blind, placebo-controlled trial of the effect of IL-2 on sputum culture conversion was conducted in 110 HIV-uninfected drug-susceptible Ugandan TB cases.[89] Contrary to expectations, the study found reduced clearance of viable M tuberculosis sputum counts and delayed sputum culture conversion in the IL-2 arm. These results suggest that IL-2 may only be beneficial when given adjunctively with MDR-TB drug regimens. A possible explanation for the lack of benefit when IL-2 is given adjunctively with bactericidal chemotherapy for drug-susceptible TB has been proposed. IL-2 may have an antagonistic effect when given adjunctively with bactericidal chemotherapy by promoting a bacteriostatic response in which M tuberculosis is sequestrated and becomes dormant within granulomas.[90] Alternatively, IL-2 may cause an excessive downregulation of some aspects of the immune response.

rh-Granulocyte-Macrophage Colony-stimulating Factor

Granulocyte-macrophage colony-stimulating factor (GM-CSF) has been shown to decrease replication of M tuberculosis within macrophages and dendritic cells.[91] Only 1 small (n = 31) randomized controlled trial of adjunctive rh-GM-CSF in patients with newly diagnosed HIV-uninfected pulmonary TB in Brazil was shown to be safe and well tolerated and showed a trend

Table 1
The role of immunotherapy forTB: objections and responses

Objection	Response
Antituberculous chemotherapy will solve the problem • MDR TB and, to some extent, XDR TB can be treated with existing drugs • New drugs will be effective in treating MDR TB and XDR TB	• The cure rate of MDR TB and XDR TB with current drugs is inadequate. In a recent study in Cape Town (K. Dheda, personal communication, 2009) only 18% of XDR TB cases ever showed sputum conversion (and more than 50% of these rapidly relapsed) • It cannot be assumed that all new drugs will reach the clinic, or that resistance will not develop, particularly when they are used in patients whose organisms are resistant to the other drugs in the regimen • Even if new drugs improve treatment outcomes of MDR TB and XDR TB, immunotherapy may still have a role to play in reducing treatment duration and reducing the risk of recurrence

Trials of immunotherapies in MDR TB and XDR TB patients are complicated by
• Heterogeneous patient group
• A high mortality rate, resulting in inadequate follow-up time for trials
• Competition for scarce participants
	• Recent results have shown that it is possible to carry out treatment trials in MDR TB patients[98]
	• The mortality rate in certain XDR TB patients is low enough to permit clinical trials
	  - 23% in HIV-uninfected XDR TB patients from Peru[99]
	  - 35% in HIV-infected XDR TB patients on antiretroviral therapy in Cape Town (K. Dheda, personal communication, 2009)

Will not work because • It is not possible to realign the immune system once it has failed • The immune system is irrelevant, as drugs work as well in HIV-infected persons • Immunotherapy would not work in HIV-infected persons due to immunosuppression	• Animal data suggest that it is possible to realign the immune response in TB disease • The immune response remains important in HIV-infected individuals, as the rate of relapse is similar to that seen in HIV-uninfected persons[100] • Immunotherapy has been shown to work in HIV disease[30]
Immunotherapy will work and therefore result in immunopathology	• Clinical trials of immunotherapy have shown immunotherapy to be well tolerated and safe
Immunology of TB and immunotherapy are not well understood • Boosting Th1/IFN-γ response is likely to be counterproductive • Animal data only, using high-dose challenge mouse models • 2–3 $\log_{10}$ reduction in CFU in mice is too small to be beneficial	• Optimizing the balance betweenTh1 and Th2 responses is more likely to be effective • High-dose challenge models are more consistent with TB in endemic areas[17] • These falls in CFU are seen in the complete absence of chemotherapy, and, moreover, take the CFU down to levels that in pre-immunized mice can remain latent. Furthermore, in humans a 2–3 $\log_{10}$ CFU reduction may lead to sterilization

toward faster sputum conversion.[92] GM-CSF may also have an adjuvant role in TB vaccines. In murine models a DNA vaccine coexpressing GM-CSF with Ag85A resulted in enhanced immunogenicity compared with Ag85A alone,[93] and bacillus Calmette-Guérin (BCG)-derived GM-CSF resulted in tenfold increased protection against disseminated TB compared with standard BCG alone.[94]

IL-12

IL-12 is a key cytokine in the response to intracellular infection with *M tuberculosis* that stimulates IFN-γ production and a Th1 response. In vitro studies have shown that recombinant IL-12 increases IFN-γ responses in *M tuberculosis*-stimulated human peripheral blood mononuclear cells and alveolar macrophages.[95,96] Continuous administration of IL-12, expressed in transgenic tomato, had therapeutic efficacy in a murine model of pulmonary TB.[97] Although IL-12 may have a role as immunotherapy for TB, there are concerns regarding its nonspecific mechanisms of action and possible toxicity. The results of a completed trial of IL-12 immunotherapy are yet to be reported.

THE FUTURE OF IMMUNOTHERAPY

Despite data from preclinical studies that have shown potential efficacy, and clinical trials showing safety, tolerability, and modest efficacy, the development of immunotherapies has been hampered by a lack of funding and interest in the potential role of these therapeutic interventions. Commonly expressed objections to immunotherapy and responses to these objections are listed in **Table 1**.

SUMMARY

Immunotherapies have the potential to improve the outcome in all TB patients including those with MDR-TB and XDR-TB. Immunotherapy for TB may shorten TB treatment and improve the immunity of individuals cured by chemotherapy, potentially preventing recurrence. Currently none of the available candidate agents have proof of efficacy for use in MDR-TB and XDR-TB, although some are registered for other indications in humans. Further development and evaluation of existing immunotherapy agents is required to find an effective agent that can be used as an adjunct to chemotherapy to shorten duration of treatment of drug-susceptible TB and improve treatment outcomes for MDR-TB and XDR-TB. With a range of potential immunotherapeutics, some of which have been produced to GMP standards, it is becoming ethically unacceptable to neglect the immunotherapy option.

REFERENCES

1. World Health Organization. Global tuberculosis control: epidemiology, strategy, financing: WHO report 2009. Geneva, Switzerland: World Health Organization; 2009. Report No.: WHO/HTM/TB/2009.411.

2. Gandhi NR, Moll A, Sturm AW, et al. Extensively drug-resistant tuberculosis as a cause of death in patients co-infected with tuberculosis and HIV in a rural area of South Africa. Lancet 2006; 368(9547):1575–80.

3. Churchyard GJ, Wallis R, Levin J, et al. Expert consultation to evaluate the potential roles of immunotherapeutic interventions for TB in TB and HIV high burden settings. Geneva, Switzerland: TDR/World Health Organization; 2007.

4. Rook GA, Lowrie DB, Hernndez-Pando R. Immunotherapeutics for tuberculosis in experimental animals: is there a common pathway activated by effective protocols? J Infect Dis 2007;196(2): 191–8.

5. van Crevel R, Karyadi E, Preyers F, et al. Increased production of interleukin 4 by CD4+ and CD8+ T cells from patients with tuberculosis is related to the presence of pulmonary cavities. J Infect Dis 2000;181(3):1194–7.

6. Kaplan G, Post FA, Moreira AL, et al. *Mycobacterium tuberculosis* growth at the cavity surface: a microenvironment with failed immunity. Infect Immun 2003;71(12):7099–108.

7. Deretic V, Singh S, Master S, et al. *Mycobacterium tuberculosis* inhibition of phagolysosome biogenesis and autophagy as a host defence mechanism. Cell Microbiol 2006;8(5):719–27.

8. Krutzik SR, Hewison M, Liu PT, et al. IL-15 links TLR2/1-induced macrophage differentiation to the vitamin D-dependent antimicrobial pathway. J Immunol 2008;181(10):7115–20.

9. Malik ZA, Denning GM, Kusner DJ. Inhibition of Ca(2+) signaling by *Mycobacterium tuberculosis* is associated with reduced phagosome-lysosome fusion and increased survival within human macrophages. J Exp Med 2000; 191(2):287–302.

10. Mariotti S, Teloni R, Iona E, et al. *Mycobacterium tuberculosis* subverts the differentiation of human monocytes into dendritic cells. Eur J Immunol 2002;32(11):3050–8.

11. Master SS, Rampini SK, Davis AS, et al. *Mycobacterium tuberculosis* prevents inflammasome activation. Cell Host Microbe 2008;3(4):224–32.

12. Fortune SM, Solache A, Jaeger A, et al. *Mycobacterium tuberculosis* inhibits macrophage responses to IFN-gamma through myeloid differentiation factor 88-dependent and -independent mechanisms. J Immunol 2004;172(10):6272–80.

13. Harris J, De Haro SA, Master SS, et al. T helper 2 cytokines inhibit autophagic control of intracellular *Mycobacterium tuberculosis*. Immunity 2007; 27(3):505–17.

14. Lewinsohn DA, Winata E, Swarbrick GM, et al. Immunodominant tuberculosis CD8 antigens preferentially restricted by HLA-B. PLoS Pathog 2007; 3(9):1240–9.

15. Chen ML, Pittet MJ, Gorelik L, et al. Regulatory T cells suppress tumor-specific CD8 T cell cytotoxicity through TGF-beta signals in vivo. Proc Natl Acad Sci U S A 2005;102(2):419–24.

16. Olver S, Groves P, Buttigieg K, et al. Tumor-derived interleukin-4 reduces tumor clearance and deviates the cytokine and granzyme profile of tumor-induced CD8+ T cells. Cancer Res 2006;66(1): 571–80.

17. Rook GA, Hernandez-Pando R, Zumla A. Tuberculosis due to high-dose challenge in partially immune individuals: a problem for vaccination? J Infect Dis 2009;199(5):613–8.

18. Hernandez-Pando R, Aguilar D, Garcia Hernandez ML, et al. Pulmonary tuberculosis in Balb/c mice with non-functional IL-4 genes; changes in the inflammatory effects of TNF-α and in the regulation of fibrosis. Eur J Immunol 2004; 34:174–83.

19. Roy E, Brennan J, Jolles S, et al. Beneficial effect of anti-interleukin-4 antibody when administered in a murine model of tuberculosis infection. Tuberculosis (Edinb) 2007;88:197–202.

20. North RJ. Mice incapable of making IL-4 or IL-10 display normal resistance to infection with Mycobaotorium tuberculosis. Clin Exp Immunol 1998; 113(1):55–8.

21. Stewart GR, Boussinesq M, Coulson T, et al. Onchocerciasis modulates the immune response to mycobacterial antigens. Clin Exp Immunol 1999;117(3):517–23.

22. Hewitson JP, Grainger JR, Maizels RM. Helminth immunoregulation: the role of parasite secreted proteins in modulating host immunity. Mol Biochem Parasitol 2009;167(1):1–11.

23. Roy E, Stavropoulos E, Brennan J, et al. Therapeutic efficacy of high-dose intravenous immunoglobulin in Mycobacterium tuberculosis infection in mice. Infect Immun 2005;73(9):6101–9.

24. Anthony RM, Nimmerjahn F, Ashline DJ, et al. Recapitulation of IVIG anti-inflammatory activity with a recombinant IgG Fc. Science 2008; 320(5874):373–6.

25. Anthony RM, Wermeling F, Karlsson MC, et al. Identification of a receptor required for the anti-inflammatory activity of IVIG. Proc Natl Acad Sci U S A 2008;105(50):19571–8.

26. Rook GA, Onyebujoh P, Wilkins E, et al. A longitudinal study of per cent agalactosyl IgG in tuberculosis patients receiving chemotherapy, with or without immunotherapy. Immunology 1994;81(1): 149–54.

27. Rademacher TW, Williams P, Dwek RA. Agalactosyl glycoforms of IgG autoantibodies are pathogenic. Proc Natl Acad Sci U S A 1994;91(13):6123–7.

28. Hernandez-Pando R, Aguilar-Leon D, Orozco H, et al. 16 alpha-Bromoepiandrosterone restores T helper cell type 1 activity and accelerates chemotherapy-induced bacterial clearance in a model of progressive pulmonary tuberculosis. J Infect Dis 2005;191(2):299–306.

29. Reading C, Dowding C, Schramm B, et al. Improvement in immune parameters and human immunodeficiency virus-1 viral response in individuals treated with 16 alpha-bromoepiandrosterone (HE2000). Clin Microbiol Infect 2006;12(11): 1082–8.

30. Stickney DR, Noveljic Z, Garsd A, et al. Safety and activity of the immune modulator HE2000 on the incidence of tuberculosis and other opportunistic infections in AIDS patients. Antimicrobial Agents Chemother 2007;51(7):2639–41.

31. Zuany-Amorim C, Sawicka E, Manlius C, et al. Suppression of airway eosinophilia by killed Mycobacterium vaccae-induced allergen-specific regulatory T-cells. Nat Med 2002;8:625–9.

32. Skinner MA, Yuan S, Prestidge R, et al. Immunization with heat-killed Mycobacterium vaccae stimulates CD8+ cytotoxic T cells specific for macrophages infected with Mycobacterium tuberculosis. Infect Immun 1997;65:4525–30.

33. Hernandez-Pando R, Pavon L, Orozco EH, et al. Interactions between hormone-mediated and vaccine-mediated immunotherapy for pulmonary tuberculosis in Balb/c mice. Immunology 2000; 100:391–8.

34. Ricklin-Gutzwiller ME, Reist M, Peel JE, et al. Intradermal injection of heat-killed Mycobacterium vaccae in dogs with atopic dermatitis: a multicentre pilot study. Vet Dermatol 2007;18(2):87–93.

35. Johnson JL, Kamya RM, Okwera A, et al. Randomized controlled trial of Mycobacterium vaccae immunotherapy in non-human immunodeficiency virus-infected Ugandan adults with newly diagnosed pulmonary tuberculosis. The Uganda-Case Western Reserve University Research Collaboration. J Infect Dis 2000;181(4):1304–12.

36. Mwinga A, Nunn A, Ngwira B, et al. Mycobacterium vaccae (SRL172) immunotherapy as an adjunct to standard antituberculosis treatment in HIV-infected adults with pulmonary tuberculosis: a randomised placebo-controlled trial. Lancet 2002;360(9339): 1050–5.

37. Dlugovitzky D, Fiorenza G, Farroni M, et al. Immunological consequences of three doses of heat-killed Mycobacterium vaccae in the immunotherapy of tuberculosis. Respir Med 2006;100(6): 1079–87 [Chinese].

38. Luo Y, Lu S, Guo S. [Immunotherapeutic effect of *Mycobacterium vaccae* on multi-drug resistant pulmonary tuberculosis]. Zhonghua Jie He He Hu Xi Za Zhi 2000;23(2):85–8 [Chinese].

39. Luo Y. [The immunotherapeutic effect of *Mycobacterium vaccae* vaccine on initially treated pulmonary tuberculosis]. Zhonghua Jie He He Hu Xi Za Zhi 2001;24(1):43–7.

40. Fan M, Chen X, Wang K, et al. Adjuvant effect of *Mycobacterium vaccae* on treatment of recurrent treated pulmonary tuberculosis: a meta-analysis. Chinese Journal of Evidence-Based Medicine 2007;7(6):449–55.

41. von Reyn CF, Arbeit RD, Mtei L, et al. [PS-81689-20] The DarDar prime-boost TB vaccine trial in HIV infection: final results. Int J Tuberc Lung Dis 2008;12(11 Suppl 2):S318.

42. Hernandez-Pando R, Orozco-Esteves H, Maldonado HA, et al. A combination of a transforming growth factor-beta antagonist and an inhibitor of cyclooxygenase is an effective treatment for murine pulmonary tuberculosis. Clin Exp Immunol 2006;144(2):264–72.

43. Lowrie DB, Tascon RE, Bonato VL, et al. Therapy of tuberculosis in mice by DNA vaccination. Nature 1999;400(6741):269–71.

44. Silva CL, Bonato VL, Coelho-Castelo AA, et al. Immunotherapy with plasmid DNA encoding mycobacterial HSP65 in association with chemotherapy is a more rapid and efficient form of treatment for tuberculosis in mice. Gene Ther 2005;12(3):281–7.

45. Nuermberger E, Tyagi S, Williams KN, et al. Rifapentine, moxifloxacin, or DNA vaccine improves treatment of latent tuberculosis in a mouse model. Am J Respir Crit Care Med 2005; 172(11):1452–6.

46. Zarate-Blades CR, Bonato VL, da Silveira EL, et al. Comprehensive gene expression profiling in lungs of mice infected with *Mycobacterium tuberculosis* following DNAHSP65 immunotherapy. J Gene Med 2009;11(1):66–78.

47. Turner OC, Roberts AD, Frank AA, et al. Lack of protection in mice and necrotizing bronchointerstitial pneumonia with bronchiolitis in guinea pigs immunized with vaccines directed against the HSP60 molecule of *Mycobacterium tuberculosis*. Infect Immun 2000;68(6):3674–9.

48. Victora GD, Socorro-Silva A, Volsi EC, et al. Immune response to vaccination with DNA-HSP65 in a Phase I clinical trial with head and neck cancer patients. Cancer Gene Ther 2009;16(7):598–608.

49. Okada M, Kita Y, Nakajima T, et al. Novel prophylactic and therapeutic vaccine against tuberculosis. Vaccine 2009;27(25-26):3267–70.

50. Yu DH, Hu XD, Cai H. Efficient tuberculosis treatment in mice using chemotherapy and immunotherapy with the combined DNA vaccine encoding Ag85B, MPT-64 and MPT-83. Gene Ther 2008;15(9):652–9.

51. Nikolaeva LG, Maystat TV, Pylypchuk VS, et al. Cytokine profiles of HIV patients with pulmonary tuberculosis resulting from adjunct immunotherapy with herbal phytoconcentrates Dzherelo and Anemin. Cytokine 2008;44(3):392–6.

52. Nikolaeva LG, Maystat TV, Pylypchuk VS, et al. Effect of oral immunomodulator Dzherelo in TB/HIV co-infected patients receiving anti-tuberculosis therapy under DOTS. Int Immunopharmacol 2008; 8(6):845–51.

53. Prihoda ND, Arjanova OV, Yurchenko LV, et al. Adjunct immunotherapy of tuberculosis in drug-resistant TB and TB/HIV co-infected patients. Int J Biomed Pharmaceut Sci 2008;2:59–64.

54. Simbirtsev A, Kolobov A, Zabolotnych N, et al. Biological activity of peptide SCV-07 against murine tuberculosis. Russ J Immunol 2003;8:11–22.

55. Orellana C. Immune system stimulator shows promise against tuberculosis. Lancet Infect Dis 2002;2:711.

56. Cardona PJ, Amat I, Gordillo S, et al. Immunotherapy with fragmented *Mycobacterium tuberculosis* cells increases the effectiveness of chemotherapy against a chronical infection in a murine model of tuberculosis. Vaccine 2005;23(11):1393–8.

57. Cardona PJ. RUTI: a new chance to shorten the treatment of latent tuberculosis infection. Tuberculosis (Edinb) 2006;86(3–4):273–89.

58. Algood HM, Lin PL, Yankura D, et al. TNF influences chemokine expression of macrophages in vitro and that of CD11b+ cells in vivo during *Mycobacterium tuberculosis* infection. J Immunol 2004; 172(11):6846–57.

59. Flynn JL, Goldstein MM, Chan J, et al. Tumor necrosis factor-alpha is required in the protective immune response against *Mycobacterium tuberculosis* in mice. Immunity 1995;2(6):561–72.

60. Corral LG, Muller GW, Moreira AL, et al. Selection of novel analogs of thalidomide with enhanced tumor necrosis factor alpha inhibitory activity. Mol Med 1996;2(4):506–15.

61. Tramontana JM, Utaipat U, Molloy A, et al. Thalidomide treatment reduces tumor necrosis factor alpha production and enhances weight gain in patients with pulmonary tuberculosis. Mol Med 1995;1(4):384–97.

62. Klausner JD, Makonkawkeyoon S, Akarasewi P, et al. The effect of thalidomide on the pathogenesis of human immunodeficiency virus type 1 and *M. tuberculosis* infection. J Acquir Immune Defic Syndr Hum Retrovirol 1996;11(3):247–57.

63. Tsenova L, Sokol K, Freedman VH, et al. A combination of thalidomide plus antibiotics protects rabbits from mycobacterial meningitis-associated death. J Infect Dis 1998;177(6):1563–72.

64. Schoeman JF, Springer P, Ravenscroft A, et al. Adjunctive thalidomide therapy of childhood tuberculous meningitis: possible anti-inflammatory role. J Child Neurol 2000;15(8):497–503.

65. Schoeman JF, Springer P, van Rensburg AJ, et al. Adjunctive thalidomide therapy for childhood tuberculous meningitis: results of a randomized study. J Child Neurol 2004;19(4):250–7.

66. Corral LG, Kaplan G. Immunomodulation by thalidomide and thalidomide analogues. Ann Rheum Dis 1999;58(Suppl 1):I107–13.

67. Gottlieb AB, Strober B, Krueger JG, et al. An open-label, single-arm pilot study in patients with severe plaque-type psoriasis treated with an oral anti-inflammatory agent, apremilast. Curr Med Res Opin 2008;24(5):1529–38.

68. Mohan VP, Scanga CA, Yu K, et al. Effects of tumor necrosis factor alpha on host immune response in chronic persistent tuberculosis: possible role for limiting pathology. Infect Immun 2001;69(3): 1847–55.

69. Kalamidas SA, Kuehnel MP, Peyron P, et al. cAMP synthesis and degradation by phagosomes regulate actin assembly and fusion events: consequences for mycobacteria. J Cell Sci 2006;119(Pt 17):3686–94.

70. Tsenova L, Mangaliso B, Muller G, et al. Use of IMiD3, a thalidomide analog, as an adjunct to therapy for experimental tuberculous meningitis. Antimicrobial Agents Chemother 2002;46(0): 1887–95.

71. de Vallire S, Barker RD. Residual lung damage after completion of treatment for multidrug-resistant tuberculosis. Int J Tuberc Lung Dis 2004;8(6): 767–71.

72. Pasipanodya JG, Miller TL, Vecino M, et al. Pulmonary impairment after tuberculosis. Chest 2007; 131(6):1817–24.

73. Verver S, Warren RM, Beyers N, et al. Rate of reinfection tuberculosis after successful treatment is higher than rate of new tuberculosis. Am J Respir Crit Care Med 2005;171(12):1430–5.

74. Wallis RS, Kyambadde P, Johnson JL, et al. A study of the safety, immunology, virology, and microbiology of adjunctive etanercept in HIV-1-associated tuberculosis. AIDS 2004;18(2):257–64.

75. Mayanja-Kizza H, Jones-Lopez E, Okwera A, et al. Immunoadjuvant prednisolone therapy for HIV-associated tuberculosis: a Phase 2 clinical trial in Uganda. J Infect Dis 2005;191(6):856–65.

76. Bilaeroglu S, Perim K, Byksirin M, et al. Prednisolone: a beneficial and safe adjunct to antituberculosis treatment? A randomized controlled trial. Int J Tuberc Lung Dis 1999;3(1):47–54.

77. Horne NW. Prednisolone in treatment of pulmonary tuberculosis: a controlled trial. Final report to the Research Committee of the Tuberculosis Society of Scotland. Br Med J 1960;2(5215):1751–6.

78. Wallis RS. Reconsidering adjuvant immunotherapy for tuberculosis. Clin Infect Dis 2005; 41(2):201–8.

79. Reljic R. IFN-gamma therapy of tuberculosis and related infections. J Interferon Cytokine Res 2007; 27(5):353–64.

80. Roy E, Lowrie DB, Jolles SR. Current strategies in TB immunotherapy. Curr Mol Med 2007;7(4): 373–86.

81. Condos R, Rom WN, Schluger NW. Treatment of multidrug-resistant pulmonary tuberculosis with interferon-gamma via aerosol. Lancet 1997; 349(9064):1513–5.

82. Giosu S, Casarini M, Ameglio F, et al. Aerosolized interferon-alpha treatment in patients with multidrug-resistant pulmonary tuberculosis. Eur Cytokine Netw 2000;11(1):99–104.

83. Surez-Mndez R, Garca-Garca I, Fernndez-Olivera N, et al. Adjuvant interferon gamma in patients with drug-resistant pulmonary tuberculosis: a pilot study. BMC Infect Dis 2004;4:44.

84. Koh WJ, Kwon OJ, Suh GY, et al. Six-month therapy with aerosolized interferon-gamma for refractory multidrug-resistant pulmonary tuberculosis. J Korean Med Sci 2004;19(2):167–71.

85. Raju B, Hoshino Y, Kuwabara K, et al. Aerosolized gamma interferon (IFN-gamma) induces expression of the genes encoding the IFN-gamma-inducible 10-kilodalton protein but not inducible nitric oxide synthase in the lung during tuberculosis. Infect Immun 2004;72(3):1275–83.

86. Johnson BJ, Estrada I, Shen Z, et al. Differential gene expression in response to adjunctive recombinant human interleukin-2 immunotherapy in multidrug-resistant tuberculosis patients. Infect Immun 1998;66(6):2426–33.

87. Johnson B, Bekker LG, Ress S, et al. Recombinant interleukin 2 adjunctive therapy in multidrug-resistant tuberculosis. Novartis Found Symp 1998;217: 99–106.

88. Johnson BJ, Bekker LG, Rickman R, et al. rhuIL 2 adjunctive therapy in multidrug resistant tuberculosis: a comparison of two treatment regimens and placebo. Tuber Lung Dis 1997;78(3–4): 195–203.

89. Johnson JL, Ssekasanvu E, Okwera A, et al. Randomized trial of adjunctive interleukin-2 in adults with pulmonary tuberculosis. Am J Respir Crit Care Med 2003;168(2):185–91.

90. Wallis RS, Johnson JL. Immunotherapy of tuberculosis. In: Schaaf HS, Zumla AI, editors. Tuberculosis. A comprehensive clinical reference. 1st edition. London: Saunders, Elsevier; 2009. p. 718–26.

91. Szeliga J, Daniel DS, Yang CH, et al. Granulocyte-macrophage colony stimulating factor-mediated innate responses in tuberculosis. Tuberculosis (Edinb) 2008;88(1):7–20.

92. Pedral-Sampaio DB, Netto EM, Brites C, et al. Use of Rhu-GM-CSF in pulmonary tuberculosis patients: results of a randomized clinical trial. Braz J Infect Dis 2003;7(4):245–52.

93. Zhang X, Divangahi M, Ngai P, et al. Intramuscular immunization with a monogenic plasmid DNA tuberculosis vaccine: enhanced immunogenicity by electroporation and co-expression of GM-CSF transgene. Vaccine 2007;25(7):1342–52.

94. Ryan AA, Wozniak TM, Shklovskaya E, et al. Improved protection against disseminated tuberculosis by Mycobacterium bovis bacillus Calmette-Guerin secreting murine GM-CSF is associated with expansion and activation of APCs. J Immunol 2007;179(12):8418–24.

95. Zhang M, Gong J, Iyer DV, et al. T cell cytokine responses in persons with tuberculosis and human immunodeficiency virus infection. J Clin Invest 1994;94(6):2435–42.

96. Fenton MJ, Vermeulen MW, Kim S, et al. Induction of gamma interferon production in human alveolar macrophages by Mycobacterium tuberculosis. Infect Immun 1997;65(12):5149–56.

97. Elas-Lpez AL, Marquina B, Gutirrez-Ortega A, et al. Transgenic tomato expressing interleukin-12 has a therapeutic effect in a murine model of progressive pulmonary tuberculosis. Clin Exp Immunol 2008;154(1):123–33.

98. Diacon AH, Pym A, Grobusch M, et al. The diarylquinoline TMC207 for multidrug-resistant tuberculosis. N Engl J Med 2009;360(23):2397–405.

99. Bonilla CA, Crossa A, Jave HO, et al. Management of extensively drug-resistant tuberculosis in Peru: cure is possible. PLoS One 2008;3(8):e2957.

100. Sonnenberg P, Murray J, Glynn JR, et al. HIV-1 and recurrence, relapse, and reinfection of tuberculosis after cure: a cohort study in South African mineworkers. Lancet 2001;358(9294):1687–93.

Biomarkers of Disease Activity, Cure, and Relapse in Tuberculosis

T. Mark Doherty, PhD[a],*, Robert S. Wallis, MD, FIDSA[b],
Alimuddin Zumla, FRCP, PhD(Lond), FRCPath[c]

KEYWORDS

• Tuberculosis • Diagnosis • Biomarkers

WHAT IS TUBERCULOSIS?

Although what actually constitutes tuberculosis might seem obvious—disease arising from infection by members of the *Mycobacterium tuberculosis* complex (primarily but not exclusively *M tuberculosis*)—the broad spectrum of clinical presentations renders this question more difficult to answer in practice. Global morbidity and mortality are estimated at 9.3 million new cases of tuberculosis and 1.8 million deaths per year, respectively.[1] However, because only approximately 10% of infections are estimated to result in clinically recognized disease,[1] this is merely the tip of the iceberg. Combined with the fact that clinical disease can manifest years or even decades after infection and that infection with *M tuberculosis* is nearly universal by adulthood in highly endemic regions,[2–5] the challenge to identifying clinically relevant biomarkers becomes apparent.

Establishing the existence of infection is not enough; most individuals become infected. The goal is to identify biomarkers that can detect tuberculosis disease status (**Fig. 1**). Currently no biomarkers meet this stringent requirement; therefore the focus of this article is not on clinical practice (which is well covered by the other reviews in this issue) but on the most promising leads from current research.

Understanding of the dynamics of *M tuberculosis* infection has changed dramatically over the past few years, and this has had major consequences for biomarker research. The gold standard for

a diagnosing active tuberculosis has long been the presence of *M tuberculosis* in patient samples, typically sputum. However, reports suggesting that an unexpectedly high number of individuals can be sputum-positive (and therefore potentially infectious) without any apparent symptoms, whereas many patients who have significant symptoms remain culture-negative, has called this simple definition into question.[6,7]

At the same time, the old model of latent tuberculosis as being caused by non- or slowly replicating bacteria has also been replaced by an appreciation that latency is a dynamic process in which the growth of metabolically active bacteria is controlled by ongoing host immune responses.[8] During infection, *M tuberculosis* is subjected to a hostile intracellular environment[9] and responds with dramatic transcriptional changes.

Of the approximately 4000 open reading frames identified in *M tuberculosis*, roughly 20% are differentially regulated during in vivo growth compared with growth during in vitro culture, and a significant subset of these genes were differentially regulated depending on whether the bacteria was located in the lesion itself, nearby involved tissue, or distal uninvolved lung tissue.[10,11] The conditions controlling regulation of these genes can be mimicked in vitro by oxygen depletion, nutrient starvation, or nitric oxide addition, allowing identification of genes that have expression believed to be essential for prolonged intracellular survival.[12] Detection of *M tuberculosis*–expressed

[a] Department of Infectious Disease Immunology, Statens Serum Institute, Artillerivej 5, 2300 København S, Denmark
[b] Pfizer Global Research & Development, MS 6025 B3149, 50 Pequot Avenue, New London, CT 06320, USA
[c] University College London Medical School, London, UK
* Corresponding author.
E-mail address: tmd@ssi.dk (T.M. Doherty).

Clin Chest Med 30 (2009) 783–796
doi:10.1016/j.ccm.2009.08.008

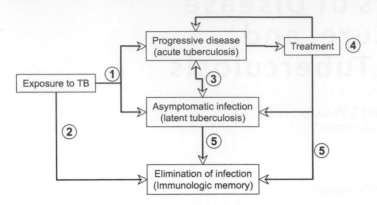

Biomarker questions

1. Can we identify those infected individuals most at risk of developing active disease?
2. Can we separate those who are latently infected from those that maintain a memory response only?
3. Can we distinguish reactivation from primary disease?
4. Can we predict likelihood of treatment failure?
5. Do infected individuals ever eliminate the pathogen?

Suggested markers

1. Magnitude of tuberculin skin test or in vitro IFN-γ response, patterns of serological epitope recognition, genetic polymorphisms
2. Antigen detection, number of Treg cells, expression of adhesion molecules like CCL1, complex biosignatures
3. Relative recognition of latency and acute phase antigens
4. Levels of cytokines such as IFN-γ, alone or relative to IL-4δ2, TNF-αR, number and phenotype of monocytes and NK T cells, levels of non-specific markers of inflammation and immune cell trafficking, presence of antigen in sputum
5. Loss of responsiveness in an IGRA

Fig. 1. A schematic indicating the broad categories used to indicate disease status. A double-ended arrow indicates two conditions that are believed to be able to revert; a single-ended arrow indicates what is believed to be an irreversible change in disease status. Circled numbers indicate where some of the most pressing questions about changes in status fall on the spectrum of disease and these. This schematic also summarizes some of the markers discussed in this article, which may give some insight into these changes.

proteins, or of host responses to them, is central to current biomarker analyses.

THE TUBERCULIN SKIN TEST: THE FIRST BIOMARKER FOR TUBERCULOSIS

The tuberculin skin test (TST) was the first biomarker for infection with *M tuberculosis*. It consists of measuring the size of a delayed-type hypersensitivity response to purified protein derivative (PPD) when injected intradermally into exposed individuals. The TST was first introduced in 1907, and the fact that it remains in clinical use a century later, despite its many shortcomings, reflects the limited options for useful biomarkers.

The shortcomings of the TST include the fact that it is a complex mixture of mycobacterial antigens, many of which are shared with nontuberculous mycobacteria.[13,14] Although levels of response are variable,[15] in countries in which Bacille Calmette-Guérin (BCG) is widely used, a substantial number of people who have no identifiable risk factors for *M tuberculosis* infection may have false-positive TSTs,[16,17] which remains a major confounder.[18]

Despite this shortcoming, the TST has clinical use. Even in regions with widespread TST positivity caused by high BCG coverage and latent tuberculosis, a clear correlation is known to exist between the size of the TST and the risk for subsequent development of active tuberculosis.[19,20] Therefore, conversion to positivity in the TST remains the single most important criterion for triggering preventive therapy among contacts. To improve the specificity of the test, various methods have been used, most typically setting different cutoff points for positivity, taking into consideration BCG vaccination status, exposure to environmental mycobacteria, and likelihood of infection.[21,22] These factors were recently reviewed in detail.[23]

One recent attempt to circumvent this problem was simply to replace PPD with a more specific reagent. The *M tuberculosis* virulence factor early-secreted antigenic target-6 (ESAT-6) effectively discriminated *M tuberculosis* infection from BCG (which lost this protein in the early stages of attenuation) when injected intradermally in various animal species.[24] A recent double-blind, randomized, Phase I study in humans indicated that it is also safe and apparently effective for the same purpose[25] and has a minimal risk for sensitization with repeated use.[26]

Despite these promising results, development of the original ESAT-6–based skin test reagent, a homodimer produced as a recombinant protein, was discontinued in favor of a heterodimer containing ESAT-6 and another protein lost in the same genetic deletion in BCG, designated *culture filtrate protein-10* (CFP10). The expectation is that the combination may increase sensitivity, because in vitro analyses indicate that peripheral blood mononuclear cells (PBMCs) from some patients who have tuberculosis respond strongly to ESAT-6 but not CFP10, and vice versa.

Moreover, in animal models of *M tuberculosis* infection the magnitude of the early response to the heterodimer correlated with later outcome, suggesting it may also have a prognostic value.[27] This test is currently in phase I clinical trials in Europe, with phase II trials in endemic countries expected to begin in late 2009, because initial results look promising (T. Mark Doherty, PhD, unpublished data, 2009). A second skin test, based on the antigen MPT64 or MPB64 (the use of *T* or *B* indicates whether the protein was cloned from *M tuberculosis* or *M bovis*, but they are functionally identical), which also has skin test potential[28] using a transdermal patch rather than injection, is also well advanced in clinical development, although the lower immunogenicity of MPT64 in humans[29] and its presence in some widely used strains of BCG vaccine[30] make it a generally less appealing candidate. Nonetheless, one or both of these tests are likely to reach the market within the next few years if their early promise can be validated.

Improved skin tests can be directly incorporated into existing clinical programs with little or no change, and should theoretically work exactly the same way but provide greater specificity. However, concerning biomarkers, although skin tests may work, disturbingly little is known about how this occurs.

A positive result in the TST is a delayed-type hypersensitivity reaction of or greater than the predefined limit, typically peaking between 48 and 72 hours after injection, although cellular infiltration may be detectable at the histopathologic level within hours. Infiltrating cells are primarily polymorph/neutrophils in the initial phases, but are mostly T cells (predominantly CD4+ CD45RO memory phenotype) and macrophages by 12 to 24 hours.[31]

What occurs at the molecular level, however, is unclear. Inflammatory cytokines such as interferon-gamma (IFN-γ), and tumor necrosis factor alpha or beta (TNF-α/β) seem to be produced in the latter stages, and these presumably activate the signaling cascade that leads to up-regulation of adhesion molecules on the endothelium and extravasation of immune cells. However, a great deal of unexplained variation occurs in human responses. Experts have suggested that an elevated number of circulating CD4+CD25+FoxP3+ regulatory T cells is associated with a decreased induration in the TST,[31] consistent with a proposed role for these cells in the down-regulation of inflammatory responses.

However, a significant number of people apparently do not respond to the TST, even after prolonged and persistent exposure to infectious individuals who have tuberculosis.[32] Whether this is because they are functionally immune or because they simply respond differently to the TST is unclear. However, recent work established that this phenotype can be mapped to two genetic regions and that it may associate with the degree of TNF-α production.[32] If this phenotype correlates with protection, it might prove a useful marker for risk. Additionally, a weak but suggestive linkage was seen with regions containing several other genes: *SLC11A1*, which is associated with skin test reactivity and susceptibility/resistance to mycobacteria in mice[33] and possibly human infants,[34] plus the cytokine/cytokine receptors interleukin (*IL-1RA*, *IL-6*, *IL12RB2*, *IL12A*, and *IFNGR2*. The latter is also linked to the region containing the *TNF-α* gene. Defects in IFN-γ and IL-12 production or signaling have been implicated in other mycobacterial infections,[35] and the same is assumed for *M tuberculosis*. However, few solid data currently link them directly to tuberculosis.

For TNF-α, however, evidence shows a role in human immunity to tuberculosis, because blocking TNF-α signaling in latently infected individuals greatly increases the risk for active disease and apparently inhibits killing of the pathogen by host macrophages.[36,37] These cytokines have been heavily studied as candidate biomarkers.

CYTOKINE EXPRESSION AS A BIOMARKER OF DISEASE STATUS

Little direct evidence exists of a role for IFN-γ in protection against mycobacterial infection. However, indirect evidence is extremely strong, including susceptibility to other mycobacterial infections of humans who have defects in IFN-γ and IL-12 signaling pathways; the extreme susceptibility of IFN-γ or IFN-γR–deficient animals to *M tuberculosis*,[38,39] and the association of IFN-γ production with successful treatment outcome in patients who have tuberculosis, but not in those experiencing relapse.[40,41]

The same is true of TNF-α. In hindsight, the effect of blocking TNF-α signaling in patients who had rheumatoid arthritis, which led to reactivation of latent *M tuberculosis* infection in some,[36,37] was predicted. Animal experiments have shown a crucial role for TNF-α in controlling *M tuberculosis* infection,[42,43] and polymorphisms in the gene for TNFR1 have been associated with the development of tuberculosis in humans.[44]

Moreover, soluble TNF-α receptors (which can bind TNF-α and thus act as competitive antagonists[45]) are elevated in the serum of patients who have tuberculosis,[46] and a combination of elevated levels of soluble TNF-α receptor 1 (sTNFR1), plus an increased total white blood cell count and absolute monocyte and neutrophil numbers, accurately identified patients whose disease responded slowly to therapy.[47]

Finally, an elevated ratio of TNF-α to sTNFR1 in bronchiolar lavage is associated with more severe pathology,[46] possibly because inhibition of TNF-α signaling increases necrosis in cells infected with *M tuberculosis*.[48]

These studies combined suggest that IFN-γ and TNF-α would make excellent biomarkers, or even surrogate end points for clinical work, because their expression has a direct and apparently causal role in immunity to *M tuberculosis*. In addition, expression of these cytokines is rapidly induced,[49] meaning that immunologic changes can often be shown in patient samples long before immunopathologic changes or the appearance of symptoms. IFN-γ has been the preferred marker because it is nonlabile and abundantly produced, and therefore pathogen-specific IFN-γ can be readily detected. It is also easily induced in PBMC or whole blood through antigenic stimulation in sufficient quantities that it can be detected using simple technologies, such as ELISA or ELISPOT.

This finding led to the development of the QuantiFERON Gold family of kits and the T.Spot.TB test. Both tests rely on detecting elevated IFN-γ production after stimulation with antigens (ESAT-6, CFP10, and TB7.7 for the former; ESAT-6 and CFP10 for the latter). Because these antigens are largely restricted to members of the *M tuberculosis* complex, the tests are not confounded by BCG or environmental mycobacteria.

As a biomarker for prior infection with *M tuberculosis*, detection of IFN-γ with these IFN-γ–release assays (IGRAs) has proved successful,[50] and they are widely used as supplements or replacements for the TST. In addition, just as an elevated TST response in tuberculosis contacts is associated with elevated risk for developing tuberculosis,[51] the same seems to be true of elevated IFN-γ responses to the antigens used in IGRAs.[52–54] Experts have suggested that the number and activity of ESAT-6/CFP10–specific IFN-γ–producing cells in circulating PBMC reflects the individual's bacterial load, and thus the relative risk for pathology and illness.

Consistent with this, isoniazid treatment of contacts with suspected latent tuberculosis infection (LTBI) reduces the number who test positive,[55] and individuals who have suspected LTBI who test positive in the IGRAs remain that way, presumably because they have a persistent, low-grade infection.[41,55] The prognostic value of a high response in the IGRAs, although potentially useful, remains to be clinically validated, and although a general correlation may exist between IFN-γ levels and bacterial activity, it is not always robust.[56]

In one prominent example, multiple reports show that IFN-γ production in response to antigenic stimulation is reduced[57] in many patients, particularly those who have advanced disease, even though their bacterial load is presumably high and their prognosis undoubtedly poor. Production of IFN-γ recovers on treatment, suggesting this recovery is caused by immunosuppression.

This phenomenon may not be unique to *M tuberculosis*, because patients who have ulcers caused by *M ulcerans* also show suppressed IFN-γ responsiveness, and this can be reversed simply through surgically excising the ulcer.[58] The mechanism involved is unclear, although increasing consensus is that it is because cytokine induction is subject to a wide array of feedback mechanisms, particularly by other cytokines.

Therefore, measuring IFN-γ–inducible protein-10 kd (IP-10), an IFN-γ–induced chemokine (also known as CXCL10) that is produced in high amounts, has been suggested as an alternative to measuring IFN-γ directly, based on the assumption that higher expression levels may increase sensitivity.[59] However, with IFN-γ as the primary driver of expression, the same problem seems to occur as with IGRAs: that although simply identifying elevated expression of a single factor may be a good measure of *M tuberculosis* infection, it tells only a little about disease status and therefore relative risk.

More promising, but also more difficult to reduce to practice, is the measurement of relative levels of multiple factors. Decreased IFN-γ in patients who have tuberculosis is often associated with increased expression of IL-4.[41,60] Healthy contacts of tuberculosis who are untreated and subsequently develop disease show elevated expression of IL-4 mRNA, which increases relative to IFN-γ over time.[60,61] At the other extreme, the ratio of IL-4 to IFN-γ mRNA decreases in patients who have successfully treated tuberculosis.[60,62]

Similar results were obtained for the IL-4 antagonistic splice variant IL-4δ2; the ratio of mRNA for IL-4δ2 to IL-4 increased over time in patients recovering from tuberculosis, whereas it decreased in contacts who developed tuberculosis-like symptoms, and stayed constant in contacts who remained healthy.[60] IL-4δ2 mRNA levels were also elevated in persons who had LTBI, consistent with their presumed ability to control disease.[63] The ratio of IL-4 to its splice variants seems to correlate with the extent of pathology in multiple diseases, not just tuberculosis.[64–66] These changes may occur over very short periods and may predict the subsequent outcome of treatment,[62] making them potentially interesting biomarkers. However, consensus is growing that measuring the level of expression of any single cytokine, or even the relative expression of several cytokines, may not be sufficient to provide an accurate picture of disease status. Therefore, the focus is shifting toward measuring what is called the *quality* of the immune response.

COMBINED RESPONSES: THE QUALITY OF THE IMMUNE RESPONSE AS A BIOMARKER

Expression of a single cytokine, even one as critical as IFN-γ or TNF-α, is likely to give only a partial picture of immune status, because the developmental stage, specificity, and location of the cytokine-producing cells are also critical determinants. Analysis of cellular function with fluorescent-activated cell sorters (FACS) allows these parameters to be studied simultaneously and has been suggested for tuberculosis diagnosis.[67] The usefulness of the technique is clear: it is highly sensitive[68] and more informative, allowing assessment of cell types not readily studied using other methods, such as non–T cells or nonconventional T cells. However, because of the technical demands of FACS analysis, it is unlikely to have wide clinical use in the immediate future. The emphasis has been on using it to identify markers that can then be measured using simpler approaches.

Recently, expression of CD11c by monocytes in the blood was shown to be elevated in patients who have tuberculosis and decline on treatment.[69] Moreover, patients whose disease responded poorly to therapy had higher absolute numbers of monocytes and elevated levels of sTNFR1.[47] Together with studies showing that tuberculosis infection was also associated with increased numbers of CD3lo/CD56+ natural killer (NK) T cells, and that patients whose tuberculosis responded poorly to therapy had a higher proportion of NK cells with this phenotype,[70] the data suggest that severe disease is associated with elevated responses by the innate and adaptive immune response, probably contributing significantly to pathology.[71,72]

The greatest focus, however, continues to be on the adaptive (T cell) response. Animal studies suggest that the presence, especially in the lung, of high numbers of polyfunctional antigen-specific T cells that simultaneously produce IL-2, IFN-γ, and TNF-α provides a more accurate picture of the protective potential of an immune response against tuberculosis.[73,74] Although only few data from patients are available, the picture seems more complex.[75,76] The presence of high proportions of polyfunctional cells may be characteristic of an enduring immune response, which can be induced by either vaccination or ongoing infection. FACS analysis is also shedding light on the potential negative regulatory responses that may define advanced, active disease.

In particular, elevated numbers of CD4+ FOXP3+ CD25hi T cells (T regulatory [Treg] cells) have been suggested as a reason for the depressed immune responsiveness in patients who have tuberculosis, because FOXP3 seems to be more highly expressed in patients who have active tuberculosis than healthy, latently infected individuals,[77] and Treg cells also can be shown to actively suppress *M tuberculosis*–specific responses.[78,79] These cells down-regulate immune responses and are believed to be essential for self-tolerance,[80] but dysregulation of this system has been associated with ineffective responses to infection.[81] Whether this reflects a pathogen virulence strategy or the attempts of the host to limit pathology is unclear, but for use as a biomarker, this finding is largely unimportant. Unfortunately, however, although data suggest that the numbers of Treg cells are elevated in active tuberculosis, this does not appear to change rapidly on treatment, suggesting that its usefulness as a biomarker may be limited to identifying active disease.[82,83]

The specificity of T cells is the last component of the quality of the immune response. The IGRAs rely on IFN-γ production by memory cells primed to ESAT-6, CFP10, or TB7.7. Unfortunately, slight evidence shows that this will distinguish between an acute or a latent infection, which, particularly in highly tuberculosis-endemic settings, limits the efficacy of the test.

However, when monitoring IFN-γ production by PBMC in response to proteins such as Rv2031c or heparin-binding hemagglutinin (HBHA), believed to be induced in *M tuberculosis* during tuberculosis latency, investigators found that the subjects who had latent infection responded more strongly to Rv2031c or HBHA[84,85] than to ESAT-6, even though their PBMC recognized both. In the case of HBHA, at least, this seemed to be caused by Treg cell suppression of the response in patients who had acute tuberculosis.[86] Large-scale proteomic screens are therefore ongoing to identify antigens produced by *M tuberculosis* specifically during the switch to the latent form of infection, with the hope of generating a simple IGRA-like test to distinguish progressive from latent disease.

SOLUBLE FACTORS AS BIOMARKERS

The FACS analyses indicate that high numbers of activated immune cells may correlate with disease, treatment outcome, and extent of pathology. Analysis of soluble factors produced by these cells confirms this. C-reactive protein (CRP) is an acute-phase protein involved in opsonizing pathogens, so they may be more easily phagocytosed and are a widely used marker of inflammation and bacterial infection. In patients undergoing treatment for tuberculosis, levels of CRP correlated with the extent of pathology, specifically the number and size of cavities[87] and the elevated levels seen in these patients declined on treatment, but only in those who had successful treatment outcomes.[88–90] Likewise, neopteri, a pteridine associated with activation of the oxidative burst and another general marker of inflammation, is present in higher concentrations in the sera of patients who have tuberculosis than of healthy controls and decreases toward normal values in patients undergoing therapy. Patients who have higher levels may be at increased risk for relapse after treatment.[91]

The chemokine IP-10 is being widely studied as a potential biomarker, and other cell migration/adhesion markers, particularly their soluble forms, are also of interest. The soluble form of uPAR (soluble urokinase-type plasminogen activator receptor, or suPAR), a receptor involved in monocyte/macrophage homing, is up-regulated by *M tuberculosis* infection of monocytes, potentially inhibiting the immune response.[92] Consistent with this, the concentrations of suPAR is correlated with bacterial positivity in patients' sputa, and patients who have tuberculosis who begin with elevated levels of suPAR in their serum or do not experience its reduction during therapy tend to show a poor response.[93–95]

Elevated suPAR levels are also predictive of poor outcome in HIV,[96] suggesting it may be a more general indicator of decreased immunity. The same is true of intercellular adhesion molecule-1 (ICAM-1) and E-selectin, two adhesion molecules crucial for the recruitment and crosstalk of immune cells. Expression of both molecules is induced by IL-1 and TNF-α, and also by *M tuberculosis* infection. Expression of ICAM-1 on the surface of immune cells seems to be beneficial.[97] However, the shed, soluble forms of these receptors (sICAM-1 and sE-Selectin) seem to act as competitive antagonists. In patients who have tuberculosis, sICAM-1 is elevated in tuberculous pleural effusions[98] and in serum,[99,100] and its concentration corresponded with estimates of bacterial load and severity of disease as assessed with radiology.[100] The soluble form of E-selectin was also elevated in these patients.[100] As with the shedding of the TNF-α receptors (which is also induced by *M tuberculosis* infection[101]), these data suggest that shedding of molecules involved in directing and activating the immune response may be a general tactic of the pathogen to interfere with recruitment and activation of lymphocytes and phagocytes.

ANTIBODIES AS BIOMARKERS

When looking for soluble biomarkers in sera or plasma, antigen-specific antibodies are an obvious target, because this approach forms the basis of diagnosis of many other diseases. This approach has not, however, been successful in tuberculosis.[102,103] *M tuberculosis* infection generates a strong humoral response,[104,105] but antigen discovery for serologic analysis has been weak, largely because antibodies are believed to play a minor role in protection against *M tuberculosis*. Therefore, the expectation was that, without a causal role, the association between antigen-specific antibodies and disease status was likely to be weak.

Despite this assumption, the appeal of simple serologic diagnostics, such as lateral flow tests, have stimulated interest in this area, and some targets have been identified.[106,107] In particular, the observation that the concentration of antibodies to ESAT-6 or the 38-kd antigen corresponds with the degree of radiologic involvement has stimulated interest. Because none of the antigens tested has shown the level of sensitivity required for clinical development, focus has shifted to cocktails of multiple antigens. Recently, a report showed that the combined response to the 38-kd antigen, MPT64, thioredoxin C, and Rv2031c was able to differentiate cavitary and noncavitary disease in patients who had tuberculosis.[108]

A proof of principle study using multiplex microbead immunoassays to screen more broadly for antibodies has highlighted some of the problems facing this approach. This pilot study in infected macaques[109] studied only six already-defined antigens (ESAT-6, CFP-10, HspX, MPT53, MPT63, and Ag85B), although the technology can theoretically screen up to 100 targets at a time. However, although strong responses were detected to all of the target antigens, the magnitude of the responses changed dramatically over time and no pattern correlated clearly with disease status.[109]

A different approach to screening involved the construction of a high-content peptide microarray. For this study, 61 M tuberculosis proteins known to have some serologic recognition were expressed as 7446 overlapping peptides and screened with sera from 34 individuals who had active pulmonary tuberculosis and 35 healthy individuals.[110] Although this study was able to segregate their cohorts based on peptide recognition, they did not find recognition of different M tuberculosis proteins between the groups, but rather differential recognition of specific epitopes at different locations within the same proteins.[110] These approaches may allow peptide-based diagnostics to be defined, wherein whole-protein approaches to serology have so far failed.

BACTERIAL PRODUCTS AS BIOMARKERS

An alternative to detecting host responses to antigens from the pathogen is to detect the antigen itself. The obvious advantage is that, theoretically, antigen should only be detectable during active infection. In contrast, immune memory may persist long after the effective control of infection,[111] although experts have suggested that this persistent response may indicate failure to eradicate the pathogen during treatment.[112]

Additionally, the presence of antigens from M tuberculosis should be detectable, perhaps even enhanced, in patients who have immunodeficiency, which is a significant concern for immunodiagnostics.[113] The presence of M tuberculosis-derived Ag85B (either as a protein or mRNA) was shown in sputum, and the concentration and length of time the protein could be detected seemed to predict subsequent relapse.[114]

Although mRNA for Ag85B seemed to be a sensitive marker for initial bacterial clearance, it did not seem to predict relapse, but this study was small.[115] However, the presence of Ag85B in sputum seemed to require the induction of new gene expression through exposure to isoniazid,[116] and could be blunted through the concomitant

administration of rifampin or the rifamycin derivative, rifalazil.[114] The practical usefulness of this marker may therefore be limited to isoniazid-sensitive infections.

Other potential targets have been found in sputum[117,118] (using ELISA or immunochromatographic assays), biopsy material,[119,120] sera or cerebrospinal fluid,[121,122] and urine.[123]

Biomarker detection in urine has attracted particular interest because of the ease and noninvasive nature of collecting specimens, even from infants and those who cannot produce sputum. However, it is usually recommended as a supplementary specimen.[124] Targets have included fragments of M tuberculosis IS6110 DNA, termed transrenal or (tr)DNA, and believed to arise from apoptosis of host cells,[125] a major glycolipid component of the outer mycobacterial cell wall called lipoarabinomannan (LAM), believed to be associated with virulence, and the M tuberculosis protein ornithine carboamyltransferase.[126]

One study involving nested polymerase chain reaction (PCR) analysis of (tr)DNA in urine from patients who had tuberculosis reported a sensitivity of 79% and clearance after 2 months of therapy,[125] but other studies have reported low sensitivity in untreated patients.[127] Although PCR-based methods for biomarker detection offer the possibility of combining diagnosis of M tuberculosis infection with identification of drug resistance mutations, the technique remains experimental.

Some studies in patients who had tuberculosis showed extremely promising results for detecting LAM in urine, with a sensitivity of 67% and specificity of 99%, whereas other studies in endemic populations found significantly lower specificity, with positive test scores among 23.5% of 800 patients who did not have tuberculosis and 8% of 50 healthy individuals.[128–130] The low accuracy of the test was suggested to be caused by formation of LAM–anti-LAM complexes, latent M tuberculosis infection, or cross-reaction with LAM from environmental mycobacterial infections. Moreover, no study established a link between disease status and the magnitude of the response, although one study found a significant correlation between the concentration of LAM in urine and the bacterial load in sputum.[128]

Finally, some groups are testing for biomarkers in exhaled breath from patients who had tuberculosis. Initial studies showed that M tuberculosis, M avium, M scrofulaceum, and Pseudomonas aeruginosa cultures could be differentiated through analyzing volatile organic compounds[131] using a 14-sensor array, or electronic nose, and identifying complex patterns or biosignatures generated by changes in the sensor's conductivity caused by the binding of organic compounds. This technique was then extended to sputum samples spiked with *M tuberculosis*, but the specificity suffered, possibly because of the complex mixture of organic volatiles released.[132] Partly as a result, attempts are being made to identify specific components[133] and, in an intriguing piece of lateral thinking, train Giant Gambian rats to recognize them, in much the way that sniffer dogs are used to identify contraband.

One study using the more conventional 14-sensor conducting array suggested that biosignatures can be identified that can distinguish between hospitalized patients whose sputum cultures were positive or negative for mycobacterial infection.[134] Although little or no data are available on the link between a positive signal to *M tuberculosis* and disease status or treatment response, this technology offers the possibility for fast, noninvasive monitoring of biomarkers.

BIOSIGNATURES

The analysis of volatile compounds relies on identifying molecules, which, although they may not necessarily be specific to the pathogen or disease individually, en masse form a pattern that is specific: a biosignature. The electronic nose analysis of patients relied on a neural network using fuzzy logic, which could be trained to recognize a complex pattern of the relative levels of more than 130 volatile compounds. A similar approach, using mass spectrometry to generate a biosignature of serum proteins, has proven capable of discriminating small panels of patients who have tuberculosis from healthy controls, with an accuracy of more than 80%.[135] Theoretically, the advantage of neural networks is that as they correctly predict more cases and are able to self-correct, thereby becoming more accurate. Even if the technology itself may not be generally applicable in the foreseeable future, these analyses can identify useful targets for further analyses. For example, the serum protein biosignature relied heavily on the relative level of just four proteins (serum amyloid A protein, transthyretin, neopterin, and CRP) for most of its classifications.

The same methodology lies behind transcriptomic scanning, using microarrays and qualitative PCR to compare gene expression among patients who have tuberculosis, healthy persons who have LTBI, and healthy controls who have had no exposure to *M tuberculosis*, with the goal of identifying combinations of gene expression unique to each group. Although the level of expression of tens of thousands of genes are being scanned in each study participant, discriminant analysis using complex computer algorithms was able to separate patients who had tuberculosis and healthy controls based on the expression of only three genes (*lactoferrin*, *CD64*, and *Rab33A*).[136]

A second microarray study comparing individuals who had active, recurrent, cured, or latent tuberculosis used discriminant analysis to separate these groups based on expression of only nine genes.[137] Although these would not necessarily have been predicted as useful biomarkers, roles for some genes identified are easily explainable: lactoferrin affects the ability of *M tuberculosis* to scavenge cations[138] and CD64 seems to be involved in activating the respiratory burst,[139] whereas *Rab33A* is a member of the Ras oncogene family, apparently involved in vesicle transport and fusion,[140] and possibly the phagosome maturation that is required for killing *M tuberculosis*.[141] However, the study identified another Ras/Rab family member (RIN3) in individuals who had active, recurrent, cured, or latent tuberculosis, suggesting a central role for this gene family that was not predicted, and indicating that members of this family may be useful biomarkers of disease status.

A more focused approach using the *M tuberculosis* virulence factor ESAT-6 to stimulate PBMC in patients who had active pulmonary or latent tuberculosis infection showed significant differences in the expression of 10 genes. However, multivariate regression analyses showed that expression of just 3 genes, IL-8, and IL-12β, plus the Treg marker FOXP3, was sufficient to distinguish the two groups, with nearly 90% specificity.[142] This finding indicates that even though both groups respond to ESAT-6, the fine specificity of that response may allow identification of current disease status.

A different group, looking at gene expression levels in ex vivo *M tuberculosis*–stimulated macrophages from patients who had latent, pulmonary, and meningeal disease, used microarray and confirmatory PCR to identify a single gene, *CCL1*, that differentiated these groups.[110] In addition, a case-control genetic association study involving 273 tuberculosis cases and 188 controls showed that single nucleotide polymorphisms in *CCL1* seemed to be associated with susceptibility to tuberculosis.[110] *CCL1* was not previously identified as a factor involved in host susceptibility to tuberculosis, indicating the power of the techniques for finding potentially important biomarkers.

BIOMARKERS: FUTURE PROGRESS

The need for biomarkers extends beyond improved diagnosis to assessment of disease status and risk for progression to disease, or of relapse are critical bottlenecks in the development of new vaccines and drugs. Although the technologies described present a wide array of potential targets, only two—the venerable TST and the IGRAs—can be considered clinically useful, and operate at the simplest level, merely detecting infection. If the plethora of potential markers described are to be converted into clinically useful tools, continuing research and improved guidance for developing and validating biomarkers are needed. One major hindrance has been difference between clinical definitions and end points used by research groups. Some steps are being made in this direction; the WHO and European Commission recently issued a guidance document including exactly this recommendation.[143] There is a long way to go to fulfill the promise of these studies, but there are also many promising leads to follow.

REFERENCES

1. Global tuberculosis control— epidemiology, strategy, financing. Geneva (Switzerland): World Health Organization; 2009. Available at: http://www.who.int/tb/publications/global_report/en/. Accessed September 18, 2009.

2. Andersen P, Doherty TM, Pai M, et al. The prognosis of latent tuberculosis: can disease be predicted? Trends Mol Med 2007;13(5):175–82.

3. Manabe YC, Dishai WR. Latent *Mycobacterium tuberculosis*—persistence, patience, and winning by waiting. Nat Med 2000;6(12):1327–9.

4. Morrison J, Pai M, Hopewell PC. Tuberculosis and latent tuberculosis infection in close contacts of people with pulmonary tuberculosis in low-income and middle-income countries: a systematic review and meta-analysis. Lancet Infect Dis 2008;8(6): 359–68.

5. Stewart GR, Robertson BD, Young DB. Tuberculosis: a problem with persistence. Nat Rev Microbiol 2003;1(2):97–105.

6. Breen RA, Leonard O, Perrin FM, et al. How good are systemic symptoms and blood inflammatory markers at detecting individuals with tuberculosis? Int J Tuberc Lung Dis 2008;12(1):44–9.

7. Marais B, Schaaf S, Hesseling A, et al. Tuberculosis case definition: time for critical re-assessment? Int J Tuberc Lung Dis 2008;12(10):1217.

8. Dietrich J, Doherty TM. Interaction of *Mycobacterium tuberculosis* with the host: consequences for vaccine development. APMIS 2009;117(5–6): 440–57.

9. Russell DG. *Mycobacterium tuberculosis*: here today, and here tomorrow. Nat Rev Mol Cell Biol 2001;2(8):569–77.

10. Rachman H, Strong M, Schaible U, et al. *Mycobacterium tuberculosis* gene expression profiling within

11. the context of protein networks. Microbes Infect 2006;8(3):747–57.

11. Rachman H, Strong M, Ulrichs T, et al. Unique transcriptome signature of *Mycobacterium tuberculosis* in pulmonary tuberculosis. Infect Immun 2006;74(2):1233–42.

12. Rustad TR, Harrell MI, Liao R, et al. The enduring hypoxic response of *Mycobacterium tuberculosis*. PLoS One 2008;3(1):e1502.

13. Edwards PQ, Edwads LB. Story of the tuberculin test from an epidemiologic viewpoint. Am Rev Respir Dis 1960;81(1 Pt 2):):1–47.

14. Judson FN, Feldman RA. Mycobacterial skin tests in humans 12 years after infection with *Mycobacterium marinum*. Am Rev Respir Dis 1974;109(5): 544–7.

15. Hill PC, Brookes RH, Adetifa IM, et al. Comparison of enzyme-linked immunospot assay and tuberculin skin test in healthy children exposed to *Mycobacterium tuberculosis*. Pediatrics 2006;117(5): 1542–8.

16. Mori T, Sakatani M, Yamagishi F, et al. Specific detection of tuberculosis infection: an interferon-gamma-based assay using new antigens. Am J Respir Crit Care Med 2004;170(1):59–64.

17. Kang YA, Lee HW, Yoon HI, et al. Discrepancy between the tuberculin skin test and the whole-blood interferon gamma assay for the diagnosis of latent tuberculosis infection in an intermediate tuberculosis-burden country. JAMA 2005;293(22): 2756–61.

18. Mack U, Migliori GB, Sester M, et al. LTBI: latent tuberculosis infection or lasting immune responses to *M. tuberculosis*? A TBNET consensus statement. Eur Respir J 2009;33(5):956–73.

19. Jeyakumar D. Tuberculin reactivity and subsequent development of tuberculosis in a cohort of student nurses. Med J Malaysia 1999;54(4):492–5.

20. Leung CC, Yew WW, Chang KC, et al. Risk of active tuberculosis among schoolchildren in Hong Kong. Arch Pediatr Adolesc Med 2006;160(3):247–51.

21. Jasmer RM, Nahid P, Hopewell PC. Clinical practice. Latent tuberculosis infection. N Engl J Med 2002;347(23):1860–6.

22. Berkel GM, Cobelens FG, de Vries G, et al. Tuberculin skin test: estimation of positive and negative predictive values from routine data. Int J Tuberc Lung Dis 2005;9(3):310–6.

23. Menzies D, Doherty TM. Diagnosis of latent tuberculosis infection. In: Raviglione M, editor. Reichman and Hershfield's tuberculosis: a comprehensive, international approach. 3rd edition. vol. 1. 2007. New York: Informa Healthcare; 2007. p. 215–51.

24. Pollock JM, McNair J, Bassett H, et al. Specific delayed-type hypersensitivity responses to ESAT-6 identify tuberculosis-infected cattle. J Clin Microbiol 2003;41(5):1856–60.

25. Arend SM, Franken WP, Aggerbeck H, et al. Double-blind randomized phase I study comparing rdESAT-6 to tuberculin as skin test reagent in the diagnosis of tuberculosis infection. Tuberculosis (Edinb) 2008;88(3):249–61.

26. Lillebaek T, Bergstedt W, Tingskov PN, et al. Risk of sensitization in healthy adults following repeated administration of rdESAT-6 skin test reagent by the Mantoux injection technique. Tuberculosis (Edinb) 2009;89(2):158–62.

27. Weldingh K, Andersen P. ESAT-6/CFP10 skin test predicts disease in M. tuberculosis-infected guinea pigs. PLoS One 2008;3(4):e1978.

28. Elhay MJ, Oettinger T, Andersen P. Delayed-type hypersensitivity responses to ESAT-6 and MPT64 from Mycobacterium tuberculosis in the guinea pig. Infect Immun 1998;66(7):3454–6.

29. Tavares RC, Salgado J, Moreira VB, et al. Interferon gamma response to combinations 38 kDa/CFP-10, 38 kDa/MPT-64, ESAT-6/MPT-64 and ESAT-6/CFP-10, each related to a single recombinant protein of Mycobacterium tuberculosis in individuals from tuberculosis endemic areas. Microbiol Immunol 2007;51(3):289–96.

30. Li H, Ulstrup JC, Jonassen TO, et al. Evidence for absence of the MPB64 gene in some substrains of Mycobacterium bovis BCG. Infect Immun 1993; 61(5):1730–4.

31. Sarrazin H, Wilkinson KA, Andersson J, et al. Association between tuberculin skin test reactivity, the memory CD4 cell subset, and circulating FoxP3-expressing cells in HIV-infected persons. J Infect Dis 2009;199(5):702–10.

32. Stein CM, Zalwango S, Malone LL, et al. Genome scan of M. tuberculosis infection and disease in Ugandans. PLoS One 2008;3(12):e4094.

33. Mortatti RC, Maia LC. Immune response to BCG-Moreau (Rio de Janeiro) strain. Spectrum of delayed hypersensitivity in genetically defined mice. FEMS Microbiol Immunol 1989;1(8–9):491–7.

34. Gallant CJ, Malik S, Jabado N, et al. Reduced in vitro functional activity of human NRAMP1 (SLC11A1) allele that predisposes to increased risk of pediatric tuberculosis disease. Genes Immun 2007;8(8):691–8.

35. Patel SY, Doffinger R, Barcenas-Morales G, et al. Genetically determined susceptibility to mycobacterial infection. J Clin Pathol 2008;61(9): 1006–12.

36. Gomez-Reino JJ, Carmona L, Valverde VR, et al. Treatment of rheumatoid arthritis with tumor necrosis factor inhibitors may predispose to significant increase in tuberculosis risk: a multicenter active-surveillance report. Arthritis Rheum 2003; 48(8):2122–7.

37. Harris J, Hope JC, Keane J. Tumor necrosis factor blockers influence macrophage responses to Mycobacterium tuberculosis. J Infect Dis 2008; 198:1842–50.

38. Ottenhoff TH, Verreck FA, Hoeve MA, et al. Control of human host immunity to mycobacteria. Tuberculosis (Edinb) 2005;85(1–2):53–64.

39. Flynn JL, Chan J, Triebold KJ, et al. An essential role for interferon gamma in resistance to Mycobacterium tuberculosis infection. J Exp Med 1993; 178(6):2249–54.

40. Hussain R, Talat N, Shahid F, et al. Longitudinal tracking of cytokines after acute exposure to tuberculosis: association of distinct cytokine patterns with protection and disease development. Clin Vaccine Immunol 2007;14(12): 1578–86.

41. Carrara S, Vincenti D, Petrosillo N, et al. Use of a T cell-based assay for monitoring efficacy of antituberculosis therapy. Clin Infect Dis 2004;38(5): 754–6.

42. Flynn JL, Goldstein MM, Chan J, et al. Tumor necrosis factor-alpha is required in the protective immune response against Mycobacterium tuberculosis in mice. Immunity 1995;2(6):561–72.

43. Jacobs M, Togbe D, Fremond C, et al. Tumor necrosis factor is critical to control tuberculosis infection. Microbes Infect 2007;9(5):623–8.

44. Stein CM, Zalwango S, Chiunda AB, et al. Linkage and association analysis of candidate genes for TB and TNFalpha cytokine expression: evidence for association with IFNGR1, IL-10, and TNF receptor 1 genes. Hum Genet 2007;121(6): 663–73.

45. Fernandez-Botran R. Soluble cytokine receptors: novel immunotherapeutic agents. Expert Opin Investig Drugs 2000;9(3):497–514.

46. Tsao TC, Hong J, Li LF, et al. Imbalances between tumor necrosis factor-alpha and its soluble receptor forms, and interleukin-1beta and interleukin-1 receptor antagonist in BAL fluid of cavitary pulmonary tuberculosis. Chest 2000;117(1): 103–9.

47. Brahmbhatt S, Black GF, Carroll NM, et al. Immune markers measured before treatment predict outcome of intensive phase tuberculosis therapy. Clin Exp Immunol 2006;146(2):243–52.

48. Clay H, Volkman HE, Ramakrishnan L. Tumor necrosis factor signaling mediates resistance to mycobacteria by inhibiting bacterial growth and macrophage death. Immunity 2008;29(2): 283–94.

49. Doherty TM, Demissie A, Menzies D, et al. Effect of sample handling on analysis of cytokine responses to Mycobacterium tuberculosis in clinical samples using ELISA, ELISPOT and quantitative PCR. J Immunol Methods 2005;298(1–2):129–41.

50. Dinnes J, Deeks J, Kunst H, et al. A systematic review of rapid diagnostic tests for the detection

of tuberculosis infection. Health Technol Assess 2007;11(3):1–196.

51. Watkins RE, Brennan R, Plant AJ. Tuberculin reactivity and the risk of tuberculosis: a review. Int J Tuberc Lung Dis 2000;4(10):895–903.

52. Diel R, Loddenkemper R, Meywald-Walter K, et al. Predictive value of a whole blood IFN-gamma assay for the development of active tuberculosis disease after recent infection with *Mycobacterium tuberculosis*. Am J Respir Crit Care Med 2008; 177(10):1164–70.

53. Doherty TM, Demissie A, Olobo J, et al. Immune responses to the *Mycobacterium tuberculosis*-specific antigen ESAT-6 signal subclinical infection among contacts of tuberculosis patients. J Clin Microbiol 2002;40(2):704–6.

54. Higuchi K, Harada N, Fukazawa K, et al. Relationship between whole-blood interferon-gamma responses and the risk of active tuberculosis. Tuberculosis (Edinb) 2008;88(3):244–8.

55. Ewer K, Millington KA, Deeks JJ, et al. Dynamic antigen-specific T Cell responses after point-source exposure to *Mycobacterium tuberculosis*. Am J Respir Crit Care Med 2006;174:831–9.

56. Wedlock DN, Denis M, Vordermeier HM, et al. Vaccination of cattle with Danish and Pasteur strains of *Mycobacterium bovis* BCG induce different levels of IFNgamma post-vaccination, but induce similar levels of protection against bovine tuberculosis. Vet Immunol Immunopathol 2007;118(1–2):50–8.

57. Winek J, Rowinska-Zakrzewska E, Demkow U, et al. Interferon gamma production in the course of *Mycobacterium tuberculosis* infection. J Physiol Pharmacol 2008;59(Suppl 6):751–9.

58. Yeboah-Manu D, Peduzzi E, Mensah-Quainoo E, et al. Systemic suppression of interferon-gamma responses in Buruli ulcer patients resolves after surgical excision of the lesions caused by the extracellular pathogen *Mycobacterium ulcerans*. J Leukoc Biol 2006;79(6):1150–6.

59. Ruhwald M, Bjerregaard-Andersen M, Rabna P, et al. IP-10, MCP-1, MCP-2, MCP-3, and IL-1RA hold promise as biomarkers for infection with *M. tuberculosis* in a whole blood based T-cell assay. BMC Res Notes 2009;2:19.

60. Wassie L, Demissie A, Aseffa A, et al. Ex vivo cytokine mRNA levels correlate with changing clinical status of Ethiopian TB patients and their contacts over time. PLoS One 2008;3(1):e1522.

61. Ordway DJ, Costa L, Martins M, et al. Increased Interleukin-4 production by CD8 and gammadelta T cells in health-care workers is associated with the subsequent development of active tuberculosis. J Infect Dis 2004;190(4):756–66.

62. Siawaya JF, Bapela NB, Ronacher K, et al. Differential expression of interleukin-4 (IL-4) and IL-4 delta 2 mRNA, but not transforming growth factor beta (TGF-beta), TGF-beta RII, Foxp3, gamma interferon, T-bet, or GATA-3 mRNA, in patients with fast and slow responses to antituberculosis treatment. Clin Vaccine Immunol 2008;15(8):1165–70.

63. Demissie A, Abebe M, Aseffa A, et al. Healthy individuals that control a latent infection with Mycobacterium tuberculosis express high levels of Th1 cytokines and the IL-4 antagonist IL-4delta2. J Immunol 2004;172(11):6938–43.

64. Orsini B, Vivas JR, Ottanelli B, et al. Human gastric epithelium produces IL-4 and IL-4delta2 isoform only upon *Helicobacter pylori* infection. Int J Immunopathol Pharmacol 2007;20(4):809–18.

65. Seah GT, Gao PS, Hopkin JM, et al. Interleukin-4 and its alternatively spliced variant (IL-4delta2) in patients with atopic asthma. Am J Respir Crit Care Med 2001;164(6):1016–8.

66. Rhodes SG, Sawyer J, Whelan AO, et al. Is interleukin-4delta3 splice variant expression in bovine tuberculosis a marker of protective immunity? Infect Immun 2007;75(6):3006–13.

67. Leung WL, Law KL, Leung VS, et al. Comparison of intracellular cytokine flow cytometry and an enzyme immunoassay for evaluation of cellular immune response to active tuberculosis. Clin Vaccine Immunol 2009;16(3):344–51.

68. Winthrop KL, Daley CL. A novel assay for screening patients for latent tuberculosis infection prior to anti-TNF therapy. Nat Clin Pract Rheumatol 2008; 4(9):456–7.

69. Rosas-Taraco AG, Salinas-Carmona MC, Revol A, et al. Expression of CDIIc in blood monocytes as biomarker for favorable response to antituberculosis treatment. Arch Med Res 2009;40(2):128–31.

70. Veenstra H, Baumann R, Carroll NM, et al. Changes in leucocyte and lymphocyte subsets during tuberculosis treatment; prominence of CD3dimCD56+ natural killer T cells in fast treatment responders. Clin Exp Immunol 2006;145(2):252–60.

71. Seiler P, Aichele P, Bandermann S, et al. Early granuloma formation after aerosol *Mycobacterium tuberculosis* infection is regulated by neutrophils via CXCR3-signaling chemokines. Eur J Immunol 2003;33(10):2676–86.

72. Tsai MC, Chakravarty S, Zhu G, et al. Characterization of the tuberculous granuloma in murine and human lungs: cellular composition and relative tissue oxygen tension. Cell Microbiol 2006;8(2):218–32.

73. Seder RA, Darrah PA, Roederer M. T-cell quality in memory and protection: implications for vaccine design. Nat Rev Immunol 2008;8(4):247–58.

74. Forbes EK, Sander C, Ronan EO, et al. Multifunctional, high-level cytokine-producing Th1 cells in the lung, but not spleen, correlate with protection against *Mycobacterium tuberculosis* aerosol challenge in mice. J Immunol 2008;181(7):4955–64.

75. Day CL, Mkhwanazi N, Reddy S, et al. Detection of polyfunctional *Mycobacterium tuberculosis*-specific T cells and association with viral load in HIV-1-infected persons. J Infect Dis 2008;197(7):990–9.

76. Mueller H, Detjen AK, Schuck SD, et al. *Mycobacterium tuberculosis*-specific CD4+, IFNgamma+, and TNFalpha+ multifunctional memory T cells co-express GM-CSF. Cytokine 2008;43(2):143–8.

77. Roberts T, Beyers N, Aguirre A, et al. Immunosuppression during active tuberculosis is characterized by decreased interferon- gamma production and CD25 expression with elevated forkhead box P3, transforming growth factor- beta, and interleukin-4 mRNA levels. J Infect Dis 2007;195(6):870–8.

78. Chen X, Zhou B, Li M, et al. CD4(+)CD25(+)FoxP3(+) regulatory T cells suppress *Mycobacterium tuberculosis* immunity in patients with active disease. Clin Immunol 2007;123(1):50–9.

79. Sharma PK, Saha PK, Singh A, et al. FoxP3+ regulatory T cells suppress effector T cell function at pathologic site in miliary tuberculosis. Am J Respir Crit Care Med 2009;179:1061–70.

80. Belkaid Y, Oldenhove G. Tuning microenvironments: induction of regulatory T cells by dendritic cells. Immunity 2008;29(3):362–71.

81. Guyot-Revol V, Innes JA, Hackforth S, et al. Regulatory T cells are expanded in blood and disease sites in patients with tuberculosis. Am J Respir Crit Care Med 2006;173(7):803–10.

82. Li L, Lao SH, Wu CY. Increased frequency of CD4(+)CD25(high) Treg cells inhibit BCG-specific induction of IFN-gamma by CD4(+) T cells from TB patients. Tuberculosis (Edinb) 2007;87(6):526–34.

83. Ribeiro-Rodrigues R, Resende Co T, Rojas R, et al. A role for CD4+CD25+ T cells in regulation of the immune response during human tuberculosis. Clin Exp Immunol 2006;144(1):25–34.

84. Demissie A, Leyten EM, Abebe M, et al. Recognition of stage-specific mycobacterial antigens differentiates between acute and latent infections with *Mycobacterium tuberculosis*. Clin Vaccine Immunol 2006;13(2):179–86.

85. Hougardy JM, Schepers K, Place S, et al. Heparin-binding-hemagglutinin-induced IFN-gamma release as a diagnostic tool for latent tuberculosis. PLoS One 2007;2(10):e926.

86. Hougardy JM, Place S, Hildebrand M, et al. Regulatory T cells depress immune responses to protective antigens in active tuberculosis. Am J Respir Crit Care Med 2007;176(4):409–16.

87. Djoba Siawaya JF, Bapela NB, Ronacher K, et al. Immune parameters as markers of tuberculosis extent of disease and early prediction of anti-tuberculosis chemotherapy response. J Infect 2008;56(5):340–7.

88. Bajaj G, Rattan A, Ahmad P. Prognostic value of 'C' reactive protein in tuberculosis. Indian Pediatr 1989;26(10):1010–3.

89. Scott GM, Murphy PG, Gemidjioglu ME. Predicting deterioration of treated tuberculosis by corticosteroid reserve and C-reactive protein. J Infect 1990;21(1):61–9.

90. Baynes R, Bezwoda W, Bothwell T, et al. The non-immune inflammatory response: serial changes in plasma iron, iron-binding capacity, lactoferrin, ferritin and C-reactive protein. Scand J Clin Lab Invest 1986;46(7):695–704.

91. Tozkoparan E, Deniz O, Cakir E, et al. The diagnostic values of serum, pleural fluid and urine neopterin measurements in tuberculous pleurisy. Int J Tuberc Lung Dis 2005;9(9):1040–5.

92. Aung H, Wu M, Johnson JL, et al. Bioactivation of latent transforming growth factor beta1 by *Mycobacterium tuberculosis* in human mononuclear phagocytes. Scand J Immunol 2005;61(6):558–65.

93. Djoba Siawaya JF, Ruhwald M, Eugen-Olsen J, et al. Correlates for disease progression and prognosis during concurrent HIV/TB infection. Int J Infect Dis 2007;11(4):289–99.

94. Eugen-Olsen J, Gustafson P, Sidenius N, et al. The serum level of soluble urokinase receptor is elevated in tuberculosis patients and predicts mortality during treatment: a community study from Guinea-Bissau. Int J Tuberc Lung Dis 2002;6(8):686–92.

95. Lawn SD, Harries AD, Anglaret X, et al. Early mortality among adults accessing antiretroviral treatment programmes in sub-Saharan Africa. AIDS 2008;22(15):1897–908.

96. Sidenius N, Sier CF, Ullum H, et al. Serum level of soluble urokinase-type plasminogen activator receptor is a strong and independent predictor of survival in human immunodeficiency virus infection. Blood 2000;96(13):4091–5.

97. Ghosh S, Saxena RK. Early effect of *Mycobacterium tuberculosis* infection on Mac-1 and ICAM-1 expression on mouse peritoneal macrophages. Exp Mol Med 2004;36(5):387–95.

98. Melis M, Pace E, Siena L, et al. Biologically active intercellular adhesion molecule-1 is shed as dimers by a regulated mechanism in the inflamed pleural space. Am J Respir Crit Care Med 2003;167(8):1131–8.

99. Demir T, Yalcinoz C, Keskinel I, et al. sICAM-1 as a serum marker in the diagnosis and follow-up of treatment of pulmonary tuberculosis. Int J Tuberc Lung Dis 2002;6(2):155–9.

100. Mukae H, Ashitani J, Tokojima M, et al. Elevated levels of circulating adhesion molecules in patients with active pulmonary tuberculosis. Respirology 2003;8(3):326–31.

101. Balcewicz-Sablinska MK, Keane J, Kornfeld H, et al. Pathogenic *Mycobacterium tuberculosis* evades apoptosis of host macrophages by release of TNF-R2, resulting in inactivation of TNF-alpha. J Immunol 1998;161(5):2636–41.

102. Steingart KR, Henry M, Laal S, et al. Commercial serological antibody detection tests for the diagnosis of pulmonary tuberculosis: a systematic review. PLoS Med 2007;4(6):e202.

103. Steingart KR, Henry M, Laal S, et al. A systematic review of commercial serological antibody detection tests for the diagnosis of extrapulmonary tuberculosis. Thorax 2007;62(10):911–8.

104. Gennaro ML, Affouf M, Kanaujia GV, et al. Antibody markers of incident tuberculosis among HIV-infected adults in the USA: a historical prospective study. Int J Tuberc Lung Dis 2007; 11(6):624–31.

105. Singh KK, Dong Y, Belisle JT, et al. Antigens of *Mycobacterium tuberculosis* recognized by antibodies during incipient, subclinical tuberculosis. Clin Diagn Lab Immunol 2005;12(2):354–8.

106. Bahk YY, Kim SA, Kim JS, et al. Antigens secreted from *Mycobacterium tuberculosis*: identification by proteomics approach and test for diagnostic marker. Proteomics 2004;4(11):3299–307.

107. Weldingh K, Rosenkrands I, Okkels LM, et al. Assessing the serodiagnostic potential of 35 *Mycobacterium tuberculosis* proteins and identification of four novel serological antigens. J Clin Microbiol 2005;43(1):57–65.

108. Sartain MJ, Slayden RA, Singh KK, et al. Disease state differentiation and identification of tuberculosis biomarkers via native antigen array profiling. Mol Cell Proteomics 2006;5(11):2102–13.

109. Khan IH, Ravindran R, Yee J, et al. Profiling antibodies to *Mycobacterium tuberculosis* by multiplex microbead suspension arrays for serodiagnosis of tuberculosis. Clin Vaccine Immunol 2008;15(3): 433–8.

110. Gaseitsiwe S, Valentini D, Mahdavifar S, et al. Pattern recognition in pulmonary tuberculosis defined by high content peptide microarray chip analysis representing 61 proteins from *M. tuberculosis*. PLoS One 2008;3(12):e3840.

111. Wu-Hsieh BA, Chen CK, Chang JH, et al. Long-lived immune response to early secretory antigenic target 6 in individuals who had recovered from tuberculosis. Clin Infect Dis 2001;33(8):1336–40.

112. Sauzullo I, Mengoni F, Lichtner M, et al. In vivo and in vitro effects of antituberculosis treatment on mycobacterial Interferon-gamma T cell response. PLoS One 2009;4(4):e5187.

113. Maher D, Harries A, Getahun H. Tuberculosis and HIV interaction in sub-Saharan Africa: impact on patients and programmes; implications for policies. Trop Med Int Health 2005;10(8):734–42.

114. Wallis RS, Phillips M, Johnson JL, et al. Inhibition of isoniazid-induced expression of *Mycobacterium tuberculosis* antigen 85 in sputum: potential surrogate marker in tuberculosis chemotherapy trials. Antimicrob Agents Chemother 2001;45(4):1302–4.

115. Desjardin LE, Perkins MD, Wolski K, et al. Measurement of sputum *Mycobacterium tuberculosis* messenger RNA as a surrogate for response to chemotherapy. Am J Respir Crit Care Med 1999; 160(1):203–10.

116. Garbe TR, Hibler NS, Deretic V. Isoniazid induces expression of the antigen 85 complex in *Mycobacterium tuberculosis*. Antimicrob Agents Chemother 1996;40(7):1754–6.

117. Chakraborty N, Bhattacharyya S, De C, et al. A rapid immunochromatographic assay for the detection of *Mycobacterium tuberculosis* antigens in pulmonary samples from HIV seropositive patients and its comparison with conventional methods. J Microbiol Methods 2009;76(1):12–7.

118. El-Masry S, El-Kady I, Zaghloul MH, et al. Rapid and simple detection of a mycobacterium circulating antigen in serum of pulmonary tuberculosis patients by using a monoclonal antibody and Fast-Dot-ELISA. Clin Biochem 2008;41(3):145–51.

119. Baba K, Dyrhol-Riise AM, Sviland L, et al. Rapid and specific diagnosis of tuberculous pleuritis with immunohistochemistry by detecting *Mycobacterium tuberculosis* complex specific antigen MPT64 in patients from a HIV endemic area. Appl Immunohistochem Mol Morphol 2008;16(6): 554–61.

120. Goel MM, Budhwar P. Species-specific immunocytochemical localization of *Mycobacterium tuberculosis* complex in fine needle aspirates of tuberculous lymphadenitis using antibody to 38 kDa immunodominant protein antigen. Acta Cytol 2008;52(4):424–33.

121. Attallah AM, Osman S, Saad A, et al. Application of a circulating antigen detection immunoassay for laboratory diagnosis of extra-pulmonary and pulmonary tuberculosis. Clin Chim Acta 2005; 356(1–2):58–66.

122. Bera S, Shende N, Kumar S, et al. Detection of antigen and antibody in childhood tuberculous meningitis. Indian J Pediatr 2006;73(8):675–9.

123. Choudhry V, Saxena RK. Detection of *Mycobacterium tuberculosis* antigens in urinary proteins of tuberculosis patients. Eur J Clin Microbiol Infect Dis 2002;21(1):1–5.

124. Gopinath K, Singh S. Urine as an adjunct specimen for the diagnosis of active pulmonary tuberculosis. Int J Infect Dis 2009;13(3):374–9.

125. Cannas A, Goletti D, Girardi E, et al. *Mycobacterium tuberculosis* DNA detection in soluble fraction of urine from pulmonary tuberculosis patients. Int J Tuberc Lung Dis 2008;12(2):146–51.

126. Napolitano DR, Pollock N, Kashino SS, et al. Iden-tification of *Mycobacterium tuberculosis* ornithine carboamyltransferase in urine as a possible molec-ular marker of active pulmonary tuberculosis. Clin Vaccine Immunol 2008;15(4):638–43.

127. Torrea G, Van de Perre P, Ouedraogo M, et al. PCR-based detection of the *Mycobacterium tuber-culosis* complex in urine of HIV-infected and uninfected pulmonary and extrapulmonary tuber-culosis patients in Burkina Faso. J Med Microbiol 2005;54(Pt 1):39–44.

128. Boehme C, Molokova E, Minja F, et al. Detection of mycobacterial lipoarabinomannan with an antigen-capture ELISA in unprocessed urine of Tanzanian patients with suspected tuberculosis. Trans R Soc Trop Med Hyg 2005;99(12):893–900.

129. Hamasur B, Bruchfeld J, Haile M, et al. Rapid diag-nosis of tuberculosis by detection of mycobacterial lipoarabinomannan in urine. J Microbiol Methods 2001;45(1):41–52.

130. Tessema TA, Bjune G, Hamasur B, et al. Circulating antibodies to lipoarabinomannan in relation to sputum microscopy, clinical features and urinary anti-lipoarabinomannan detection in pulmonary tuberculosis. Scand J Infect Dis 2002;34(2): 97–103.

131. Pavlou AK, Magan N, Jones JM, et al. Detection of *Mycobacterium tuberculosis* (TB) in vitro and in situ using an electronic nose in combination with a neural network system. Biosens Bioelectron 2004;20(3):538–44.

132. Fend R, Kolk AH, Bessant C, et al. Prospects for clinical application of electronic-nose technology to early detection of *Mycobacterium tuberculosis* in culture and sputum. J Clin Microbiol 2006; 44(6):2039–45.

133. Syhre M, Chambers ST. The scent of *Mycobacte-rium tuberculosis*. Tuberculosis (Edinb) 2008; 88(4):317–23.

134. Phillips M, Cataneo RN, Condos R, et al. Volatile biomarkers of pulmonary tuberculosis in the breath. Tuberculosis (Edinb) 2007;87(1):44–52.

135. Agranoff D, Fernandez-Reyes D, Papadopoulos MC, et al. Identification of diagnostic markers for tubercu-losis by proteomic fingerprinting of serum. Lancet 2006;368(9540):1012–21.

136. Kaufmann SH, Parida SK. Tuberculosis in Africa: learning from pathogenesis for biomarker identifi-cation. Cell Host Microbe 2008;4(3):219–28.

137. Mistry R, Cliff JM, Clayton CL, et al. Gene-expres-sion patterns in whole blood identify subjects at risk for recurrent tuberculosis. J Infect Dis 2007; 195(3):357–65.

138. Schaible UE, Collins HL, Priem F, et al. Correction of the iron overload defect in beta-2-microglobulin knockout mice by lactoferrin abolishes their increased susceptibility to tuberculosis. J Exp Med 2002;196(11):1507–13.

139. Barth E, Fischer G, Schneider EM, et al. Peaks of endogenous G-CSF serum concentrations are fol-lowed by an increase in respiratory burst activity of granulocytes in patients with septic shock. Cyto-kine 2002;17(5):275–84.

140. Schimmoller F, Simon I, Pfeffer SR. Rab GTPases, directors of vesicle docking. J Biol Chem 1998; 273(35):22161–4.

141. Brumell JH, Scidmore MA. Manipulation of rab GTPase function by intracellular bacterial path-ogens. Microbiol Mol Biol Rev 2007;71(4): 636–52.

142. Wu B, Huang C, Kato-Maeda M, et al. Messenger RNA expression of IL-8, FOXP3, and IL-12beta differentiates latent tuberculosis infection from disease. J Immunol 2007;178(6): 3688–94.

143. Doherty M, Wallis RS, Zumla A. Biomarkers for tuberculosis disease status and diagnosis. Curr Opin Pulm Med 2009;15(3):181–7.

Tuberculosis-associated Immune Reconstitution Inflammatory Syndrome and Unmasking of Tuberculosis by Antiretroviral Therapy

Graeme Meintjes, MBChB, MRCP(UK), FCP(SA), Dip HIV Man(SA)[a,b,c,]*,
Helena Rabie, MBChB, FCPaed(SA), MMed Paed[d],
Robert J. Wilkinson, MA, BM, BCh, PhD, DTM&H[a,b,c,e,f],
Mark F. Cotton, MMed(Paed), FCPaed(SA), DCH(SA), DTM&H, PhD[d]

KEYWORDS

- Immune reconstitution inflammatory syndrome
- HIV • Tuberculosis • Antiretroviral therapy

HIV-1 substantially increases the risk of developing active tuberculosis (TB) and the HIV-1 epidemic is undermining TB control efforts in many regions of the world.[1,2] Sub-Saharan Africa is now severely affected by the dual epidemic of HIV-1 and TB, with TB incidence rates increasing by up to fivefold in many countries in the region over the last 2 decades.[1] The diagnosis of TB is a common reason for HIV-1 testing and entry into HIV-1 care in these settings. As a consequence, a substantial proportion of patients starting combined antiretroviral therapy (ART) globally, and particularly in sub-Saharan Africa, are under treatment of active TB (up to 25%), or have undiagnosed active TB.[3] ART dramatically improves survival in people infected with HIV-1,[4] and reduces TB risk by 70% to 90%,[5–8] but high TB incidence rates have been noted in the first 3 months of ART in developing countries.[3,9,10]

After initiating ART, the CD4+ T lymphocyte count rises rapidly in the first month, representing redistribution of memory cells from sites of immune activation, followed by a more gradual recovery of naive cells.[11] Other components of the immune system also recover quantitatively and functionally.

It was recognized before the HIV-1 era that the immune response to TB contributes to pathology and protection. During the early period of rapid immune recovery on ART, immunopathology in

GM and RJW are supported by the Wellcome Trust (072070, 084323, 088316, 081667).

[a] Institute of Infectious Diseases and Molecular Medicine, Faculty of Health Sciences, University of Cape Town, Anzio Road, Observatory 7925, South Africa

[b] Division of Infectious Diseases and HIV Medicine, Department of Medicine, University of Cape Town, Anzio Road, Observatory 7925, South Africa

[c] Infectious Diseases Unit, GF Jooste Hospital, Duinefontein Road, Manenberg, 7764, South Africa

[d] Children's Infectious Diseases Clinical Research Unit, Department of Paediatrics and Child Health, Faculty of Health Science, University of Stellenbosch, Tygerberg Academic Hospital, PO Box 19063, Tygerberg 7505, South Africa

[e] Division of Medicine, Wright Fleming Institute, Imperial College London, London, W2 1PG, UK

[f] National Institute for Medical Research, Mill Hill, London, NW7 1AA, UK

* Corresponding author. Institute of Infectious Diseases and Molecular Medicine, Faculty of Health Sciences, University of Cape Town, Anzio Road, Observatory 7925, South Africa.

E-mail address: graemein@mweb.co.za (G. Meintjes).

Clin Chest Med 30 (2009) 797–810
doi:10.1016/j.ccm.2009.08.013

the form of the immune reconstitution inflammatory syndrome (IRIS) has emerged as an important clinical entity altering the clinical presentation and course of TB infection. IRIS is believed to result from dysregulated recovering immune responses driving exaggerated inflammation directed at the antigens of opportunistic pathogens.[12,13] IRIS may occur in the context of treated or untreated infections, and has been most frequently described in association with mycobacterial, fungal, and herpes virus infections.

In the case of TB, 2 forms of IRIS are recognized.[14] Paradoxical TB-IRIS occurs in patients diagnosed with TB and established on TB treatment before ART, who then manifest with recurrent or new TB symptoms and clinical manifestations after ART initiation. Unmasking TB-IRIS occurs in patients who are not on TB treatment when they start ART, and who then have an unusually inflammatory presentation of TB in the first 3 months of ART (**Fig. 1**).

PARADOXICAL REACTIONS IN PATIENTS NOT ON ART

Paradoxical reactions during TB treatment (new or recurrent TB symptoms, or signs occurring after initial response to treatment) occur in patients not infected with HIV-1 and patients infected with HIV-1 and not on ART. Up to 25% of patients with TB lymphadenitis will experience a paradoxical reaction, usually manifesting as enlargement of the nodes.[15,16] Other manifestations include recurrent fevers, worsening pulmonary infiltrates, enlarging pleural effusions, the development of tuberculous meningitis (TBM), new or enlarging tuberculomas, or tuberculous lesions developing at other anatomic sites.[17–19] In a South African case series, reported before widespread availability of ART, 23% of TBM in patients infected with HIV-1

was diagnosed in patients already on TB treatment, so-called "breakthrough" TBM.[20]

These paradoxical reactions are believed to reflect an immunologically mediated deterioration rather than TB treatment failure. The pathogenesis has variably been attributed to a combination of the following factors: persistence of lipid-rich insoluble cell wall antigen in infected tissue,[16] exposure and release of new antigen targets during mycobacterial killing,[21] hypersensitivity to such antigens,[21] and exaggerated immune restoration (following TB-induced immunosuppression) occurring on TB treatment.[18] The development of paradoxical reactions in patients not infected with HIV-1 is associated with greater increases in total lymphocyte count on TB treatment.[18] There is also the phenomenon of paradoxical reactions occurring after withdrawal of iatrogenic immunosuppression, particularly tumor necrosis factor-α receptor inhibitors.[22,23]

PARADOXICAL TB-IRIS

As a form of deterioration during TB therapy, paradoxical TB-IRIS often seems more severe, and frequently involves multiple organ systems. Paradoxical reactions are also far more frequent in the period after ART initiation than in patients not infected with HIV-1 and patients infected with HIV-1 and not on ART (36% vs 2% vs 7%, respectively, in one study).[24]

Paradoxical TB-IRIS occurs in 8% to 43% of patients starting ART while on TB treatment (**Table 1**).[24–35] The median interval from ART initiation to onset of paradoxical TB-IRIS is typically 2 to 4 weeks,[24–26,30,31,35] but cases may occur within a few days and, rarely, onset may be months after ART is started.[36] The median duration of symptoms is reported to be 2 to 3 months.[29,32,36] A minority of cases have manifestations that last for more than a year[14,32,36] and

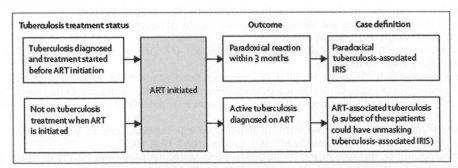

Fig. 1. Different forms of TB-IRIS and ART-associated TB. (*From* Meintjes G, Lawn SD, Scano F, et al. Tuberculosis-associated immune reconstitution inflammatory syndrome: case definitions for use in resource-limited settings. Lancet Infect Dis 2008;8(8):516–23; with permission.)

Table 1
Cohort studies reporting the incidence, treatment, and outcome of paradoxical TB-IRIS in adult patients[a]

First Author (Country and Year of Publication)	Incidence of Paradoxical TB-IRIS (%)	Treatment of IRIS Episode	Duration (Symptom Onset to Resolution of IRIS Episode)	Number of Deaths (% of IRIS Cases)
Narita (United States, 1998)[24]	12/33 (36)	Corticosteroids (2) ART interruption (1)	NR	NR
Breen (United Kingdom, 2004)[25]	8/28 (29)	Prednisone (8 of 14)[b]	NR	NR
Breton (France, 2004)[26]	16/37 (43)	Corticosteroids (6) NSAIDs (2) ART interruption (7) Surgery (1)	NR	NR
Kumarasamy (India, 2004)[27]	11/144 (8)	Corticosteroids (6) NSAIDs (5) Aspiration (1)	NR	0 (0)
Michailidis (United Kingdom, 2005)[29]	9/28 (32)	Corticosteroids (11) Interleukin-2 and granulocyte-macrophage colony-stimulating factor (1) Aspiration (10)[c]	Median 2.5 months (range 0.5–15 months)[c]	NR
Manosuthi (Thailand, 2006)[30]	21/167 (13)	Corticosteroids (11)	NR	2 (10)
Lawn (South Africa, 2007)[31]	19/160 (12)	Corticosteroids (2) Laporotomy (1)	NR	2 (11)
Burman (United States, 2007)[32]	19/109 (17)	Corticosteroids (4) Aspirations (11) Surgical drainage (6)[d]	Median 60 days (range 11–442 days)[d]	1 (5)
Tansuphasawadikul (Thailand, 2007)[34]	15/101 (15)	Corticosteroids (6)	NR	0 (0)
Serra (Brazil, 2007)[35]	10/84 (12)[e]	Prednisone (8) NSAIDs (2)	Mean 91 days ±30 days	0 (0)
Baalwa (Uganda, 2008)[33]	13/45 (29)	NR	NR	NR

Abbreviations: NR, not reported; NSAIDs, nonsteroidal anti-inflammatory drugs.

[a] This table is restricted to cohort studies that assessed the incidence and outcomes of paradoxical TB-IRIS in adult patients starting ART while on TB treatment, and in which 8 or more cases of TB-IRIS were documented. Cohorts in which all-cause IRIS was assessed are not included.

[b] This study reported 14 paradoxical reactions in patients infected with HIV-1, 8 of them in patients who started ART after TB treatment (paradoxical TB-IRIS). Among the 14, 8 were treated with corticosteroids.

[c] This study reported 14 cases of paradoxical reaction, 9 of which were paradoxical TB-IRIS. Data regarding treatment and duration relate to all 14 patients.

[d] Burman et al reported 25 cases of paradoxical reaction in patients infected with HIV-1, 19 of which were in patients starting ART after TB treatment. Data regarding treatment and duration are for all 25 cases.

[e] Of these 10 patients who had paradoxical reactions, 9 were on ART when the paradoxical reaction occurred, and 1 was not.

recurrent episodes are described up to 4 years after ART initiation.[37]

The most frequent clinical features are recurrent symptoms, fever, enlarging inflammatory lymph nodes, and new or enlarging serous effusions. In addition, worsening of radiographic pulmonary infiltrate is seen in up to 45% of TB patients starting ART, and patterns observed include consolidation, cavitation, miliary infiltrates, and cystic changes.[38,39] Subcutaneous and deep tissue abscesses may form.[14,32]

Abdominal manifestations of TB-IRIS are frequent, but not widely reported. Hepatic and splenic involvement may occur together with intestinal lesions, peritonitis, ascites, enlargement of intraabdominal lymphadenopathy (**Fig. 2**), and formation of abscesses including psoas abscesses.[40,41] Abdominal symptoms include abdominal pain, nausea, vomiting, and diarrhea.[30,40] Hepatic involvement, which occurs in 21% to 56% of TB-IRIS cases, can be difficult to differentiate from drug-induced hepatitis.[40,42] Hepatic TB-IRIS manifests with tender liver enlargement, cholestatic liver function derangement, with or without jaundice, and frequently there is evidence of TB-IRIS at other sites. Granulomatous hepatitis is found on liver biopsy.[42] Such patients may have had subclinical abdominal involvement at the time of TB diagnosis and only manifest with abdominal features at the time of IRIS.

Neurologic deterioration has been reported as 12% of paradoxical TB-IRIS cases.[43] Manifestations include new or recurrent meningitis, enlarging tuberculomas, and radiculomyelopathy. In the case series of neurologic TB-IRIS reported by Pepper and colleagues,[43] only 70% of patients were known to be alive at 6 months; of the survivors, 6 of 16 had long-term neurologic disability. Other life-threatening manifestations of paradoxical TB-IRIS include pericardial tamponade,[44]

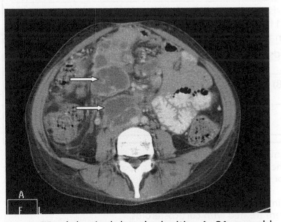

Fig. 2. TB abdominal lymphadenitis. A 21-year-old woman infected with HIV-1, with a CD4 count of 77 cells/μL, was diagnosed with pulmonary TB (*Mycobacterium tuberculosis* isolated from sputum, susceptible to rifampicin and isoniazid). She commenced ART (stavudine, lamivudine, and efavirenz) 5 weeks after starting 5-drug antituberculosis therapy as an inpatient. After 2 weeks on ART, she developed progressively worsening abdominal pain and severe vomiting. The pain required opiate analgesia. A contrasted computed tomography scan of her abdomen revealed mesenteric and retroperitoneal rim enhancing, coalescent lymph nodes with necrotic centers (*arrows*) that were thought to be the cause of her symptoms and the consequence of paradoxical TB-IRIS. A percutaneous aspirate of one of these nodes grew drug-susceptible *M tuberculosis*.

acute renal failure,[45] splenic rupture,[26,46] intestinal perforation,[47] airway compromise due to compression by enlarging nodes,[26] and respiratory failure. Overall, however, reports of death from paradoxical TB-IRIS are rare (see **Table 1**), although this may represent publication bias. Although many cases are self-limiting, paradoxical TB-IRIS results in considerable morbidity, and places considerable burden on the health services. Patients frequently require hospitalization, involving diagnostic and therapeutic procedures.

The most consistently identified risk factors for paradoxical TB-IRIS are: disseminated TB, low CD4 count before ART, and shorter interval from TB treatment to ART.[25,26,28–32] Should ART therefore be delayed to reduce the risk of TB-IRIS? The risk that delaying ART confers in terms of increased HIV-1 disease progression, and the associated additional opportunistic infections and mortality, need to be considered. A further complication is that patients at highest risk for TB-IRIS are those with low CD4 counts who are most at risk of HIV-1 complications if ART is delayed. In addition, delaying ART until after 2 months of TB treatment does not necessarily prevent paradoxical TB-IRIS. In a Ugandan study, 22% of patients starting ART within 2 months developed TB-IRIS, whereas 31% of those starting after 2 months developed TB-IRIS.[33] Several randomized clinical trials are underway that address the optimal time to initiate ART in TB patients.[48] A modeling study favored early introduction of ART in TB patients with advanced HIV-1 infection, provided mortality due to TB-IRIS is less than 5% in the cohort of patients under consideration.[49] Currently, expert opinion and clinical guidelines suggest introducing ART between 2 weeks and 2 months after starting TB treatment in patients with low CD4 counts.[50]

Paradoxical TB-IRIS is diagnosed on the basis of a characteristic clinical presentation, temporal relationship to the initiation of ART, and exclusion of alternative explanations for clinical deterioration. It is important to factor and investigate for other opportunistic infections and malignancies, TB treatment failure (due to nonadherence, TB drug resistance, or malabsorption of TB drugs), or drug reaction. In addition, TB-IRIS may develop in patients with undiagnosed rifampicin resistance, clinically indistinguishable from TB-IRIS which occurs in patients with drug-susceptible disease.[40] If possible, drug susceptibility testing, preferably a rapid diagnostic assay, should be performed in all patients presenting with paradoxical TB-IRIS. Other investigations in a particular case will depend on the nature of the clinical presentation. Consensus case definitions for use in resource-limited settings have recently been developed.[14]

Mild cases require reassurance and symptomatic treatment. In cases with more significant symptoms, nonsteroidal anti-inflammatory drugs (NSAIDs) and corticosteroids have been used. Corticosteroid therapy will exacerbate other untreated infection or drug-resistant TB, so should only be considered for TB-IRIS when alternative diagnoses have been excluded. Breen[25] reported 8 patients infected with HIV-1 with paradoxical reactions or paradoxical TB-IRIS who all responded to prednisone at a range of dosages (10–80 mg/d). A randomized placebo-controlled trial of prednisone for the treatment of paradoxical TB-IRIS demonstrated a significant reduction in a combined end point of days hospitalized plus outpatient therapeutic procedures in prednisone-treated cases. Significant benefit was also demonstrated for symptom improvement. Patients received prednisone or placebo at a dosage of 1.5 mg/kg/d for 2 weeks followed by 0.75 mg/kg/d for 2 weeks. Cases with life-threatening manifestations were excluded from this trial.[51] Corticosteroid use is associated with risks such as reactivations of herpes virus infections, Kaposi sarcoma, and metabolic side effects.[52,53] Some patients require corticosteroids for several months,[54] resulting in a greater likelihood of side effects. There is a case report of successful treatment with the tumor necrosis factor-α receptor antagonist, infliximab, of a TB paradoxical reaction involving the central nervous system,[55] and the role of these agents in life-threatening TB-IRIS requires further investigation. Needle aspiration to provide symptom relief, and for esthetic reasons, for suppurative lymphadenitis or cold abscesses may be required.[32] ART interruption should be considered in life-threatening cases such as those with depressed levels of consciousness due to neurologic involvement.

PATHOGENESIS OF PARADOXICAL TB-IRIS

The frequent occurrence of TB-IRIS in rapidly expanding ART programs in TB endemic environments has again brought into focus the importance of pathologic immunity in TB and how poorly it is understood in humans. Whether TB-IRIS arises as a purely quantitative imbalance ("too much of a good thing"), or whether there is specific activation of tissue damaging mechanisms ("the wrong sort of immunity"), or both, is at present unknown. Clues come from the risk factors for paradoxical IRIS: disseminated TB, low CD4 count before ART, and shorter interval from TB treatment to ART.[25,26,28–32] Low CD4 is

associated with disseminated TB; no analysis has been sufficiently powered to identify low CD4 independently as a factor in multivariate analysis. It seems that TB-IRIS is therefore driven by increased recognition of TB antigens. It seems improbable that a disease that requires 2 infections, and 2 treatments for those infections, can be modeled in animals.

Most human studies have hitherto been anecdotal or underpowered, which is particularly important considering the highly heterogenous nature of the condition. An early feature associated with TB-IRIS was conversion of a negative tuberculin skin test (TST) to strongly positive after ART.[24] Hengel and colleagues[56] noted remarkable expansion of terminally differentiated tuberculin protein purified derivative (PPD)-specific CD4 T cells by flow cytometric analysis in TST positive patients during ART in the absence of TB-IRIS. Subsequent work described such PPD-specific Th1 expansions as the cause of TB-IRIS.[57] The authors[58] have also found that TB-IRIS is associated with large peripheral expansions of terminally differentiated activated Th1 expansions and contractions, but, like Hengel and colleagues, found that similar expansions also occur frequently in patients who develop no symptoms, bringing into question whether these striking expansions are truly causal. Another area of interest has been the hypothesis that TB-IRIS is associated with defective restoration of regulatory T cell function. However patients with TB-IRIS actually have increased numbers of $CD4^+FoxP3^+$ compared with similar patients who did not develop the syndrome.[58] These observations have subsequently been replicated by others.[59,60] Many questions regarding the pathogenesis of TB-IRIS remain to be answered.

UNMASKING TB-IRIS AND UNMASKING OF TB BY ART

High TB incidence rates (5.6–23 TB cases per 100 person years) in the first 3 months of ART have been reported from developing country ART programs.[3,9,10] It is likely that several factors account for this. Patients may seek medical attention and enter HIV-1 care because of the symptoms of TB. Many such patients have TB diagnosed before ART, but, because of the insensitivity of sputum smear[61] and chest radiography[62] in patients with advanced immunosuppression, the diagnosis may be missed before ART initiation. Alternatively, when they start ART, patients may have subclinical TB that becomes clinically apparent on ART, or patients may reactivate latent TB, or be infected or reinfected with TB around the time of ART initiation. Increased clinical surveillance in patients attending for clinical care likely also plays a role.

There is a spectrum of clinical presentations among such TB cases occurring during early ART that is postulated to be influenced by the complex interplay between the infectious load of mycobacterial organisms and immune recovery (which tends to result in TB becoming more clinically overt).[63] The dynamics of this interplay may result in TB remaining subclinical, a typical clinical presentation, or an exaggerated inflammatory presentation. The effect of ART-mediated immune restoration, particularly in the presence of a high mycobacterial load, may be threefold: the timing of onset of TB symptoms may be brought forward, there may be more rapid symptom onset, and it may result in heightened inflammatory clinical manifestations.[63] Lawn and colleagues[63] proposed that only the latter category should be regarded as IRIS, and be termed unmasking TB-IRIS.

Some investigators have regarded any presentation of TB diagnosed while patients are on ART as TB-IRIS provided there was a CD4 increase and viral load reduction.[64] However, there is increasing consensus that IRIS plays a role in presentation in only a subset of patients presenting with TB on ART.[14,63] A nomenclature has been proposed[63]: all TB diagnosed while on ART should be termed "ART-associated TB." TB that presents soon after ART initiation due to restoration of TB antigen-specific immune responses should be termed "unmasking TB." As stated previously, a subset of these cases presenting with heightened intensity of clinical manifestations, particularly when there is evidence of a marked inflammatory component, during the first 3 months of ART should be termed "unmasking TB-IRIS."

Unmasking TB-IRIS is less well characterized than paradoxical TB-IRIS, with fewer cases reported. Cases described include patients presenting with rapid onset of severe respiratory presentations,[14,65–67] one of whom required mechanical ventilation for adult respiratory distress syndrome associated with miliary TB.[65] A fatal case of unmasking TB-IRIS presenting after 6 weeks on ART was shown at postmortem to have extensive infiltrate of the upper lobe of the right lung, with histologic appearance compatible with bronchiolitis obliterans organizing pneumonia.[66] Complicated neurologic involvement in unmasking TB-IRIS cases has been described,[68,69] as has pyomyositis.[70]

Breen and colleagues[71] reported 13 patients diagnosed with active TB in the first 3 months of ART. These patients developed paradoxical reactions more frequently (62%) than patients who were diagnosed with TB later on ART, none of whom had paradoxical reactions. They conclude that an "inflammatory phenotype" associated with early ART may have resulted in these paradoxical reactions, perhaps another manifestation of IRIS.[71] Lawn and colleagues[72] noted in a South African cohort that, during the first 4 months of ART, the adjusted TB incidence rate for those with a CD4 cell count of less than 200 cells/μL was 1.7-fold higher than the incidence rate for patients with an updated CD4 cell count of less than 200 cells/μL during long-term ART. This excess adjusted risk was attributed to "unmasking" of active TB by recovering immunity.[72] The proportion of these cases whose presentation was suggestive of unmasking TB-IRIS was not quantified. In Haiti, a threefold increase in mortality in those diagnosed with TB in the first 3 months on ART (27% mortality) compared with other patients with AIDS and TB (8% mortality) was noted.[73] This higher mortality may in part be attributable to unmasking TB-IRIS.

Clinicians should screen for TB symptoms before ART, investigate those with symptoms, be aware that a subset of patients with advanced HIV-1 infection may have subclinical TB, and be vigilant for the development of unmasking TB and TB-IRIS during early ART. It has been reported that around 50% to 70% of patients diagnosed with TB in the first 3 months of ART had TB symptoms at the time of ART initiation.[71,73] A simple screening tool for active TB in patients entering ART programs, or on ART in resource-poor settings, has been proposed.[74] The diagnosis of TB may be difficult to prove in patients with advanced HIV-1 infection given the insensitivity of sputum smears, and empirical treatment based on strong clinical suspicion and compatible radiography should be considered, particularly in patients whose condition is rapidly deteriorating.[75]

Further research to characterize the clinical manifestations and immunologic mechanisms of unmasking TB-IRIS will help in refining the proposed clinical case definition for this condition in the future.[14]

TB-IRIS AND UNMASKING OF TB IN CHILDREN

Diagnostic criteria for IRIS in children, similar to those used in adults, have been proposed.[76] Although there are fewer data on incidence and clinical manifestations of IRIS in children than in adults, IRIS has most frequently been described in association with bacille Calmette-Guérin (BCG) immunization and TB.[76]

TB in Children Infected with HIV-1

TB incidence rates of up to 53 cases/100 patient years have been reported among African children attending an HIV clinic before starting ART.[77] Young age and degree of immunosuppression are risk factors for TB in children infected with HIV-1. High rates of exposure to potentially infectious source cases of TB are well documented in infants of mothers infected with HIV-1.[78] Contact with a source case has been documented in 30% to 54% of children infected with HIV-1 with TB.[77,79] Recurrent episodes of TB in children infected with HIV-1 are well documented and are caused by relapse and reinfection. Thirty percent of children with HIV-1 and culture-confirmed TB had received prior TB therapy in a study antedating widespread availability of ART.[79]

Up to 30% of African children initiating ART are on TB treatment.[77,80] Cohort data from resource-limited settings indicate that a large proportion of children initiate ART at low CD4 counts and with clinically advanced HIV-1 disease.[81] These children are therefore at risk for paradoxical TB-IRIS, unmasking TB-IRIS, and TB disease from new exposure to M tuberculosis.

The diagnosis of TB in children infected with HIV-1 is difficult. Signs and symptoms overlap with those of HIV-1 itself and other HIV-1-related morbidities, especially when there is associated chronic lung disease. Clinical scoring tools for TB have poor specificity in children infected with HIV-1.[82] Sputa are difficult to collect in young children.[83] Culture yields from gastric washings and induced sputa are low in children, although yields of up to 40% are reported in research settings.[84] In sub-Saharan Africa, less than 3% of patients have access to TB culture.[85] Chest radiographs are difficult to interpret because of the high prevalence of radiographic changes related to chronic HIV-1-associated lung disease, and TSTs have a low sensitivity even when the extent of induration is adjusted from 10 to 5 mm.[86] The diagnostic usefulness of interferon-γ release assays (IGRAs) in children infected with HIV-1 is still being studied. Negative results do not exclude TB.[87] Difficulties in diagnosing TB in children add to the clinical complexities when pediatric patients present with suspected paradoxical TB-IRIS and suspected TB after starting ART. As the diagnosis of TB in children is seldom confirmed by culture, and drug susceptibility test results are often unavailable, differentiating paradoxical TB-IRIS from an incorrect TB diagnosis or drug-resistant TB is often difficult.

Paradoxical TB-IRIS in Children

Few data exist on the risk of paradoxical TB-IRIS in children, and only a few studies have reported clinical details. No IRIS cases occurred in a cohort of 18 children coinfected with TB and HIV-1 in the United Kingdom, 7 of whom initiated ART.[88] A Ugandan study reported 2 cases of paradoxical TB-IRIS.[89] Zampoli and colleagues[90] reported 4 cases of paradoxical TB-IRIS in children between 6 and 105 days after starting ART. TST conversion was documented in 1 child, and was positive at the time of IRIS in another. Two children presented with deterioration of pulmonary TB, 1 developed local adenitis, and another abdominal adenitis. One child died of suspected TB-IRIS pneumonitis.[90] Walters and colleagues[77] did not report the number of paradoxical TB-IRIS cases in their cohort, but did report that, in 4 children who died, this may have been partly attributable to TB-IRIS. All 4 patients had good immune recovery on ART. Three died 5 months or more after starting ART: 1 had an intestinal perforation, 1 had acute upper airway obstruction and the other had multidrug-resistant TB (MDR-TB) and TBM that was complicated by hydrocephalus. The fourth patient also had MDR-TB and developed multiple TB abscesses 3 weeks after starting ART and died soon afterwards.[77] A case of paradoxical TB-IRIS in a child is shown in **Fig. 3**.

The workup of suspected cases of paradoxical TB-IRIS involves reviewing adherence to TB treatment and ART, a careful history of exposure to drug-resistant TB, sending appropriate specimens for TB culture and drug susceptibility testing, when possible, and excluding alternative opportunistic infections. Clinical judgment should guide clinicians as to the investigations required to exclude alternative diagnoses such as acute bacterial infections, drug reactions, and other opportunistic infections or malignancies. **Fig. 4**A presents a diagnostic algorithm that could be used to evaluate children presenting with suspected paradoxical TB-IRIS. The diagnosis of IRIS may often only be made retrospectively. The proposed case definitions for paradoxical TB-IRIS, although appropriate for well-resourced settings, are problematic in lower-resourced settings.[76] This is due to the diagnostic uncertainty of TB in children infected with HIV-1, the difficulties in excluding alternative diagnoses, and the lack of access to CD4 counts or viral load measurements to confirm a response to ART.

Children are at high risk of death and hospitalization in the immediate period after ART initiation. Mortality rates of up to 17.4/100 patient years in the first 3 months of ART are reported.[91] Up to 30% require hospitalization in the first 6 months, and two-thirds of these admissions are related to bacterial infections including pneumonia.[92] It is therefore prudent to prescribe broad-spectrum antibiotic therapy to any deteriorating child

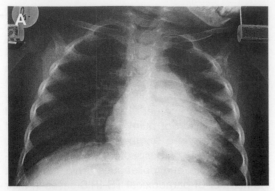

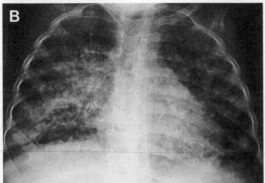

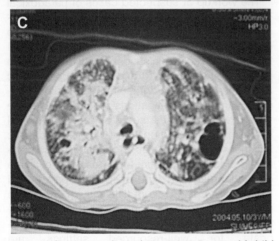

Fig. 3. Pediatric paradoxical TB-IRIS. A 3-year-old child infected with HIV-1, with severe immunosuppression, was diagnosed with drug-susceptible pulmonary TB and started on rifampicin, isoniazid, ethambutol, and pyrazinamide. Two weeks later the child started ART. Ten days after initiation of ART the child developed fever, respiratory failure, and exacerbation of pulmonary infiltrate with formation of multiple cavities. The first chest radiograph (A) was taken at the time of diagnosis of TB. The second chest radiograph (B), and the chest CT-scan (C), were performed 3 weeks after ART initiation, demonstrating dramatic worsening of the pulmonary infiltrate due to paradoxical TB-IRIS.

whenever a bacterial illness is considered in the differential diagnosis, even if TB-IRIS is believed to be most likely. In children with paradoxical TB-IRIS, TB treatment and ART can usually be continued. If TB-IRIS is considered to be life threatening or likely to cause permanent disability (eg, TBM worsening on ART), temporary interruption of ART may be considered. Immunomodulatory therapies such as corticosteroids and NSAIDs have been used, but have not been systematically studied in children. Clinicians should consider the likelihood of drug-resistant TB before considering corticosteroid therapy to treat paradoxical TB-IRIS.[40] Despite the lack of data, a reasonable approach might be to prescribe NSAIDs for mild to moderate disease and corticosteroids for severe disease. A trial of NSAIDs for prevention of paradoxical TB-IRIS is currently in the late planning phase.

Delaying the initiation of ART may reduce the risk of paradoxical TB-IRIS, but, in TB cases with severe immunodeficiency, this delay may be associated with increased HIV-1–related mortality. Currently the World Health Organization recommends that children with severe immune suppression or stage 4 disease should begin ART 2 to 8 weeks after the initiation of TB treatment.[93]

Unmasking TB-IRIS and Unmasking of TB by ART in Children

The incidence of TB during early ART varies by location according to risk of incident TB, screening policy used, and use of isoniazid preventive therapy. There are no published studies on the usefulness of TB screening strategies before ART in children, and there are no validated screening algorithms. Not all cases of TB diagnosed in the first 6 months of ART present as TB-IRIS. Severity of clinical presentation is an important factor in identifying a case of unmasking TB-IRIS. However, besides the general principles of IRIS diagnosis proposed by Boulware and colleagues,[76] there are no established diagnostic criteria for distinguishing unmasking TB-IRIS from incident TB on ART in children. Adult clinicians have suggested that only cases occurring in the first 3 months with heightened clinical features be classified as unmasking TB-IRIS.[14] An algorithm for assessing patients who present with TB after ART initiation or regimen change is shown in **Fig. 4**B.

Data from cohort studies report that the proportion of children who develop TB in Africa after initiating ART is 3.4% to 6.2%.[77,94] Walters and colleagues[77] described a cohort of 290 children initiating ART at a median age of 23 months. The number of TB cases per 100 patient years

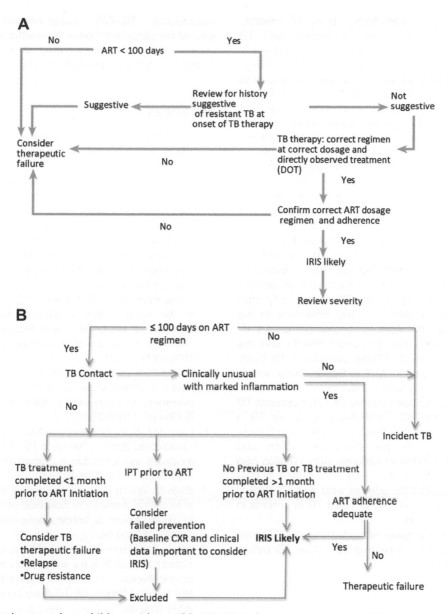

Fig. 4. Clinical approach to children with possible TB-IRIS in low resource settings. (*A*) Suspected paradoxical TB-IRIS. (*B*) Suspected unmasking TB-IRIS.

decreased from 53.3 before ART to 6.4 after ART. The number of microbiologically confirmed TB cases similarly decreased from 18.3 to 1.8/100 patient years. Fourteen children were diagnosed with TB in the first 6 months of ART; 6 of these had been treated for TB before ART. Ten cases occurred in children with a good clinical and immunologic response to ART and were considered to be unmasking TB-IRIS. All 10 children had pulmonary TB diagnosed between 2 weeks and 4 months after initiation of ART, and 5 of the cases were confirmed by culture. However, none

of the children had remarkable clinical or radiological findings, and none had extrapulmonary TB.[77] Thus, using the suggested adult definitions given previously, many may have had ART-associated TB or unmasking TB rather than TB-IRIS.[63]

Smith and colleagues[95] documented 34 IRIS events in 162 infants enrolled in the NEVEREST study in South Africa. Of IRIS events, TB was the second most common (35%) and BCG was the most common (71%). Bakeera-Kitaka and colleagues[94] described a large cohort of 1806 Ugandan children and adolescents initiating

ART, with a median follow-up of 14 months. Seventeen percent were diagnosed with TB following ART initiation. They documented a 2.7-fold increase in risk for TB in the first 100 days after ART initiation, which may be attributable to unmasking of TB by ART.[94] Zampoli and colleagues[90] described 7 children diagnosed with TB 8 to 54 days after commencing ART; all had pulmonary involvement and 1 also had extrapulmonary disease. Three had a prior history of TB treatment. Chest radiographs showed significant lymphadenopathy with airway compression, extensive parenchymal infiltration, and pleural reactions.[90] Although IRIS cases are defined by a significant and clinically apparent inflammatory response, radiological findings in most children diagnosed with TB on ART are similar to children infected with HIV-1 diagnosed with TB but not on ART.[79] Studies thus demonstrate a clustering of new TB cases early after the initiation of ART.[77,94] The difference in the rates between the Walters[77] and Bakeera-Kitaka[94] studies may be due to cohort effects and the large proportion of children already on TB treatment when initiating ART in South Africa, where the Walters study was conducted.

In BCG-vaccinated infants, BCG far exceeds TB as a cause for IRIS.[96] IRIS due to BCG and TB in the same patient has been documented in 2 pediatric cohorts. In the study by Smith and colleagues,[96] 50% of children with TB also had BCG-IRIS. In the CHER study cohort, 19% of children with BCG-IRIS adenitis also had TB-IRIS.[96] Mortality due to ART-associated TB in cohorts in this study was low.

It is likely that cases of unmasking TB-IRIS may be prevented by screening for active TB before ART initiation.

SUMMARY

TB-IRIS, a clinical syndrome that results from exaggerated inflammatory responses toward the antigens of *M tuberculosis*, is a frequent early complication of ART in adult and pediatric patients, especially in regions where TB is prevalent. Two forms of TB-IRIS are recognized: paradoxical and unmasking. Although mortality from paradoxical TB-IRIS seems rare, life-threatening forms may occur, and patients who develop paradoxical TB-IRIS frequently need hospitalization and diagnostic and therapeutic procedures. Unmasking TB-IRIS may account for a proportion of the high mortality associated with TB that is diagnosed in the initial months of ART.[3,73] Treatment of both forms of TB-IRIS includes TB treatment and continuation of ART in most patients. In

paradoxical TB-IRIS, corticosteroid therapy should be considered once alternative diagnoses have confidently been excluded, and particularly in patients with more severe manifestations.

REFERENCES

1. Corbett EL, Marston B, Churchyard GJ, et al. Tuberculosis in sub-Saharan Africa: opportunities, challenges, and change in the era of antiretroviral treatment. Lancet 2006;367(9514):926–37.
2. Maartens G, Wilkinson RJ. Tuberculosis. Lancet 2007;370(9604):2030–43.
3. Lawn SD, Myer L, Bekker LG, et al. Burden of tuberculosis in an antiretroviral treatment programme in sub-Saharan Africa: impact on treatment outcomes and implications for tuberculosis control. AIDS 2006;20(12):1605–12.
4. Palella FJ Jr, Baker RK, Moorman AC, et al. Mortality in the highly active antiretroviral therapy era: changing causes of death and disease in the HIV outpatient study. J Acquir Immune Defic Syndr 2006;43(1):27–34.
5. Girardi E, Antonucci G, Vanacore P, et al. Tuberculosis in HIV-infected persons in the context of wide availability of highly active antiretroviral therapy. Eur Respir J 2004;24(1):11–7.
6. Lawn SD, Badri M, Wood R. Tuberculosis among HIV-infected patients receiving HAART: long term incidence and risk factors in a South African cohort. AIDS 2005;19(18):2109–16.
7. Badri M, Wilson D, Wood R. Effect of highly active antiretroviral therapy on incidence of tuberculosis in South Africa: a cohort study. Lancet 2002; 359(9323):2059–64.
8. Jones JL, Hanson DL, Dworkin MS, et al. HIV-associated tuberculosis in the era of highly active antiretroviral therapy. The Adult/Adolescent Spectrum of HIV Disease Group. Int J Tuberc Lung Dis 2000; 4(11):1026–31.
9. Brinkhof MW, Egger M, Boulle A, et al. Tuberculosis after initiation of antiretroviral therapy in low-income and high-income countries. Clin Infect Dis 2007; 45(11):1518–21.
10. Moh R, Danel C, Messou E, et al. Incidence and determinants of mortality and morbidity following early antiretroviral therapy initiation in HIV-infected adults in West Africa. AIDS 2007;21(18):2483–91.
11. Lederman MM. Immune restoration and CD4+ T-cell function with antiretroviral therapies. AIDS 2001; 15(Suppl 2):S11–5.
12. Dhasmana DJ, Dheda K, Ravn P, et al. Immune reconstitution inflammatory syndrome in HIV-infected patients receiving antiretroviral therapy: pathogenesis, clinical manifestations and management. Drugs 2008;68(2):191–208.

13. French MA, Price P, Stone SF. Immune restoration disease after antiretroviral therapy. AIDS 2004; 18(12):1615–27.

14. Meintjes G, Lawn SD, Scano F, et al. Tuberculosis-associated immune reconstitution inflammatory syndrome: case definitions for use in resource-limited settings. Lancet Infect Dis 2008;8(8):516–23.

15. Campbell IA, Dyson AJ. Lymph node tuberculosis: a comparison of various methods of treatment. Tubercle 1977;58(4):171–9.

16. Hawkey CR, Yap T, Pereira J, et al. Characterization and management of paradoxical upgrading reactions in HIV-uninfected patients with lymph node tuberculosis. Clin Infect Dis 2005;40(9): 1368–71.

17. Afghani B, Lieberman JM. Paradoxical enlargement or development of intracranial tuberculomas during therapy: case report and review. Clin Infect Dis 1994;19(6):1092–9.

18. Cheng VC, Yam WC, Woo PC, et al. Risk factors for development of paradoxical response during anti-tuberculosis therapy in HIV-negative patients. Eur J Clin Microbiol Infect Dis 2003;22(10):597–602.

19. Al-Majed SA. Study of paradoxical response to chemotherapy in tuberculous pleural effusion. Respir Med 1996;90(4):211–4.

20. Karstaedt AS, Valtchanova S, Barriere R, et al. Tuberculous meningitis in South African urban adults. QJM 1998;91(11):743–7.

21. Reiser M, Fatkonhouor G, Diehl V. Paradoxical expansion of intracranial tuberculomas during chemotherapy. J Infect 1997;35(1):88–90.

22. Belknap R, Reves R, Burman W. Immune reconstitution to Mycobacterium tuberculosis after discontinuing infliximab. Int J Tuberc Lung Dis 2005;9(9): 1057–8.

23. Wallis RS, van Vuuren C, Potgieter S. Adalimumab treatment of life-threatening tuberculosis. Clin Infect Dis 2009;48(10):1429–32.

24. Narita M, Ashkin D, Hollender ES, et al. Paradoxical worsening of tuberculosis following antiretroviral therapy in patients with AIDS. Am J Respir Crit Care Med 1998;158(1):157–61.

25. Breen RA, Smith CJ, Bettinson H, et al. Paradoxical reactions during tuberculosis treatment in patients with and without HIV co-infection. Thorax 2004; 59(8):704–7.

26. Breton G, Duval X, Estellat C, et al. Determinants of immune reconstitution inflammatory syndrome in HIV type 1-infected patients with tuberculosis after initiation of antiretroviral therapy. Clin Infect Dis 2004;39(11):1709–12.

27. Kumarasamy N, Chaguturu S, Mayer KH, et al. Incidence of immune reconstitution syndrome in HIV/tuberculosis-coinfected patients after initiation of generic antiretroviral therapy in India. J Acquir Immune Defic Syndr 2004;37(5):1574–6.

28. Shelburne SA, Visnegarwala F, Darcourt J, et al. Incidence and risk factors for immune reconstitution inflammatory syndrome during highly active antiretroviral therapy. AIDS 2005;19(4):399–406.

29. Michailidis C, Pozniak AL, Mandalia S, et al. Clinical characteristics of IRIS syndrome in patients with HIV and tuberculosis. Antivir Ther 2005;10(3):417–22.

30. Manosuthi W, Kiertiburanakul S, Phoorisri T, et al. Immune reconstitution inflammatory syndrome of tuberculosis among HIV-infected patients receiving antituberculous and antiretroviral therapy. J Infect 2006;53(6):357–63.

31. Lawn SD, Myer L, Bekker LG, et al. Tuberculosis-associated immune reconstitution disease: incidence, risk factors and impact in an antiretroviral treatment service in South Africa. AIDS 2007;21(3): 335–41.

32. Burman W, Weis S, Vernon A, et al. Frequency, severity and duration of immune reconstitution events in HIV-related tuberculosis. Int J Tuberc Lung Dis 2007;11(12):1282–9.

33. Baalwa J, Mayanja-Kizza H, Kamya MR, et al. Worsening and unmasking of tuberculosis in HIV-1 infected patients after initiating highly active antiretroviral therapy in Uganda. Afr Health Sci 2008; 8(3):190–5.

34. Tansuphasawadikul S, Saito W, Kim J, et al. Outcomes in HIV-infected patients on antiretroviral therapy with tuberculosis. Southeast Asian J Trop Med Public Health 2007;38(6):1053–60.

35. Serra FC, Hadad D, Orofino RL, et al. Immune reconstitution syndrome in patients treated for HIV and tuberculosis in Rio de Janeiro. Braz J Infect Dis 2007;11(5):462–5.

36. Olalla J, Pulido F, Rubio R, et al. Paradoxical responses in a cohort of HIV-1-infected patients with mycobacterial disease. Int J Tuberc Lung Dis 2002;6(1):71–5.

37. Huyst V, Lynen L, Bottieau E, et al. Immune reconstitution inflammatory syndrome in an HIV/TB co-infected patient four years after starting antiretroviral therapy. Acta Clin Belg 2007;62(2):126–9.

38. Fishman JE, Saraf-Lavi E, Narita M, et al. Pulmonary tuberculosis in AIDS patients: transient chest radiographic worsening after initiation of antiretroviral therapy. AJR Am J Roentgenol 2000;174(1): 43–9.

39. Richardson D, Rubinstein L, Ross E, et al. Cystic lung lesions as an immune reconstitution inflammatory syndrome (IRIS) in HIV-TB co-infection? Thorax 2005;60(10):884.

40. Meintjes G, Rangaka MX, Maartens G, et al. Novel relationship between tuberculosis immune reconstitution inflammatory syndrome and anti-tubercular drug resistance. Clin Infect Dis 2009;48(5):667–76.

41. Lawn SD, Bekker LG, Miller RF. Immune reconstitution disease associated with mycobacterial

infections in HIV-infected individuals receiving anti-retrovirals. Lancet Infect Dis 2005;5(6):361–73.

42. Lawn SD, Wood R. Hepatic involvement with tuberculosis-associated immune reconstitution disease. AIDS 2007;21(17):2362–3.

43. Pepper DJ, Marais S, Maartens G, et al. Neurologic manifestations of paradoxical tuberculosis-associated immune reconstitution inflammatory syndrome: a case series. Clin Infect Dis 2009;48(11):e96–107.

44. Wang SH, Menon A, Hyslop NE. Cardiac tamponade: an unusual complication of simultaneous treatment of tuberculosis and HIV. South Med J 2008;101(5):558–60.

45. Salliot C, Guichard I, Daugas E, et al. Acute kidney disease due to immune reconstitution inflammatory syndrome in an HIV-infected patient with tuberculosis. J Int Assoc Physicians AIDS Care (Chic Ill) 2008;7(4):178–81.

46. Weber E, Gunthard HF, Schertler T, et al. Spontaneous splenic rupture as manifestation of the immune reconstitution inflammatory syndrome in an HIV type 1 infected patient with tuberculosis. Infection 2009;37(2):163–5.

47. Guex AC, Bucher HC, Demartines N, et al. Inflammatory bowel perforation during immune restoration after one year of antiretroviral and antituberculous therapy in an HIV-1-infected patient: report of a case. Dis Colon Rectum 2002;45(7):977–8.

48. Blanc FX, Havlir DV, Onyebujoh PC, et al. Treatment strategies for HIV-infected patients with tuberculosis: ongoing and planned clinical trials. J Infect Dis 2007;196(Suppl 1):S46–51.

49. Schiffer JT, Sterling TR. Timing of antiretroviral therapy initiation in tuberculosis patients with AIDS: a decision analysis. J Acquir Immune Defic Syndr 2007;44(2):229–34.

50. World Health Organization. Antiretroviral therapy for HIV infection in adults and adolescents: recommendations for a public healthy approach: 2006 revision. Geneva: WHO Press; 2006.

51. Meintjes G, Wilkinson RJ, Morroni C, et al. Randomised placebo-controlled trial of prednisone for the TB immune reconstitution inflammatory syndrome. Abstract 34. 16th Conference on Retroviruses and Opportunistic Infections. Montreal (QC); February 8–11, 2009.

52. Elliott AM, Halwiindi B, Bagshawe A, et al. Use of prednisolone in the treatment of HIV-positive tuberculosis patients. QJM 1992;85(307–8): 855–60.

53. Elliott AM, Luzze H, Quigley MA, et al. A randomized, double-blind, placebo-controlled trial of the use of prednisolone as an adjunct to treatment in HIV-1-associated pleural tuberculosis. J Infect Dis 2004;190(5):869–78.

54. Manabe YC, Campbell JD, Sydnor E, et al. Immune reconstitution inflammatory syndrome: risk factors and treatment implications. J Acquir Immune Defic Syndr 2007;46(4):456–62.

55. Blackmore TK, Manning L, Taylor WJ, et al. Therapeutic use of infliximab in tuberculosis to control severe paradoxical reaction of the brain and lymph nodes. Clin Infect Dis 2008;47(10):e83–5.

56. Hengel RL, Allende MC, Dewar RL, et al. Increasing CD4+ T cells specific for tuberculosis correlate with improved clinical immunity after highly active antiretroviral therapy. AIDS Res Hum Retroviruses 2002; 18(13):969–75.

57. Bourgarit A, Carcelain G, Martinez V, et al. Explosion of tuberculin-specific Th1-responses induces immune restoration syndrome in tuberculosis and HIV co-infected patients. AIDS 2006;20(2):F1–7.

58. Meintjes G, Wilkinson KA, Rangaka MX, et al. Type 1 helper T cells and FoxP3-positive T cells in HIV-tuberculosis-associated immune reconstitution inflammatory syndrome. Am J Respir Crit Care Med 2008;178(10):1083–9.

59. Tan DB, Yong YK, Tan HY, et al. Immunological profiles of immune restoration disease presenting as mycobacterial lymphadenitis and cryptococcal meningitis. HIV Med 2008;9(5):307–16.

60. Seddiki N, Sasson SC, Santner-Nanan B, et al. Proliferation of weakly suppressive regulatory CD4+ T cells is associated with over-active CD4+ T-cell responses in HIV-positive patients with mycobacterial immune restoration disease. Eur J Immunol 2009;39(2):391–403.

61. Colebunders R, Bastian I. A review of the diagnosis and treatment of smear-negative pulmonary tuberculosis. Int J Tuberc Lung Dis 2000;4(2):97–107.

62. Mtei L, Matee M, Herfort O, et al. High rates of clinical and subclinical tuberculosis among HIV-infected ambulatory subjects in Tanzania. Clin Infect Dis 2005;40(10):1500–7.

63. Lawn SD, Wilkinson RJ, Lipman MC, et al. Immune reconstitution and "unmasking" of tuberculosis during antiretroviral therapy. Am J Respir Crit Care Med 2008;177(7):680–5.

64. Park WB, Choe PG, Jo JH, et al. Tuberculosis manifested by immune reconstitution inflammatory syndrome during HAART. AIDS 2007;21(7): 875–7.

65. Goldsack NR, Allen S, Lipman MC. Adult respiratory distress syndrome as a severe immune reconstitution disease following the commencement of highly active antiretroviral therapy. Sex Transm Infect 2003;79(4):337–8.

66. Lawn SD, Wainwright H, Orrell C. Fatal unmasking tuberculosis immune reconstitution disease with bronchiolitis obliterans organizing pneumonia: the role of macrophages. AIDS 2009;23(1):143–5.

67. John L, Baalwa J, Kalimugogo P, et al. Response to 'Does immune reconstitution promote active tuberculosis in patients receiving highly active

antiretroviral therapy?' AIDS 22 July 2005. AIDS 2005;19(17):2049–50.

68. Tahir M, Sinha S, Sharma SK, et al. Immune reconstitution inflammatory syndrome manifesting as disseminated tuberculosis, deep venous thrombosis, encephalopathy and myelopathy. Indian J Chest Dis Allied Sci 2008;50(4):363–4.

69. Crump JA, Tyrer MJ, Lloyd-Owen SJ, et al. Miliary tuberculosis with paradoxical expansion of intracranial tuberculomas complicating human immunodeficiency virus infection in a patient receiving highly active antiretroviral therapy. Clin Infect Dis 1998; 26(4):1008–9.

70. Chen WL, Lin YF, Tsai WC, et al. Unveiling tuberculous pyomyositis: an emerging role of immune reconstitution inflammatory syndrome. Am J Emerg Med 2009;27(2):251, e251–2.

71. Breen RA, Smith CJ, Cropley I, et al. Does immune reconstitution syndrome promote active tuberculosis in patients receiving highly active antiretroviral therapy? AIDS 2005;19(11):1201–6.

72. Lawn SD, Myer L, Edwards D, et al. Short-term and long-term risk of tuberculosis associated with CD4 cell recovery during antiretroviral therapy in South Africa. AIDS 2009;23:1717–25.

73. Koenig SP, Riviere C, Leger P, et al. High mortality among patients with AIDS who received a diagnosis of tuberculosis in the first 3 months of antiretroviral therapy. Clin Infect Dis 2009;48(6):829–31.

74. Were W, Moore D, Ekwaru P, et al. A simple screening tool for active tuberculosis in HIV-infected adults receiving antiretroviral treatment in Uganda. Int J Tuberc Lung Dis 2009;13(1):47–53.

75. World Health Organization. Improving the diagnosis and treatment of smear-negative pulmonary and extrapulmonary tuberculosis among adults and adolescents. Recommendations for HIV-prevalent resource-constrained settings. Geneva: WHO Press; 2006.

76. Boulware DR, Callens S, Pahwa S. Pediatric HIV immune reconstitution inflammatory syndrome. Curr Opin HIV AIDS 2008;3(4):461–7.

77. Walters E, Cotton MF, Rabie H, et al. Clinical presentation and outcome of tuberculosis in human immunodeficiency virus infected children on anti-retroviral therapy. BMC Pediatr 2008;8:1.

78. Cotton MF, Schaaf HS, Lottering G, et al. Tuberculosis exposure in HIV-exposed infants in a high-prevalence setting. Int J Tuberc Lung Dis 2008;12(2): 225–7.

79. Schaaf HS, Marais BJ, Whitelaw A, et al. Culture-confirmed childhood tuberculosis in Cape Town, South Africa: a review of 596 cases. BMC Infect Dis 2007;7:140.

80. Moultrie H, Yotebieng M, Kuhn L, et al. Mortality and virological outcomes of 2105 HIV-infected children receiving ART in Soweto, South Africa. 16th Conference on Retroviruses and Opportunistic Infections. Abstract 97. Montreal (QC); February 8–11, 2009.

81. Sutcliffe CG, van Dijk JH, Bolton C, et al. Effectiveness of antiretroviral therapy among HIV-infected children in sub-Saharan Africa. Lancet Infect Dis 2008;8(8):477–89.

82. Marais BJ, Graham SM, Cotton MF, et al. Diagnostic and management challenges for childhood tuberculosis in the era of HIV. J Infect Dis 2007; 196(Suppl 1):S76–85.

83. Eamranond P, Jaramillo E. Tuberculosis in children: reassessing the need for improved diagnosis in global control strategies. Int J Tuberc Lung Dis 2001;5(7):594–603.

84. Zar HJ, Hanslo D, Apolles P, et al. Induced sputum versus gastric lavage for microbiological confirmation of pulmonary tuberculosis in infants and young children: a prospective study. Lancet 2005; 365(9454):130–4.

85. Cohen GM. Access to diagnostics in support of HIV/AIDS and tuberculosis treatment in developing countries. AIDS 2007;21(Suppl 4):S81–7.

86. Madhi SA, Gray GE, Huebner RE, et al. Correlation between CD4+ lymphocyte counts, concurrent antigen skin test and tuberculin skin test reactivity in human immunodeficiency virus type 1-infected and -uninfected children with tuberculosis. Pediatr Infect Dis J 1999;18(9):800–5.

87. Davies MA, Connell T, Johannisen C, et al. Detection of tuberculosis in HIV-infected children using an enzyme-linked immunospot assay. AIDS 2009; 23(8):961–9.

88. Cohen JM, Whittaker E, Walters S, et al. Presentation, diagnosis and management of tuberculosis in HIV-infected children in the UK. HIV Med 2008;9(5):277–84.

89. Bakeera-Kitaka S, Kekitiinwa A, Dhabangi A, et al. Tuberculosis immune reconstitution syndrome among Ugandan children. Int J Infect Dis 2008;12: e63–4.

90. Zampoli M, Kilborn T, Eley B. Tuberculosis during early antiretroviral-induced immune reconstitution in HIV-infected children. Int J Tuberc Lung Dis 2007;11(4):417–23.

91. Bolton-Moore C, Mubiana-Mbewe M, Cantrell RA, et al. Clinical outcomes and CD4 cell response in children receiving antiretroviral therapy at primary health care facilities in Zambia. JAMA 2007; 298(16):1888–99.

92. Puthanakit T, Aurpibul L, Oberdorfer P, et al. Hospitalization and mortality among HIV-infected children after receiving highly active antiretroviral therapy. Clin Infect Dis 2007;44(4):599–604.

93. World Health Organization. Antiretroviral therapy of HIV infection in infants and children: towards universal access. Recommendations for a public health approach. Geneva: WHO Press; 2006.

94. Bakeera-Kitaka S, Dhabangi A, Namulema E, et al. Immune reconstitution inflammatory syndrome and post-antiretroviral tuberculosis among HIV-infected Ugandan children. Abstract 921. Infectious Diseases Society of America Annual Conference. San Diego (CA); October 4–7, 2007.

95. Smith K, Kuhn L, Coovadia A, et al. Immune reconstitution inflammatory syndrome among HIV-infected South African infants initiating antiretroviral therapy. AIDS 2009;23(9):1097–107.

96. Rabie H, Violari A, Madhi S, et al. Complications of BCG vaccination in HIV-infected and uninfected children: evidence from the Children with HIV Early Antiretroviral Therapy (CHER) study. Abstract 600. 15th Conference on Retroviruses and Opportunistic Infections. Boston (MA); February 3–6, 2008.

New Vaccines Against Tuberculosis

Paul-Henri Lambert, MD[a],*, Tony Hawkridge, MBChB[b],
Willem A. Hanekom, MBChB, DCH, FCP[c]

KEYWORDS

- Tuberculosis • Vaccine • Prophylaxis • Adjuvant
- Trial • BCG • HIV • Latency • Infection

About 1 in 3 of the world's inhabitants is infected with *Mycobacterium tuberculosis*. Major challenges to tuberculosis (TB) control include TB-human immunodeficiency virus (HIV) coinfection and strains of *M tuberculosis* that are resistant to 1 or more anti-TB drugs.[1] Children are particularly susceptible to severe TB and death following infection, and those who do not develop disease may become reservoirs for future transmission, following disease reactivation in adulthood.[2] Although the global burden of TB is slowly decreasing, it is likely that neither the World Health Organization (WHO) epidemiologic impact targets set for 2015, nor the TB elimination target set for 2050, will be met without new tools for TB control, including new vaccines or vaccination strategies.[3,4]

BACILLE CALMETTE GUÉRIN VACCINE

The only licensed vaccine against TB, bacille Calmette Guérin (BCG) vaccine, was first given to a human infant in 1921. The vaccine has been administered to more than 90% of the world's children; 4 billion persons have received BCG to date.[5] More than 120 million doses are given each year, making BCG one of the most widely used vaccines in the world.[6]

Efficacy

BCG has shown consistent efficacy against childhood TB meningitis and miliary TB, but only variable efficacy against adult pulmonary TB.[1,7–9]

Several meta-analyses of the efficacy of BCG have been conducted.[10–12] The overall efficacy against infant TB in randomized controlled trials was 74% (95% confidence interval [CI] 62%–83%), and in case-control studies 52% (95% CI 38%–64%). In infants, the protective effect against death from TB was 65% (95% CI 12%–86%), against TB meningitis 64% (95% CI 0.30%–0.82%), against disseminated TB 78% (95% CI 58%–88%) and against laboratory-confirmed TB 83% (95% CI 58%–93%). It was concluded that BCG vaccination of newborns and infants reduces the risk of TB by 50%, on average. Conferred protection was across populations, study designs, and across different forms of TB.[10–12] Another meta-analysis found that the protective effect against pulmonary disease was too heterogeneous for a summary measure of protection to be calculable.[13] The protective effect against miliary or meningeal TB in randomized controlled trials was 86% (95% CI 65%–95%), and in case-control studies 75% (95% CI 61%–84%).[13]

Although there has been widespread BCG vaccination for many years, 9.3 million people develop TB disease each year, and 1.8 million die.[4] Administering 2 doses of BCG does not confer added protection; in Malawi, neither 1 nor 2 doses of BCG protected against adult pulmonary TB.[14] Brazilian studies have confirmed that a second dose of BCG does not increase protective efficacy.[8]

Reasons for the partial and variable efficacy of BCG may include exposure of individuals to

---

[a] Centre of Vaccinology, CMU, 1 rue Michel-Servet, 1211 Geneva 4, Switzerland University of Geneva, Switzerland
[b] Aeras Global TB Vaccine Foundation, Africa Office, South Africa
[c] South African TB Vaccine Initiative, University of Cape Town Health Sciences, Anzio Road, Observatory, 7925, South Africa, South Africa
* Corresponding author.
E-mail address: paul.lambert@unige.ch (P-H. Lambert).

Clin Chest Med 30 (2009) 811–826
doi:10.1016/j.ccm.2009.08.014
0272-5231/09/$ – see front matter © 2009 Elsevier Inc. All rights reserved.

environmental mycobacteria, masking the effects of the vaccine.[14] Distance from the equator is associated with higher BCG efficacy. Factors that vary with latitude that may contribute include socioeconomic conditions, genetic background, climate, exposure to sunlight, diet and nutrition, environmental nontuberculous mycobacterial exposure, virulence of prevalent M tuberculosis strains, storage and viability of BCG vaccine, and quality of the BCG vaccine studies from which data were generated.[15]

Another hypothesis for the variability of BCG is that different strains of BCG vary in protective efficacy, and evolutionarily early strains are more efficacious than the more attenuated evolutionarily late strains, which lack region of deletion.[2] Horwitz and colleagues[5] tested 6 widely used BCG strains (the "early" strain BCG Japanese, 2 "late" strains in DU2 Group III [Danish and Glaxo], and 3 "late" strains in DU2 Group IV [Connaught, Pasteur, and Tice]) in the guinea pig model of pulmonary TB. With the exception of BCG Glaxo, which had poor efficacy, they found no substantial differences in efficacy between the early strains and the late strains, and only small differences in efficacy among late strains. Currently, there are insufficient data to favor or recommend one particular BCG strain compared with another.[6]

Finally, protection induced by BCG may wane,[16] but it may persist for up to 10 years after infant vaccination.[11]

Safety

There are concerns surrounding the safety of BCG in immune-compromised individuals. WHO has previously recommended that BCG be given to all asymptomatic infants, irrespective of HIV exposure at birth. It was recommended that the vaccine be withheld in infants with symptomatic HIV infection. This approach has led to some HIV-infected neonates, who were asymptomatic at birth, developing severe vaccine-related complications.[17] This disease may present as lymph node swelling in the region of vaccination or as more distant or even disseminated disease that may affect multiple organs.[18] In areas with high prevalence, the incidence of BCGosis may be similar to that of TB disease in HIV-infected infants.[19] Although data on the protective effect of BCG in HIV-infected children are lacking,[20] the vaccine induces a poor immune response in infected infants.[21] The revised WHO guidelines have therefore made HIV infection a full contraindication to BCG vaccination.[22] Ideally, BCG vaccination should be delayed in infants born to mothers infected with HIV, until the diagnosis of HIV infection has been excluded with a viral amplification test. This strategy is difficult to implement in the developing world.[21]

Other Issues with BCG

The tuberculin skin test (TST) is a low-cost and simple diagnostic test for M tuberculosis infection. Its interpretation is based on extensive published literature; however, specificity is reduced by BCG vaccination. The age of BCG vaccination may determine its effect on the TST; BCG given in infancy is believed to have a minimal effect, although the effect is greater if BCG is given after infancy.[23,24] Regardless, positive skin tests with indurations of 15 mm or more are more likely to be the result of M tuberculosis infection than of BCG vaccination.[24]

NEW VACCINES AGAINST TB: GENERAL STRATEGIES
Potential Uses of a New TB Vaccine

New vaccination strategies should significantly improve on BCG and have a noticeable effect on the global TB burden. This expectation implies the need for vaccines or vaccine combinations that induce more "optimal" immunity, compared with BCG, not only in infants, but also in adolescents and adults. Pre- and postexposure vaccines are needed.

In infancy, the optimal vaccine would be expected to fully prevent initial infection. So far, this has been an unachievable objective, which reflects the exceptional resistance of extracellular mycobacteria to antibody-mediated, or cytokine-mediated, bacteriolytic mechanisms. Soon after infection, mycobacteria hide and grow inside macrophages and may be destroyed or their growth contained only through cell-mediated immunity. Most vaccination strategies target this early phase, with the goal of drastically reducing the initial mycobacterial burden and ensuring containment of escaping bacteria.

An optimal vaccine might be expected to clear all remaining organisms; however, it is likely that some mycobacteria escape because of imperfect immune control. Immunologically contained M tuberculosis is believed to enter a stage of latency, characterized by a reduced metabolism and a different gene expression profile, compared with early after infection. A vaccine that targets latent M tuberculosis would therefore be required to act via immunologic mechanisms that may be distinct from those required to tackle the pathogen early after infection. This process may include targeting of antigens predominantly expressed during latency.

Prevention of reactivation of latent *M tuberculosis*, with resulting disease, may also depend on host capacity to interfere quickly with this change in the pathogen's metabolic status, including its set of reactivation gene products. Vaccines that specifically prevent reactivation should considerably reduce the risk of TB relapse.

Target Product Profiles

Four types of vaccines have to be considered in a comprehensive TB vaccination strategy.

First, BCG would still have its place in a re-shuffled prevention strategy. This vaccine should prime the immune system, in preparation for subsequent complementary vaccines. BCG could also be replaced by vaccines with a better safety profile, particularly in the context of immune compromise. In TB exposure, the vaccine would reduce the initial bacterial burden as much as possible, slow down bacterial growth, and protect against early disease. Although live vectors or subunit vaccines could be used, live mycobacteria (BCG or others) remain the most appropriate prime vaccines of a new global vaccination strategy.

A second vaccine should be capable of boosting and possibly redirecting the immune response induced by the first vaccine. Its role would be to boost immunologic memory, increase the duration of immunity, and improve the protection conferred by the priming event. Such boosting vaccines may have to be administered repeatedly during an individual's lifespan.

A third vaccine should target healthy adolescents or adults already infected with mycobacteria, to be administered post exposure. The vaccine would be expected either to clear persistent latent bacteria or to prevent reactivation.

Finally, therapeutic vaccines would complement chemotherapy to contribute to reducing treatment duration, and increasing treatment efficacy, particularly in the context of antibiotic resistance or relative immune deficiency (**Fig. 1**).

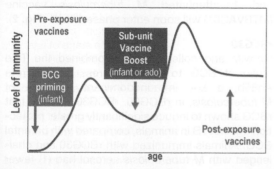

Fig. 1. New TB vaccination strategies.

Targeted Immune Profile for New Vaccines

The immunologic mechanisms that mediate protection at different stages of *M tuberculosis* infection remain incompletely understood. There is evidence that cell-mediated immune mechanisms are essential, as shown by the high incidence of TB in conditions associated with T-cell deficiencies. It is also recognized that interferon-gamma (IFN-γ) producing CD4 T cells are needed, but are not sufficient to control the infection. CD8 T cells might be critical for clearance of the pathogen. Other cells, for example, natural killer cells, may also play a role in protective mechanisms. It seems as if antibodies are not a major component of immune control, but may contribute to limiting bacterial dissemination.

New vaccines therefore aim to induce or boost T-cell-mediated responses. Such responses should be directed at antigens expressed by intracellular bacteria, and presented as peptide-major histocompatibility complexes at the cell surface. Effector cells must be generated for early protection, but immunologic memory is essential for long-term protection. From animal data, it seems that effective vaccines have to induce polyfunctional T cells, that is, cells that can respond to specific antigens through the concomitant production of several types of cytokines (eg, IFN-γ, interleukin [IL]-2, tumor necrosis factor [TNF]-α). Although the role of mucosal immunity in the prevention of lung infection is still controversial, several vaccines aim to induce local responses after aerosol administration.

In addition, new vaccines should avoid the triggering of regulatory T cells that may hamper the persistence of protective mechanisms.

Therefore, it is difficult to define a single optimal target profile. Present development aims at vaccination strategies that can induce potent IFN-γ responses within a multifunctional T-cell context, and with a specificity directed at antigens relevant to targeted stages of infection. The availability of better indicators of protection would greatly help the clinical assessment of new candidate vaccines (see later discussion).

Antigen Discovery

Although several candidate vaccines are already at a clinical development stage, their protective efficacy remains to be demonstrated, and continued upstream research is essential for the identification of key antigens. Particular attention is now given to antigens that are expressed during the phase of latency, to antigens that are not classically identified by genetic approaches of bacterial proteome screening and to nonpeptidic antigens (eg, glycolipids).

Many latency-associated antigens have been described. Their expression in "dormant" mycobacteria reflects a distinct metabolic state.[25] The identification of M tuberculosis stage specific genes has been facilitated by genome-wide expression arrays. For example, the dosR regulon of M tuberculosis was shown to be upregulated during conditions encountered by intracellular mycobacteria. Many of the dosR-encoded antigens are recognized by individuals with latent TB, and cumulative responses to dosR antigens are higher in latently infected individuals, compared with responses in TB patients. Remarkably, BCG vaccination does not induce immunity to dormancy antigens. Latency vaccines may target dormant M tuberculosis and help eliminate the pathogen during its dormant or slowly replicating phase of infection. Subunit vaccines based on dormancy antigens might also be combined with such vaccines containing antigens expressed early after M tuberculosis infection, in multiphase vaccines. Such vaccines would offer the advantage of immune protection against early and late stages of infection. Alternatively, one can develop recombinant BCG strains that would constitutively express selected latency-associated antigens.

Another line of discovery is targeting antigens not identified by classic genetic approaches of bacterial proteome screening. A typical example is heparin-binding hemagglutinin (HBHA), an antigen that undergoes posttranslation modifications apparently essential for immune recognition.[26] These modifications consist of a complex methylation pattern in the C-terminal region, which plays roles in B- and T-cell activation.

Nonpeptidic antigens may also be involved in protection and they are investigated for their potential value as vaccine components. CD1-restricted lipid-specific T lymphocytes are primed during infection with M tuberculosis. Some of these lipids, for example, diacylated sulfoglycolipids and glycerol monomycolate, seem promising as potential vaccines or vaccine components.[27,28]

Vaccine Design

The portfolio of candidate TB vaccines reflects the diversity of new approaches in vaccinology. It comprises live attenuated candidates (eg, recombinant or recombinant attenuated M tuberculosis), live vectored subunits (eg, modified vaccinia Ankara [MVA] or adenovirus), recombinant proteins in adjuvants, DNA vaccines, and whole cell killed mycobacteria (eg, M vaccae). It seems important for vaccines to target the appropriate

antigen-presenting cells to generate desired protective responses and to avoid serious adverse events. For example, recent studies with a subunit TB vaccine have demonstrated that, using appropriate formulations, immune cellular activation can be restricted to these dendritic cells that have captured the vaccine antigen, which may result in reduction of risks associated with broad nonspecific stimulation of the immune system.[29]

Preclinical Studies

Preclinical studies of candidate vaccines are largely based on animal models. Although appropriate models exist for assessing safety and immunogenicity of new vaccines, the main challenge is the estimation of the potential protective capacity of candidate products. The present approach is first to screen candidates in murine challenge models, then to move to guinea pigs challenged by the aerosol route and finally to perform challenge studies in nonhuman primates. In principle, the latter model is expected to reflect the human situation better in immunogenicity and disease susceptibility. However, limited amounts of nonhuman primates are available for study, and genetic diversity and ethical issues may prove to be hampering factors.

VACCINES CURRENTLY IN DEVELOPMENT
Live Mycobacterial Vaccines in Clinical Development

These vaccine candidates are based either on improvement of BCG, through addition of relevant genes, or on attenuation of M tuberculosis, through deletion of virulence or other essential genes. The aim would be to replace BCG, and the vaccines should therefore induce a better primary protective response than BCG, and adequately prime for a subsequent boost vaccine. For success, such vaccines must be safer than BCG in immune-compromised patients. Two improved BCG vaccines have already entered clinical trials: rBCG30, and rBCG-δUreC:Hly+, and 1 attenuated M tuberculosis vaccine (MTBVAC01) will soon enter phase 1 trials (**Fig. 2**).

rBCG30

Horwitz and colleagues[30] recombined the Tice strain of BCG to stably express and secrete Ag85b, a key immunodominant molecule of M tuberculosis, in rBCG30. rBCG30 was the first rBCG shown to induce significantly greater protection against TB in animals, compared with parental BCG. Animals immunized with rBCG30 and challenged with M tuberculosis aerosol had (1) fewer TB bacilli in their lungs and spleens, (2) fewer

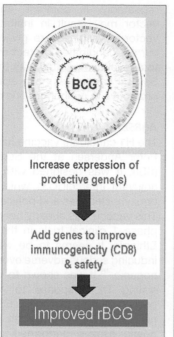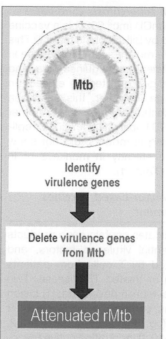

Fig. 2. Rationale used in development of live mycobacterial vaccines.

and smaller lesions in their lungs, spleens, and livers, (3) significantly less lung pathology, and (4) survived significantly longer. The parental and recombinant vaccine strains were comparably avirulent in guinea pigs, and were susceptible to the same antimycobacterial antibiotics. The limited replication of rBCG30 in vivo renders the vaccine safer than BCG in SCID mice; this may also translate to better safety in individuals infected with HIV. Intradermal rBCG30 and Tice BCG were compared in a double-blind phase 1 clinical trial involving 35 adults. Clinical reactogenicity was similar, although immunogenicity was significantly increased in the rBCG30 group.[31]

rBCG-δUreC:Hly+ (VPM1002)

This vaccine is a recombinant, urease C-deficient, listeriolysin-expressing BCG.[32] The listeriolysin (Hly) of *Listeria monocytogenes* incorporated into VPM1002 enables escape from the phagosome of infected host cells, by perforating the membrane of this organelle. Omitting the urease C gene was necessary to ensure an acidic phagosomal environment, optimal for Hly activity. Perforation promotes antigen translocation into the cytoplasm and facilitates cross-priming, as the infected cell is more likely to die from apoptosis.[33] This process mimics the immune induction of *M tuberculosis* effectively. The mode of action is expected to result in an efficacious and well-tolerated vaccine against TB, which should be at least as potent as the classic

BCG strain that is currently used and should cause fewer adverse events. Preclinical studies in mice, guinea pigs, nonhuman primates, and in immune-deficient animals indicate that this target profile has been achieved. A first clinical trial was initiated in 2008 and this vaccine seems so far to be safe (Leander Grode, personal communication, 2009).

Other live vaccines expected to be in clinical trials soon

MTBVAC01

MTBVAC01 is an attenuated live *M tuberculosis* double mutant deficient for phoP and fadD26. The rationale for disrupting phoP is that overexpression of this transcriptional regulator seems to be associated with a high virulence phenotype.[34] PhoP mutants proved to be safe in SCID mice, and to confer better protective efficacy than BCG, in various animal models.[35] MTBVAC01 was shown to protect rhesus macaques against virulent *M tuberculosis* challenge,[36] and to be sensitive to first-line anti-TB drugs.

The addition of an independent fadD26 mutation did not change the immunogenicity profile of the vaccine, but conferred additional safety. FadD is an essential gene for phthiocerol dimycocerosate biosynthesis, a complex lipid implicated in *M tuberculosis* virulence.[37] The vaccine is now moving to good manufacturing practice production, and should enter clinical trials in 2011.

Other attenuated M tuberculosis candidates

Mtb H37Rv δlysA δpanCD (mc^2 6020) is a vaccine candidate developed by Bill Jacobs's team.[35] This nonreplicating double mutant seems to be safe in SCID and IFN-γ-deficient mice, guinea pigs, and monkeys. It delivers good protective efficacy in mice and guinea pigs; however, this has been more variable in nonhuman primates. Another candidate, H37Rv δRD1 δpanCD (mc^2 6030, replicating), also promising in rodents, did not show significant protective efficacy in monkeys or in neonatal calves[36,37] (Table 1).

Subunit and Live Vector-based Vaccines in Clinical Development

These vaccine candidates contain gene products recognized as potential virulence factors, and which are recognized by T cells from patients with latent infection or treated TB disease. Two types of products have been developed: (1) fusion recombinant proteins, comprising 2 or 3 major TB or BCG antigens (eg, Ag85A, Ag85B, Mtb32, Mtb39, ESAT-6, TB-10.4), or purified native mycobacterial antigens (eg, HBHA), and, (2) live vectors that express one or several of these mycobacterial proteins. The vaccines are designed primarily to boost responses induced by a BCG prime, and possibly to induce additional responses to M tuberculosis specific antigens like ESAT-6. Recombinant protein vaccines require an adjuvant that drives Th1 responses (CD4 T cells that make IFN-γ, IL-2 and TNF-α), and which may be given

repeatedly. In contrast, immunity against the vector may result in inhibition when live virus vectored vaccines are given repeatedly. All the current candidates protect mice and guinea pigs to a level comparable with that induced by BCG. Several candidates have also been shown to be protective in nonhuman primates[26,38–44] (Fig. 3).

Ag85B-ESAT-6 (H1)

The H1 candidate vaccine has been developed by Peter Andersen at the Statens Serum Institute (SSI). It was designed with a strong novel Th1 adjuvant, Intercell IC31, which is a mixture of oligodeoxynucleotides and polycationic amino acids.[45] This vaccine has already been assessed in several phase 1 clinical trials in the Netherlands and in Ethiopia. It seems to be well tolerated, without inducing serious adverse events, and highly immunogenic.[46] It was shown to induce a strong, persisting Th1 response to Ag85B. The modest primary T-cell response to ESAT-6 did not persist, nor seem to interfere with ESAT-6-based diagnostic assays performed a few months after immunization.

Ag85B-TB-10.4 (H4, AERAS-404)

This vaccine was also developed by the SSI team, as an alternative to H1. In this fusion protein, ESAT-6 was replaced by TB-10.4, a protein also in BCG, to reduce the theoretic risk of interference with ESAT-6-based diagnostic assays. It is now in joint development by SSI, Aeras and

---

Table 1
Leading live mycobacterial vaccine candidates

	Profile	Developers	Sponsors	Status
rBCG30	Increased expression of 30-kDa protein	M Horwitz	University of California at Los Angeles and AERAS	In phase 1 clinical trials
rBCG-δUreC:Hly+	Expression of *Listeria* cytolysin	S. Kaufmann and VPM	TBVI	In phase 1 clinical trials
rBCG-AERAS	Expression of perfringolysin + Ag85& Tb-10.4	AERAS	AERAS	Planned to be in a phase 1 clinical trial before end of 2009
Mtb PhoP mutant	Deletion PhoP virulence genes	C. Martin	TBVI	Preclinical
Mtb mc^2 6020/30 mutant	Deletion LysA + panCD or panCD + RD1 virulence genes	W. Jacobs	Albert Einstein College of Medicine	Preclinical

Abbreviations: TBVI, tuberculosis vaccine initiative; VPM, vakzine projekt management GmbH.

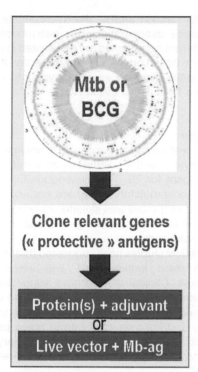

Fig. 3. Rationale used in development of subunit and live vector-based vaccines.

Sanofi-Pasteur, and is in phase 1 clinical trials in Finland and South Africa.

M72

Two proteins contained in this vaccine, Mtb32 and Mtb39, were identified through screening T-cell and antibody responses in latently infected humans. The proteins were expressed as a recombinant fusion polyprotein designated Mtb72F.[47] This protein was developed as a candidate vaccine by GSK Biologicals, formulated in 2 different adjuvant systems, AS01B and AS02A. This vaccine was shown to induce good T-cell responses in various animal models and to protect mice, guinea pigs, rabbits and nonhuman primates after M tuberculosis challenge.[48,49] Several phase 1 and initial phase 2 clinical trials have now been completed. Results from the first phase 1 trial with Mtb72F/ ASO2A have recently been reported.[50] The vaccines induced good production of IL-2 and IFN-γ in the enzyme-linked immunosorbent spot (ELISPOT) assay, and CD4+ T cells expressing at least 2 activation markers (mainly CD40-L and IL-2 but also TNF-α and IFN-γ) were observed with an intracellular cytokine assay. The induced cell-mediated immune response persisted for at least 6 months post vaccination. Anti-Mtb72F antibodies were induced in all recipients. The tolerability profile was acceptable.

Vaccinia-based live-vectored vaccine: MVA85A

Viral vectors are attractive as TB vaccines as a Th1-dominated immune response to the expressed "foreign" antigen may be induced. In some cases, CD8 T-cell responses are also induced. The first live viral vectored TB vaccine to be tested in humans was MVA85A, a recombinant, replication-deficient vaccinia virus expressing Ag85A. Many clinical trials have already been completed with this vaccine, developed at the University of Oxford. It induces strong Th1 responses, and in BCG-vaccinated individuals, even those vaccinated many years earlier, MVA85A boosts previous immunity.[51] Only mild adverse events have been observed. Similar results were obtained in persons with latent M tuberculosis infection.[52] Some data suggest that previous exposure to vaccinia may reduce the efficacy of vaccinia-vectored vaccines.[53] MVA85A is now undergoing multiple phase 1/2 trials in Africa, including trials in patients infected with HIV, and a phase 2b trial in infants has recently started (July 2009) in Cape Town.

Adenovirus based live-vectored vaccine: AERAS-402 Ad35

The second virally vectored vaccine is AERAS-402 Ad35, a replication-deficient (E1-deleted) recombinant adenovirus-35 expressing Ag85A, Ag85B, and Tb-10.4, as a single fusion polyprotein.[54] The expressed antigens are present in BCG. This vaccine seems of particular interest for its ability to induce CD8 T-cell responses. Successful propagation of an rAd35 vector has been achieved on existing cell lines, such as PER.C6 cells, important for large-scale manufacturing of rAd35-based vaccines.[55] The first clinical trial started in 2007 and it is currently in several phase 1 clinical trials in the United States, Europe, and Africa, with phase 2b trials planned to start in 2009. Although there was evidence that previous natural exposure to a homologous or cross-reacting strain of adenovirus may hamper responses to adenovirus-based vaccines,[56] the first dose of Ad35-vectored vaccines may escape this limitation because this adenovirus serotype has a low prevalence (ranging from 3% to 5% in developed countries, to 20% in Africa).

Other subunit vaccines expected to be in clinical trials soon

HBHA HBHA is an interesting but challenging vaccine candidate. It is a mycobacterial surface protein that interacts specifically with nonphagocytic cells, expresses hemagglutination activity, and binds to sulfated glycoconjugates.[57] HBHA-deficient strains of *M tuberculosis* are significantly impaired in their ability to disseminate from the lungs to other tissues. This finding suggests that HBHA interaction with nonphagocytic cells, such as pulmonary epithelial cells, may play an important role in the extrapulmonary dissemination of *M tuberculosis*, a key step that may lead to latency.[58] Latently infected humans mount a strong T-cell response to HBHA, whereas patients with active disease do not.[26] Good HBHA-mediated protection has been shown in mouse challenge models. HBHA is a methylated protein and its antigenicity in latently infected patients, and its protective immunogenicity in animal models, strongly depends on the methylation pattern. In mice and man, HBHA-specific IFN-γ is produced by CD4 and CD8 T cells. BCG-derived HBHA is now produced and processed. It should enter clinical trials in 2011 (**Table 2**).

Therapeutic Vaccines

Vaccines that could accelerate or complement the effects of chemotherapy against TB would be welcome. Many attempts have been made, but particular caution against the Koch phenomenon (ie, disease exacerbation) has been in place.[59] Two different approaches are now tested in clinical trials: one based on the killed *Mycobacterium vaccae*, and the other on selected myobacterium antigens in a formulation called RUTI.

M vaccae

Whole heat-killed *M vaccae*, an environmental saprophyte, has been tested as an immunotherapeutic agent for TB. The compounds that trigger its immunostimulatory ability are not known, but elements of the cell wall skeleton may be responsible. The vaccine is usually given intradermally as a multidose series.

Preclinical studies have suggested that vaccination in mice induces Th1 and inhibits Th2 responses. Clinical studies have suggested that vaccination may improve radiological and clinical outcomes, decrease time to negative sputum culture, and improve cure rate in some patients with sputum culture-positive pulmonary TB, including patients with multidrug-resistant strains.[60]

Table 2
Leading subunit and vectored vaccine candidates

Leading Subunit and Vectored Vaccine Candidates	Profile	Adjuvant	Developers	Sponsors	Status
Ag85B-ESAT6 (H1)	Fusion recombinant protein	IC31	P. Andersen and SSI	TBVI	In phase 1 clinical trials
Ag85B-Tb-10.4 (H4)	Fusion recombinant protein	IC31	P. Andersen and SSI	Sanofi-Pasteur & AERAS	In phase 1 clinical trials
M72	Fusion recombinant protein (34 and 39 Kda)	AS01	GSK	GSK, AERAS and TBVI	In phase 1 clinical trials
HBHA	Methylated protein (latency antigen)	Tbd	Institut Pasteur Lille	TBVI	In preclinical studies
MVA85A (AERAS-485)	Live vectored antigens (MVA modified vaccinia)	None	A. Hill and University of Oxford	AERAS, WT and TBVI	In phase 2 clinical trials
Adeno35-Ag85A-B-TB-10.4 (AERAS-402)	Live vectored antigens (Adenovirus 35)	None	Crucell	AERAS	In phase 2 clinical trials

Geographic variations in the results have been striking. Three major randomized, placebo-controlled and partially blinded trials have been performed in Africa. The first, in South Africa, showed no M vaccae-related effects. The second trial, in Uganda, confirmed earlier observations of faster sputum conversion and better radiological clearance. The third trial, in Zambia and Malawi, showed a trend toward benefits in the treatment of HIV-seronegative patients but failed to show beneficial effects in HIV-seropositive patients.[61]

In the Tanzanian "DarDar" phase 3 trial, a randomized, placebo-controlled, double-blind study of 5 intradermal doses of M vaccae in 1975 HIV-infected BCG-exposed Tanzanian patients with CD4 counts less than or equal to 200/μL and no active TB, the rate of culture-confirmed TB was significantly lower and the time to development of definite TB significantly prolonged in vaccine recipients. There was no adverse effect on CD4 count, HIV viral load, or nontuberculosis clinical events. The trial found a significant reduction in cases of definite TB ($P = .027$); 33 occurred in the vaccine recipients compared with 52 in the placebo group, indicating a vaccine efficacy of 37%.[62]

RUTI

RUTI is a therapeutic vaccine developed in Spain.[63] M tuberculosis is grown under stress conditions and bacilli are then fragmented, detoxified, and formulated into liposomes. The therapeutic effect of the vaccine may be linked to the induction of a Th1 response, and stimulation of specific immunity against structural and growth-related antigens. Immunotherapy with RUTI following chemotherapy is designed to prevent reactivation of latent bacilli in the tissues, where local specific immunity may be suppressed. RUTI-treated mice and guinea pigs, infected with M tuberculosis showed (1) lower bacillary load, (2) less pulmonary infiltration, and (3) stronger immune responses, compared with controls given BCG. RUTI is now in phase 1 clinical trials.

ASSESSMENT OF NEW TB VACCINES: SAFETY AND REACTOGENICITY

Development plans for new TB vaccine candidates generally take longer than 10 years to complete, and include multiple clinical trials before licensure for use in the general public. This is an arduous, complex, expensive, and lengthy process. Safety is vital, and is a theme that runs throughout the plan. Some regulatory bodies have recognized the need for expedited development and approval pathways for new vaccines of

global importance.[64] The US Food and Drug Administration (FDA) can grant priority review of applications for the treatment and prevention of specified tropical diseases, including TB.[65]

Early phases of trials involve healthy volunteers who agree to undergo any medical testing necessary to assess the safety of the vaccine.[66] Enrolling healthy volunteers dictates a low tolerance for risk in these trials.[67]

The severity of clinical and laboratory abnormalities among these volunteers is best assessed using toxicity grading scales, which classify severity of specific clinical and laboratory adverse events. Stopping rules provide specific criteria for halting or stopping the trial. The use of uniform criteria for categorizing toxicities would improve comparisons of safety data within a study, and between different studies.[67]

Local, systemic, and potential end-organ toxicity are monitored. At clinic visits, symptoms and diary cards are reviewed and clinical examinations are performed. These examinations may be supplemented by photographs of vaccination sites to assess reactogenicity. Periodic laboratory studies monitor hematologic, biochemical, and endocrine parameters such as hepatic and renal function tests. Other tests may be required based on the results of preclinical toxicology studies and previous experience with similar vaccines.

Phase 1 Trials

Phase 1 clinical trials are designed primarily to investigate safety and identify common adverse events. They usually involve 20 to 100 volunteers who are followed for between 6 and 12 months. Immunogenicity is often measured, as a secondary outcome.

Concern about the possibility of inducing the so-called Koch phenomenon has meant that trials of new TB vaccines have generally started in participants who have been naive, or near-naive, for mycobacterial exposure, such as persons who are BCG naive, with no evidence of latent M tuberculosis infection, or living in areas with little exposure to TB or nontuberculous mycobacteria. The next step involves progressing to individuals vaccinated with BCG, next to individuals known to be latently infected with M tuberculosis, and ultimately to those with TB disease. Given that HIV-infected individuals are at highest risk of developing TB, it is important that the safety (and efficacy) of all new TB vaccines is also demonstrated in this group.

Even though most vaccines are destined for use in infants and children, trials always start in healthy adult volunteers. Some regulatory authorities insist on age de-escalation through all categories: adults to adolescents to older children to younger children to toddlers to infants. An ethical argument can be made against this de-escalation, because some of these groups which are being put at risk in the trials do not stand to benefit directly from the product.

Other phase 1 trials require test interference between the novel TB vaccine and existing vaccines in the extended program of immunization schedule, in safety and immunogenicity, from both sides. Trials may need to be done specifically to establish the optimum interval between prime vaccines (BCG or rBCG) and boost vaccines.

Phase 2 Trials

Phase 2 trials target populations that will be vaccinated in an efficacy trial, and again aim to assess safety, primarily, and immunogenicity.

Phase 2 trials involve several hundred participants, last from several months to 2 years, and usually also collect information on efficacy. Data gained from phase 2 trials can be used to decide on the final composition of the vaccine, how many doses are necessary, and to produce a profile of common adverse events.

Because of the huge cost of phase 3 trials, so-called proof of concept phase 2b trials may be planned to allow extended safety/immunogenicity and preliminary efficacy evaluation. Populations targeted for these trials need to have exceptionally high TB incidence rates (eg, 2%–5% per annum). The sample size is determined with a low power to detect a difference between a vaccine and placebo; if no trend toward a vaccine effect is shown, progress to a phase 3 trial is unlikely. Such trials are currently being planned for adults infected with HIV (n ~ 1000) and for infants (n ~ 3000).

Monitoring Vaccine Safety Postlicensure

Rare adverse events and delayed reactions of a new TB vaccine may not be evident until the vaccine is administered to millions of people. Postlicensure safety monitoring is essential to detect these and surveillance systems similar to the US Vaccine Adverse Event Reporting System (VAERS) may need to be devised and set up in countries with a high TB burden.

ASSESSING IMMUNOGENICITY IN NOVEL TB VACCINE TRIALS

As biomarkers of a protective immune response against TB are not known, the immune response induced by a novel vaccine should best be termed "vaccine take." Current assessment of vaccine take focuses on T-cell immunity believed to be important for protection. Specific CD4 T cells able to produce IFN-γ are critical for protection against TB, as shown in congenital and acquired human immune deficiency,[68,69] and in experimental models of mycobacterial disease. Therefore, specific IFN-γ production by CD4 T cells is measured in all current phase 1 trials of novel TB vaccines, either by an IFN-γ ELISPOT assay or by an intracellular cytokine staining (ICS) assay.

The IFN-γ ELISPOT detects production of cellular production of IFN-γ as "spots" in a well (Fig. 4).[70] Each spot represents cytokine production by a single cell, following incubation of peripheral blood mononuclear cells (PBMCs) with specific vaccine antigens within the well. It is likely that most spots originate from specific CD4 T cells, although natural killer cells may contribute. In contrast, flow cytometric ICS assays detect IFN-γ production specific to CD4 T cells, following incubation of whole blood or PBMC with specific antigens.[70] Multiparameter ICS assays allow assessment of multiple complementary T-cell outcomes. For example, CD4 T-cell production of IL-2 and TNF, and of the proinflammatory cytokine IL-17,[71,72] cytokines that may contribute to protection against TB, may be measured within the same sample (Fig. 5). In addition, activation of CD8 T cells, which may also be important for protection,[70] may be measured by ability to produce IFN-γ, IL-2, or TNF, following specific stimulation.

ELISPOT and ICS assays are classic examples of shorter-term assays, in which cells do not have time to proliferate, allowing a more quantitative assessment of outcome. Many other assays may be used to measure the T-cell response (recently summarized by Hanekom and colleagues[73]). Some assays have longer periods of incubation (5–7 days), which may allow better assessment of cells that require longer periods for activation, such as central memory T cells. The lymphocyte proliferation assay is a classic longer-term assay: PBMC are prestained with a dye such as carboxyfluorescein succinimidyl ester (CFSE), incubated with specific antigens for 5 to 7 days, and proliferation of CD4 or CD8 T cells measured by flow cytometry.[74] Every time the cell replicates it loses 50% of the original fluorescence intensity of the CFSE, allowing easy detection of expanded specific cells (Fig. 6).

Multiple variables determine assay success (summarized by Hanekom and colleagues[73]). For example, following blood collection, delay of incubation into assays or of PBMC isolation may compromise outcome. Use of freshly isolated PBMC allows greater sensitivity in measuring an immune response, compared with use of thawed PBMC after cryopreservation. Selecting peptide

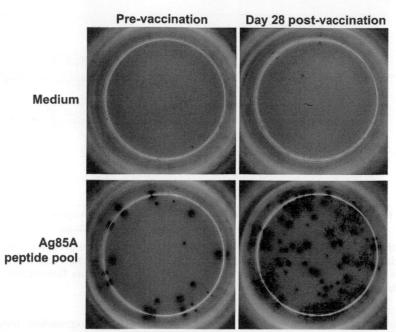

Fig. 4. Example of an IFN-γ ELISPOT assay to assess responses to a novel TB vaccine, MVA85A. PBMC were isolated from a healthy adult immediately before and 28 days after vaccination with MVA85A. The cells were incubated with medium alone or with Ag85A peptide pools for 20 hours. Each dark spot in the well represents a single cell making IFN-γ.

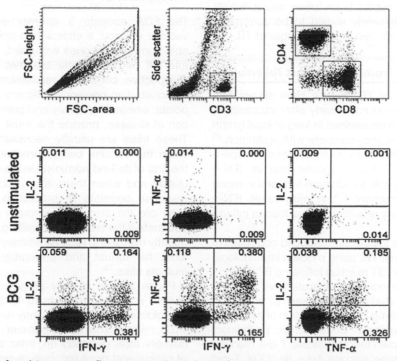

Fig. 5. Example of multiparameter flow cytometric analysis of BCG-induced immunity. Whole blood from a 10-week old infant, routinely vaccinated with BCG at birth, was left unincubated (unstimulated) or incubated with BCG for 12 hours. The gating strategy to detect CD4 and CD8 T cells is shown in the top row, and CD4 T cell-specific expression of IFN-γ, IL-2 an TNF-α is shown below that.

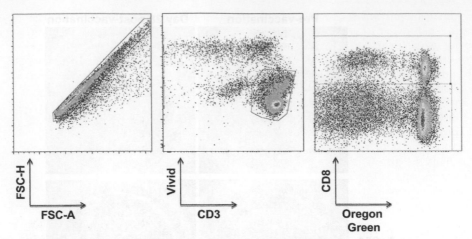

Fig. 6. Example of flow cytometric detection of proliferation, after incubation of Oregon Green-prestained PBMC with BCG for 5 days. On the left plot, singlet cells were gated, followed by CD3+ T cells in the middle plot. The right plot shows proliferating CD8 T and CD4 (CD8−) T cells, as cells with low fluorescence intensity for the Oregon Green dye.

versus recombinant protein versus whole bacterial (eg, BCG) antigen, and the dose of the antigen may significantly affect assay results. In most trials of novel TB vaccines, the choice of assay system depends largely on preferences of sponsors and local investigators; however, short-term ELISPOT and ICS assays are the most commonly used. A complementary strategy may involve cryopreservation of blood products for future measurement of outcomes ultimately shown to be surrogates of vaccination-induced protection against TB.

Biomarkers of Protection Against Tuberculosis

Animal models of TB disease have shown that specific IFN-γ production early after vaccination, particularly when determined in lung or local lymph node CD4 T cells, may correlate with protection.[75] However, results from multiple recent experimental studies caution against use of IFN-γ production as a sole vaccination-induced immune correlate of protection[76–78]: in many cases, IFN-γ production merely reflects bacterial load or inflammatory status.

In humans, no vaccination-induced correlates of protection against TB, using modern immunologic tools, exist. The TST reaction following BCG vaccination is a poor correlate of protection. The only large, ongoing study of biomarkers of protection against TB following BCG vaccination of newborns is currently ongoing in South Africa; preliminary results have shown that the classic T-cell markers used to determine vaccine take (ie, CD4 T-cell production of IFN-γ) do not correlate with protection. Other preliminary results suggest unbiased screening methods, such as DNA microarray

analysis of gene expression, may yield patterns that associate with protection; these approaches may ultimately allow discovery of novel correlates. These correlates may only be validated in a phase 3 trial of new TB vaccine that effectively protects against lung TB.

ASSESSMENT OF NEW TB VACCINES: EFFICACY

The FDA accepts 3 approaches to showing vaccine efficacy: a clinical end point, an acceptable immune response end point, or the "animal rule," if certain criteria are met. It is felt that prospective, controlled, randomized clinical trials demonstrating preventive efficacy for clinical end points, where the primary end point is the prevention of disease, provide the most scientific rigor. These trials are usually necessary in situations when the vaccine being considered is novel or the first of its kind administered to the target population and when there is no accepted immune response correlate of protection. Two efficacy trials are the standard, although 1 trial may be adequate if the result is compelling, as is not infrequently the case in vaccine efficacy trials. The data must be robust and preferably generated in multiple sites.[79]

Phase 3 trials of new TB vaccines will likely involve several thousands to tens of thousands of volunteers. Each trial may cost more than $100 million. The exact number of participants (sample size) depends on, inter alia, the choice of clinical end point (eg, culture-positive disease), the annual incidence rate of that end point in target populations at participating sites (eg, 2%), the predicted efficacy of the test vaccine (eg, 70%), and the length of follow-up envisaged. These trials likely take at least a year to enrol, and follow-up continues for a minimum of 18 to 24 months. This follow-up is particularly relevant to trials in infants and young children, in which the peak incidence of TB disease is expected to occur between 12 and 24 months of age. The prime BCG or rBCG vaccination likely occurs at birth, and the boost vaccine is given at around 3 to 4 months. Apart from providing an estimate of vaccine efficacy, these large trials are also able to detect adverse events that occur at low frequency (eg, <0.1%); control arms allow determination of whether these events are truly related to the test vaccine.

The necessity of using clinical end points raises some issues. In infants, TB disease is poorly characterized and consequently difficult to diagnose. Clinical signs and symptoms are nonspecific, radiographic findings are difficult to interpret (particularly in early disease, which is likely in a population under intense observation as in a clinical trial), a positive TB culture is obtained in only 30% to 40% of cases, and tests of TB infection (TST, interferon-gamma release assays) are unreliable and subject to confounding. It has therefore been difficult to construct a robust case definition for these trials. Similar problems beset trials planned for HIV-infected adult populations. The timely advent of a novel, more specific TB diagnostic would be most helpful. If the vaccine is being developed "under IND (Investigational New Drug Application)" with the FDA, as some of the new candidates are, which allows for ongoing dialog between regulator and developer concerning, inter alia, acceptable trial design, potential trial issues, subject selection, choice of control group, trial end points, vaccine dose, trial duration, concomitant medications, concomitant vaccines, and methods to be used in assessing safety, then some or most of these issues will be addressed (but not necessarily solved) in presubmission meetings.[80]

The preference by regulators for multicenter trials and the need for large numbers of participants has prompted groups such as the Aeras Global TB Vaccine Foundation and the European Developing Countries Trials Partnership (EDCTP) to sponsor development at multiple sites in sub-Saharan Africa and Asia in preparation for their involvement in phase 3 TB vaccine trials. Large epidemiologic cohort studies ("mock trials") are undertaken in likely target populations at the sites (eg, infants or adolescents). These studies allow for infrastructure and capacity to be built and more precise estimates of disease rates to be obtained. Site development is taking place or is planned at Worcester (South Africa), Palamaner (India), Syaya (Kenya), Iganga (Uganda), Manhica (Mozambique), and Svay Rieng (Cambodia) in partnership with local academic or research institutions or, in 1 case, a nongovernmental organization. All of these areas have an appreciable incidence of TB.

If the phase 2b trials started in or planned to start in 2009 or 2010 show encouraging results, the first phase 3 trial of a new TB vaccine could start as early as 2012.

SUMMARY

Decades after the discovery of M tuberculosis, a test for M tuberculosis infection, a vaccine against TB, and drugs to treat disease, TB remains a major cause of morbidity and mortality in many developing countries. The disease also poses a considerable risk in many developed countries. Efforts to control TB are seriously hampered by escalating rates of drug-resistant TB and the TB/HIV syndemic. Without improved tools, including a safer and more effective vaccine regimen, TB rates are unlikely to decline in high-burden countries. The field is not without significant challenges, including the lack of good animal models of disease, the absence of immune correlates of protection, the chronic nature of the disease itself, and the difficulties in making an accurate and reliable diagnosis of TB disease in vaccine target groups. Despite this, significant progress has been made. Several candidate vaccines have shown promise in preclinical studies and are now entering phase 1 to 2b clinical trials. More resources are being put into TB vaccine development now than at any time in the past. There is at least a reasonable prospect for a safer, more effective vaccination schedule to become standard of care within a decade.

REFERENCES

1. Ly LH, McMurray DN. Tuberculosis: vaccines in the pipeline. Expert Rev Vaccines 2008;7(5):635–50.
2. Newton SM, Brent AJ, Anderson S, et al. Paediatric tuberculosis. Lancet Infect Dis 2008;8(8):498–510.
3. Lönnroth K, Raviglione M. Global epidemiology of tuberculosis: prospects for control. Semin Respir Crit Care Med 2008;29(5):481–91.
4. Hoft DF. Tuberculosis vaccine development: goals, immunological design, and evaluation. Lancet 2008;372(9633):164–75 [Review].
5. Horwitz MA, Harth G, Dillon BJ, et al. Commonly administered BCG strains including an evolutionarily early strain and evolutionarily late strains of disparate genealogy induce comparable protective immunity against tuberculosis. Vaccine 2009;27(3):441–5.

6. Ritz N, Hanekom WA, Robins-Browne R, et al. Influence of BCG vaccine strain on the immune response and protection against tuberculosis. FEMS Microbiol Rev 2008;32(5):821–41.

7. Comstock GW. Field trials of tuberculosis vaccines: how could we have done them better? Control Clin Trials 1994;15(4):247–76.

8. Barreto ML, Pereira SM, Ferreira AA. BCG vaccine: efficacy and indications for vaccination and revaccination. J Pediatr (Rio J) 2006;82(3):S45–54.

9. Trunz BB, Fine P, Dye C. Effect of BCG vaccination on childhood tuberculous meningitis and miliary tuberculosis worldwide: a meta-analysis and assessment of cost-effectiveness. Lancet 2006; 367(9517):1173–80.

10. Colditz GA, Brewer TF, Berkey CS. Efficacy of BCG vaccine in the prevention of tuberculosis. Meta-analysis of the published literature. JAMA 1994;271(9): 698–702.

11. Colditz GA, Berkey CS, Mosteller F, et al. The efficacy of bacillus Calmette-Guérin vaccination of newborns and infants in the prevention of tuberculosis: meta-analyses of the published literature. Pediatrics 1995;96(1):29–35.

12. Brewer TF. Preventing tuberculosis with bacillus Calmette-Guérin vaccine: a meta-analysis of the literature. Clin Infect Dis 2000;31(3):S64–7.

13. Rodrigues LC, Diwan VK, Wheeler JG. Protective effect of BCG against tuberculous meningitis and miliary tuberculosis: a meta-analysis. Int J Epidemiol 1993;22(6):1154–8.

14. Crampin AC, Glynn JR, Fine PE. What has Karonga taught us? Tuberculosis studied over three decades. Int J Tuberc Lung Dis 2009;13(2):153–64.

15. Wilson ME, Fineberg HV, Colditz GA. Geographic latitude and the efficacy of bacillus Calmette-Guérin vaccine. Clin Infect Dis 1995;20(4):982–91.

16. Sterne JA, Rodrigues LC, Guedes IN. Does the efficacy of BCG decline with time since vaccination? Int J Tuberc Lung Dis 1998;2(3):200–7.

17. Karpelowsky JS, Alexander AG, Peek SD, et al. Surgical complications of bacille Calmette-Guérin (BCG) infection in HIV-infected children: time for a change in policy. S Afr Med J 2008;98(10):801–4.

18. Hesseling AC, Rabie H, Marais BJ, et al. Bacille Calmette-Guérin vaccine-induced disease in HIV-infected and HIV-uninfected children. Clin Infect Dis 2006;42(4):548–58.

19. Hesseling AC, Cotton MF, Marais BJ, et al. BCG and HIV reconsidered: moving the research agenda forward. Vaccine 2007;25(36):6565–8.

20. Mansoor N, Scriba TJ, de Kock M, et al. HIV-1 infection in infants severely impairs the immune response induced by Bacille Calmette-Guérin vaccine. J Infect Dis 2009;199(7):982–90.

21. Hesseling AC, Cotton MF, Fordham von Reyn C, et al. Consensus statement on the revised World Health Organization recommendations for BCG vaccination in HIV-infected infants. Int J Tuberc Lung Dis 2008;12(12):1376–9.

22. Hesseling AC, Marais BJ, Gie RP, et al. The risk of disseminated Bacille Calmette-Guerin (BCG) disease in HIV-infected children. Vaccine 2007; 25(1):14–8.

23. Farhat M, Greenaway C, Pai M, et al. False-positive tuberculin skin tests: what is the absolute effect of BCG and non-tuberculous mycobacteria? Int J Tuberc Lung Dis 2006;10(11):1192–204.

24. Wang L, Turner MO, Elwood RK, et al. A meta-analysis of the effect of Bacille Calmette Guérin vaccination on tuberculin skin test measurements. Thorax 2002;57(9):804–9.

25. Lin MY, Ottenhoff TH. Not to wake a sleeping giant: new insights into host-pathogen interactions identify new targets for vaccination against latent Mycobacterium tuberculosis infection. Biol Chem 2008; 389(5):497–511.

26. Locht C, Hougardy JM, Rouanet C, et al. Heparin-binding hemagglutinin, from an extrapulmonary dissemination factor to a powerful diagnostic and protective antigen against tuberculosis. Tuberculosis (Edinb) 2006;86(3–4):303–9.

27. Gilleron M, Stenger S, Mazorra Z, et al. Diacylated sulfoglycolipids are novel mycobacterial antigens stimulating CD1-restricted T cells during infection with Mycobacterium tuberculosis. J Exp Med 2004; 199(5):649–59.

28. Layre E, Collmann A, Bastian M, et al. Mycolic acids constitute a scaffold for mycobacterial lipid antigens stimulating CD1-restricted T cells. Chem Biol 2009; 16(1):82–92.

29. Kamath AT, Valenti MP, Rochat AF, et al. Protective anti-mycobacterial T cell responses through exquisite in vivo activation of vaccine-targeted dendritic cells. Eur J Immunol 2008;38(5):1247–56.

30. Horwitz MA, Harth G, Dillon BJ, et al. A novel live recombinant mycobacterial vaccine against bovine tuberculosis more potent than BCG. Vaccine 2006; 24(10):1593–600.

31. Hoft DF, Blazevic A, Abate G, et al. A new recombinant bacille Calmette-Guérin vaccine safely induces significantly enhanced tuberculosis-specific immunity in human volunteers. J Infect Dis 2008; 198(10):1491–501.

32. Grode L, Seiler P, Baumann S, et al. Increased vaccine efficacy against tuberculosis of recombinant Mycobacterium bovis bacille Calmette-Guérin mutants that secrete listeriolysin. J Clin Invest 2005;115(9):2472–9.

33. Winau F, Weber S, Sad S, et al. Apoptotic vesicles crossprime CD8 T cells and protect against tuberculosis. Immunity 2006;24(1):105–17.

34. Soto CY, Menendez MC, Perez E, et al. IS6110 mediates increased transcription of the phoP virulence

gene in a multidrug-resistant clinical isolate responsible for tuberculosis outbreaks. J Clin Microbiol 2004;42:212–9.

35. Martin C, Williams A, Hernandez-Pando R, et al. The live *Mycobacterium tuberculosis* phoP mutant strain is more attenuated than BCG and confers protective immunity against tuberculosis in mice and guinea pigs. Vaccine 2006;24(17):3408–19.

36. Larsen MH, Biermann K, Chen B, et al. Efficacy and safety of live attenuated persistent and rapidly cleared *Mycobacterium tuberculosis* vaccine candidates in non-human primates. Vaccine 2009;27(34):4709–17.

37. Waters WR, Palmer MV, Nonnecke BJ, et al. Failure of a *Mycobacterium tuberculosis* DeltaRD1 DeltapanCD double deletion mutant in a neonatal calf aerosol *M bovis* challenge model: comparisons to responses elicited by *M. bovis* bacille Calmette Guerin. Vaccine 2007;25(45):7832–40.

38. Verreck FA, Vervenne RA, Kondova I, et al. MVA85A boosting of BCG and an attenuated, phoP deficient *M tuberculosis* vaccine both show protective efficacy against tuberculosis in rhesus macaques. PLoS One 2009;4(4):e5264.

39. Camacho LR, Constant P, Raynaud C, et al. Analysis of the phthiocerol dimycocerosate locus of *Mycobacterium tuberculosis*. Evidence that this lipid is involved in the cell wall permeability barrier. J Biol Chem 2001;276(23):19845–54.

40. Sambandamurthy VK, Derrick SC, Hsu T, et al. *Mycobacterium tuberculosis* DeltaRD1 DeltapanCD: a safe and limited replicating mutant strain that protects immunocompetent and immunocompromised mice against experimental tuberculosis. Vaccine 2006;24(37–39):6309–20.

41. Weinrich Olsen A, van Pinxteren LAH, Meng Okkels L, et al. Protection of mice with a tuberculosis subunit vaccine based on a fusion protein of antigen 85b and esat-6. Infect Immun 2001;69:2773–8.

42. Reed S, Lobet Y. Tuberculosis vaccine development; from mouse to man. Microbes Infect 2005; 7(5–6):922–31.

43. Langermans JA, Doherty TM, Vervenne RA, et al. Protection of macaques against *Mycobacterium tuberculosis* infection by a subunit vaccine based on a fusion protein of antigen 85B and ESAT-6. Vaccine 2005;23:2740–50.

44. Williams A, Hatch GJ, Clark SO, et al. Evaluation of vaccines in the EU TB Vaccine Cluster using a guinea pig aerosol infection model of tuberculosis. Tuberculosis (Edinb) 2005;85(1–2):29–38.

45. Lingnau K, Riedl K, von Gabain A. IC31 and IC30, novel types of vaccine adjuvant, based on peptide delivery systems. Expert Rev Vaccines 2007;6: 741–6.

46. Aagaard C, Dietrich J, Doherty M, et al. TB vaccines: current status and future perspectives. Immunol Cell Biol 2009;87(4):279–86.

47. Skeiky YA, Lodes MJ, Guderian JA, et al. Cloning, expression, and immunological evaluation of two putative secreted serine protease antigens of *Mycobacterium tuberculosis*. Infect Immun 1999;67: 3998–4007.

48. Skeiky YA, Alderson MR, Ovendale PJ, et al. Differential immune responses and protective efficacy induced by components of a tuberculosis polyprotein vaccine, Mtb72F, delivered as naked DNA or recombinant protein. J Immunol 2004; 172:7618–28.

49. Reed SG, Coler RN, Dalemans W, et al. Defined tuberculosis vaccine, Mtb72F/AS02A, evidence of protection in cynomolgus monkeys. Proc Natl Acad Sci U S A 2009;106(7):2301–6.

50. Von Eschen K, Morrison R, Braun M, et al. The candidate tuberculosis vaccine Mtb72F/AS02A: Tolerability and immunogenicity in humans. Hum Vaccin 2009;5:7.

51. McShane H, Pathan AA, Sander CR, et al. Recombinant modified vaccinia virus Ankara expressing antigen 85A boosts BCG-primed and naturally acquired antimycobacterial immunity in humans. Nat Med 2004;10:1240–4.

52. Sander CR, Pathan AA, Beveridge NE, et al. Safety and immunogenicity of a new TB vaccine, MVA85A, in *M tuberculosis* infected individuals. Am J Respir Crit Care Med 2009;179(8):724–33.

53. Rooney JF, Wohlenberg C, Cremer KJ, et al. Immunization with a vaccinia virus recombinant expressing herpes simplex virus type 1 glycoprotein D: long-term protection and effect of revaccination. J Virol 1988;62:1530–4.

54. Radosevic K, Wieland CW, Rodriguez A, et al. Protective immune responses to an rAd35 TB vaccine in two mouse strains (H-2d vs H-2b): CD4 and CD8 T-cell epitope mapping and role of IFNγ. Infect Immun 2007;75:4105–15.

55. Havenga M, Vogels R, Zuijdgeest D, et al. Novel replication-incompetent adenoviral B-group vectors: high vector stability and yield in PER.C6 cells. J Gen Virol 2006;87(8):2135–43.

56. Bangari DS, Mittal SK. Development of nonhuman adenoviruses as vaccine vectors. Vaccine 2006; 24(7):849–62.

57. Menozzi FD, Rouse JH, Alavi M, et al. Identification of a heparin-binding hemagglutinin present in mycobacteria. J Exp Med 1996;184:993–1001.

58. Pethe K, Alonso S, Biet F, et al. The heparin-binding haemagglutinin of *M tuberculosis* is required for extrapulmonary dissemination. Nature 2001;412: 190–4.

59. Rook GA, Stanford JL. The Koch phenomenon and the immunopathology of tuberculosis. Curr Top Microbiol Immunol 1996;215:239–62.

60. Dlugovitzky D, Fiorenza G, Farroni M, et al. Immunological consequences of three doses of heat-killed

M vaccae in the immunotherapy of tuberculosis. Respir Med 2006;100(6):1079–87.

61. Stanford J, Stanford C, Grange J. Immunotherapy with *Mycobacterium vaccae* in the treatment of tuberculosis. Front Biosci 2004;9:1701–19.

62. Von Reyn CF, et al. The DarDar prime-boost TB vaccine trial in HIV infection: final results [abstract PS-81689-20] in conference abstract book: 39th World Conference on Lung Health of the International Union against Tuberculosis and Lung Disease, Paris. Int J Tuberc Lung Dis 2008;12(11 S 2):S318.

63. Cardona PJ. RUTI: a new chance to shorten the treatment of latent tuberculosis infection. Tuberculosis (Edinb) 2006;86(3–4):273–89.

64. Tiernan R. Regulatory perspective on development of preventive vaccines for global infectious diseases review. Available at: http://www.fda.gov/downloads/BiologicsBloodVaccines/NewsEvents/WorkshopsMeetingsConferences/UCM106632.pdf. Accessed March 21, 2009.

65. US Food and Drug Administration, Center for Biologics Evaluation and Research. Guidance for industry. General principles for the development of vaccines to protect against global infectious diseases. Available at: http://www.fda.gov/cber/gdlns/gidvacc.htm; Aug 2008. Accessed March 22, 2009.

66. Centers for Disease Control and Prevention. History of vaccine safety. 28 Feb 2008. Available at: http://www.cdc.gov/vaccinesafety/basic/history.htm%237. Accessed May 24, 2009.

67. US Food and Drug Administration, Center for Biologics Evaluation and Research. Guidance for industry toxicity grading scale for healthy adult and adolescent volunteers enrolled in preventive vaccine clinical trials. Available at: http://www.fda.gov/cber/gdlns/toxvac.htm. Accessed March 22, 2009.

68. Al-Muhsen S, Casanova JL. The genetic heterogeneity of Mendelian susceptibility to mycobacterial diseases. J Allergy Clin Immunol 2008;122:1043–51.

69. Lawn SD, Myer L, Edwards D, et al. Short-term and long-term risk of tuberculosis associated with CD4 cell recovery during antiretroviral therapy in South Africa. AIDS 2009 Aug 24;23(13):1717–25.

70. Hawkridge T, Scriba TJ, Gelderbloem S, et al. Safety and immunogenicity of a new tuberculosis vaccine,

MVA85A, in healthy adults in South Africa. J Infect Dis 2008;198:544–52.

71. Scriba TJ, Kalsdorf B, Abrahams DA, et al. Distinct, specific IL-17- and IL-22-producing CD4+ T cell subsets contribute to the human anti-mycobacterial immune response. J Immunol 2008;180:1962–70.

72. Chen CY, Huang D, Wang RC, et al. A critical role for CD8 T cells in a nonhuman primate model of tuberculosis. PLoS Pathog 2009;5(4):e1000392.

73. Hanekom WA, Dockrell HM, Ottenhoff TH, et al. Immunological outcomes of new tuberculosis vaccine trials: WHO panel recommendations. PLoS Med 2008;5(7):e145.

74. Beveridge NE, Price DA, Casazza JP, et al. Immunisation with BCG and recombinant MVA85A induces long-lasting, polyfunctional *Mycobacterium tuberculosis*-specific CD4+ memory T lymphocyte populations. Eur J Immunol 2007;37(11):3089–100.

75. Hanekom WA, Ernst JD. Maintenance of latent infection, with correlates of protective immunity. In: Kaufmann SHE, Britton WJ, editors. Handbook of tuberculosis: immunology and cell biology. Weinheim: Wiley-VCH; 2008. p. 279.

76. Bennekov T, Dietrich J, Rosenkrands I, et al. Alteration of epitope recognition pattern in Ag85B and ESAT-6 has a profound influence on vaccine-induced protection against *Mycobacterium tuberculosis*. Eur J Immunol 2006;36(12):3346–55.

77. Forbes EK, Sander C, Ronan EO, et al. Multifunctional, high-level cytokine-producing Th1 cells in the lung, but not spleen, correlate with protection against *Mycobacterium tuberculosis* aerosol challenge in mice. J Immunol 2008;181(7):4955–64.

78. Mittrucker HW, Steinhoff U, Kohler A, et al. Poor correlation between BCG vaccination-induced T cell responses and protection against tuberculosis. Proc Natl Acad Sci U S A 2007;104(30):12434–9.

79. US Food and Drug Administration. Center for Biologics Evaluation and Research: Guidance for industry: providing clinical evidence of effectiveness for human drugs and biological products. May 1998. Available at: http://www.fda.gov/BiologicsBloodVaccines/GuidanceComplianceRegulatoryInformation/Guidances/Vaccines/ucm074762.htm.

80. Brennan MJ, Sizemore C, Morris SL. Tuberculosis vaccine development: research, regulatory and clinical strategies. Expert Opin Biol Ther 2004;4(9):1493–504.

Screening and Preventive Therapy for Tuberculosis

Ben J. Marais, MMed Paed, FCPaed(SA), PhD[a],*,
Helen Ayles, MD, PhD[b,c], Stephen M. Graham, MD, PhD[d,e],
Peter Godfrey-Faussett, MD, PhD[b,c]

KEYWORDS

• Tuberculosis • Screening • Preventive therapy
• Prophylaxis • Latent infection

The tuberculosis (TB) epidemic is well controlled in most developed countries and the focus in these areas has shifted to TB eradication. Transmission within nonendemic areas is limited and most cases of TB result from reactivation of distant (latent) infection. With adequate resources, wide-scale use of preventive therapy can assist to eliminate the pool of latent infection that is required for TB eradication. In contrast, TB control remains poor in many developing countries, especially those worst affected by poverty and the human immunodeficiency virus (HIV) epidemic.

This dichotomy demonstrates the need for rational approaches tailored to the situation in TB-endemic areas where epidemic control and morbidity/mortality reduction are the primary aims. Differences in transmission dynamics and the availability of resources imply careful consideration of feasibility and prioritization of interventions. High rates of ongoing transmission persist in TB-endemic areas making it impossible to eliminate the pool of latent infection. Poor epidemic control and limited resources require TB-endemic areas to focus preventive therapy strategies on those individuals who are at greatest risk of progressing to active disease.

In this review the authors critically assess the approach to TB preventive therapy in children and adults, focus on the underlying treatment rationale, discuss available data, and identify issues of concern. There is strong evidence of efficacy and tolerance of preventive therapy in these populations. Preventive therapy for all high-risk individuals following documented exposure to TB should be regarded as the standard of care. However, there is limited evidence of effectiveness because implementation and adherence are often poor. In resource-limited settings, excluding active disease in HIV-infected individuals and the additional burden on health care services are particular challenges. There is a need to implement and evaluate preventive therapy strategies in various settings to better inform policy and practice.

BACKGROUND

It is difficult to grasp the full scale of the global TB epidemic. An estimated 10.4 million cases (new and recurrent) and 1.8 million deaths were attributed to TB in 2007.[1] Great strides have been made in the last 15 years to scale up diagnostic and treatment services, but the effect on the

Conflicts of interest: None to declare.
[a] Department of Paediatrics and Child Health, Faculty of Health Sciences, Stellenbosch University, PO Box 19063, Tygerberg 7505, South Africa
[b] Clinical Research Unit, Department of Infectious and Tropical Disease, London School of Hygiene and Tropical Medicine (LSHTM), London, UK
[c] ZAMBART Project, University of Zambia, Lusaka, Zambia
[d] Department of Paediatrics, Centre for International Child Health, Murdoch Children's Research Institute, Royal Children's Hospital, University of Melbourne, Victoria, Australia
[e] International Union Against Tuberculosis and Lung Disease, Paris, France
* Corresponding author.
E-mail address: bjmarais@sun.ac.za (B.J. Marais).

Clin Chest Med 30 (2009) 827–846
doi:10.1016/j.ccm.2009.08.012
0272-5231/09/$ – see front matter © 2009 Published by Elsevier Inc.

epidemic remains limited in poor countries where TB is most prevalent. Although incidence rates per capita are starting to decrease, the absolute number of cases continues to increase because of increases in population size.[1] Incidence rates in HIV-endemic countries are also showing a slow decline, but rates remain at very high levels.[1,2] The dichotomy that exists between high-income countries where incidence rates are less than 10/100,000 and low-income TB-endemic countries where incidence rates exceed 100/100,000 justifies critical assessment of current approaches and the identification of optimal strategies tailored to specific situations. Strategies need to consider feasibility issues and how different levels of epidemic control influence the rationale that guides the implementation of effective screening and preventive therapy programs.

Nonendemic Areas

Transmission within these areas is limited and most cases of TB disease occur among immigrant populations, the socially destitute, and the elderly.[3] Immune-compromised individuals are at increased risk for TB but their risk of TB exposure is low. Therefore, most cases of TB disease result from reactivation of distant (latent) infection. With adequate resources, preventive therapy can assist to eliminate the pool of latent infection. Comprehensive screening of all contacts of active TB cases is often feasible. Methods to identify those infected by the index case, such as the tuberculin skin test (TST), are more specific as an indicator of recent infection in nonendemic settings where TB transmission is uncommon and bacillus Calmette-Guérin (BCG) vaccination often not used. Low rates of transmission imply limited risk of future reinfection. These factors provide a strong rationale for the treatment of all cases with latent infection. To reduce the risk of transmission from imported TB cases, new immigrant control measures require screening and treatment of TB disease in the country of origin.

Endemic Areas

High rates of transmission persist in TB-endemic areas. Directly observed therapy, short-course (DOTS)-based programs failed to report an estimated 3.7 million cases of TB in 2007, including 1.5 million with sputum smears positive for TB representing 40% of incident cases.[1] Although some of these estimated cases may have received undocumented care, ongoing transmission in TB-endemic areas is sustained by a high prevalence of undiagnosed TB and prolonged diagnostic delay. The level of ongoing transmission equates to the infection pressure that exists within communities.

The TST has traditionally been used in surveys on TB infection to provide an estimation of the annual risk of TB infection (ARTI) in a population. ARTI studies provide a good assessment of accumulated primary (first time) TB infection rates and infection pressure among children despite sensitivity and specificity constraints using the TST. However, a major limitation of ARTI studies is that they typically enroll primary school children. This age restriction introduces selection bias and ARTI surveys probably represent a significant underestimate of the infection pressure experienced by adolescents and adults within the same community, especially among those with high-risk social behavior. The selection of primary school children is necessitated by the inability of the TST to register a reinfection event. Because many adolescents and adults in TB-endemic areas are already infected with *Mycobacterium tuberculosis*, it is impossible to determine their risk of reinfection or quantify the infection pressure that they are exposed to. Confirmation of the high infection pressure that exists in endemic areas is provided by molecular epidemiology studies, which demonstrated that exogenous reinfection is the most common cause of recurrent TB in some settings.[4,5] The risk of reinfection has relevance because it determines the ability to eliminate the pool of latent infection and the duration of benefit derived from the treatment of latent infection.

Contrary to most diseases preventable by vaccine, previous TB infection or disease offers no protection against future infection or disease. In fact, TB patients are at increased risk of recurrent TB compared with those who never had TB before,[6] which may reflect increased vulnerability and/or increased likelihood of repeat exposure. Comstock[7] demonstrated that it is possible to break the reinfection cycle with a successful TB eradication program among the Inuit population in northern Canada. The intervention was able to eliminate the pool of latent infection (by provision of preventive therapy) and terminate ongoing transmission (by treating all TB cases) at the same time, which explains its long-lasting impact. However, although this public health intervention provides proof of principle, it is important to emphasize that it was achieved in a geographically remote area where the entire population was screened in a short period of time and provided with either TB treatment or preventive therapy. It seems impossible to replicate these findings in less isolated TB-endemic areas where continuous population mixing would facilitate reinfection even if the pool of latent infection were successfully eradicated in 1 part of the population.

These differences between and within settings of varying TB endemicity explain why achievable aims should be carefully formulated. The provision of preventive therapy to all infected individuals may be warranted in nonendemic areas, but limited resources and ongoing transmission require endemic areas to focus on populations at greatest risk of progression to disease. This review provides a comprehensive overview of preventive therapy strategies in children and adults, and the different variables to consider in endemic versus nonendemic areas.

Clarification of Terminology

Terms such as "treatment of latent infection," "chemoprophylaxis," and "preventive therapy" are often used interchangeably, which obscures some important differences. Controlled trials have largely focused on preventing progression to active disease in those already infected, an approach referred to as "treatment of latent infection." The exact meaning of "latent infection" remains a topic of discussion and debate.[8,9] The treatment rationale is to provide a limited course (either in duration or number of drugs) of chemotherapy with the main aim of sterilizing existing subclinical lesions and preventing future progression to disease. "Chemoprophylaxis" (genuine primary prevention) aims to prevent new infections from becoming established and only provides protection during the period of exposure. Recurrent TB may be prevented by "secondary prophylaxis," which is provided after successful completion of TB treatment and may serve a dual function. First, secondary prophylaxis may reduce relapse disease as a result of improved sterilization achieved with prolonged duration of therapy. Second, it may reduce reinfection disease by preventing reinfection events from becoming established (analogous to primary chemoprophylaxis) during the period of secondary prophylaxis. "Preventive therapy" is a blanket term that incorporates chemoprophylaxis, treatment of latent infection, and secondary prophylaxis.

PEDIATRIC PERSPECTIVE

In TB control, the treatment of children is not considered a priority in endemic areas, as they rarely transmit disease and contribute little to the maintenance of the TB epidemic. Given the diagnostic difficulties and poor reporting systems in endemic areas, accurate quantification of the global pediatric TB disease burden is impossible.[10] In a community-based survey from South Africa, children (<13 years of age) contributed 13.7% of the total disease burden with a calculated incidence of TB of 408/100,000/y (about 50% of the total adult incidence of TB of 840/100,000/y).[11] Childhood TB is generally a mild disease if diagnosed early. However, autopsy results from Zambia demonstrated that advanced TB rivals bacterial pneumonia as a major cause of death from respiratory disease in children; these findings probably reflect the reality in most TB-endemic areas.[12] A major part of this disease burden is preventable if feasible and effective preventive therapy strategies can be implemented. Children in HIV-affected areas are experiencing increased exposure at a young and vulnerable age as a result of changing TB epidemiology. HIV infection introduced a pronounced age and gender shift with more young adults and especially women of child-bearing age developing TB, which increases the risk of exposure in young children.[13–15]

Risk of Infection

M tuberculosis is usually acquired by inhalation, following exposure to an index case with infectious TB. The risk of infection (TST positivity) among child contacts is associated with the proximity and duration of contact, and the degree of lung involvement and/or sputum smear positivity of the index case.[16–19] Cases with positive sputum smears pose the greatest transmission risk, although patients with pulmonary TB with negative sputum smears can also transmit disease, albeit at a reduced rate. Higher infection rates have been reported in child contacts of primary caregivers with TB, such as mothers or grandmothers.[18,20] This may have particular relevance in HIV-affected communities, where the transmission risk posed by a primary caregiver with a negative sputum smear should be taken into consideration.[15,21] Other studies demonstrated a relationship with crowding and sleeping arrangements.[19] The level of transmission within a community determines the rate at which TST positivity increases with age, and the potential value of the TST as a measure of recent infection. TB-endemic countries such as India, Indonesia, and Malawi report ARTIs of around 1% to 2%,[22–24] and ARTIs in excess of 4% have been reported in some hyper-endemic South African communities.[25,26]

In endemic areas transmission frequently occurs outside of the household, especially in older children.[27–29] This is different from nonendemic areas where TB infection usually occurs in an identifiable setting such as the home or school.[17,30] Irrespective of the setting, TB infection and/or disease in young children is associated with an identifiable adult index case in most instances, because social contact is restricted during the first years of life. The risk of TB infection in children from families affected by HIV/AIDS is likely to be substantially increased, because TB is the most common opportunistic infection in TB-endemic areas and most cases of TB/HIV coinfection occur in young adults (20–40 years of age) who are often parents themselves.[14] This is confirmed by the exceptionally high rates of TB exposure recorded among South African infants born to HIV-infected mothers.[15] Other modes of transmission include in utero transplacental infection, which presents as congenital TB in the newborn.[31] TB during and shortly after pregnancy is increasingly being described in HIV-infected mothers, which poses a risk of pre- and postpartum infection to the baby[14,31]; the risk also extends to other mothers and newborns cared for in the same facility.[32]

Risk of Disease

Once infected, the risk of a child developing TB is related to the maturation and competence of the immune system, especially of cell-mediated immunity. Natural history data indicate that young age is a major risk factor for the development of TB disease following primary infection. The risk for disease following documented infection was 40% to 50% during infancy, 25% if infected in the second year of life, less than 10% for the 2- to 5-year age group, and only 2% for those 5 to 10 years of age.[33] The routine use of neonatal BCG vaccination has reduced the risk of severe disseminated disease, such as TB meningitis and miliary TB, but the risk in endemic areas remains high and BCG has failed to reduce the prevalence of adult-type TB, which sustains the TB epidemic.[34] Most children who are infected with TB remain asymptomatic and never progress to disease. Of those who do develop disease, the vast majority (>95%) do so in the first year after infection and develop progressive symptoms suggestive of disease.[33] However, HIV infection is an important risk factor for TB disease in all age groups that was not reflected in the early pre-chemotherapy studies. Immune-compromised HIV-infected children are at the same high risk as very young children, and are vulnerable to developing disease following primary infection, reinfection, or reactivation of distant latent infection.[14,35]

Prospective data from South Africa indicate that the risk of culture-confirmed and disseminated TB is around 20 times higher among HIV-infected compared with uninfected infants[36]; a similar magnitude of risk was calculated in a previous retrospective study.[37] Clinical data from settings endemic for TB/HIV indicate that HIV infection is common in children with culture-confirmed TB. However, the ratio of HIV-infected children is generally lower than in adults because relatively fewer children are infected with HIV and young children are highly vulnerable to develop TB irrespective of their HIV status.[14,35] The relationship between malnutrition and TB is difficult to quantify because of overlapping epidemiologic associations, cause-effect confounding, and frequent inability to confirm TB in settings where these co-morbidities occur.

Rationale for Preventive Therapy

The most effective means to prevent TB infection in children is to improve epidemic control. Early detection and cure of infectious cases reduces transmission, which should reduce the high reproductive rate that sustains the epidemic. This explains why a well-functioning National TB Control Programme (NTP) with a strong focus on early diagnosis and effective management of the most infectious cases is critical to protect children.[21,22] However, with poor epidemic control and ongoing transmission TB will remain an important preventable cause of childhood morbidity and mortality.[35,38] Therefore, opportunities to prevent TB disease in susceptible children should form an important part of efforts to reduce mortality in children less than 5 years of age in TB-endemic areas. The high risk of infection and disease in children exposed to TB provides the rationale for recommendations from the World Health Organization (WHO), the International Union Against TB and Lung Disease (IUATLD) and the Centers for Disease Control and Prevention (CDC) to make preventive therapy available to all high-risk close contacts.[39–41]

Screening for Disease

Contact screening represents an important opportunity to identify new cases of TB and educate people about the disease. All close contacts, irrespective of age, should be informed of their exposure and encouraged to return for formal evaluation should they develop symptoms suspicious of TB in the coming months and years. The long delay between TB exposure and subsequent development of disease often obscures exposure-disease relationships and may induce a false sense of security among contacts in whom active disease has been ruled out. Screening is rarely performed in endemic areas, because of limited awareness of its benefits and inability to perform prerequisite screening tests.[42] The natural history of TB in children demonstrates that transient hilar adenopathy is a common finding following recent primary infection, with only a small percentage of these children developing progressive disease. This suggests that asymptomatic hilar adenopathy is a natural component of the primary (Ghon) complex, reflecting recent M tuberculosis infection rather than TB disease.[33,43] By convention, asymptomatic hilar adenopathy is currently treated as TB disease in most countries, but experience during public health trials in the United States in the 1950s demonstrated that isoniazid (INH) monotherapy should be sufficient.[44]

Lack of capacity to perform TST and chest radiograph-based screening is a barrier to the provision of preventive therapy. Symptom-based screening (**Fig. 1**) may offer a feasible alternative and has been promoted by the WHO for initial screening in resource-limited settings.[39] In a recent survey in South Africa, about 70% of child TB contacts were completely asymptomatic at the

time of screening.[45] The TST result did not influence patient management and none of the asymptomatic children had signs of complicated or progressive disease on chest radiography, indicating likely adequacy of preventive therapy in all asymptomatic children. This suggests that asymptomatic high-risk contacts should be offered immediate access to preventive therapy even if additional screening tests are unavailable. Additional investigations could be reserved for the minority with symptoms suggestive of TB and those who may develop these symptoms while receiving preventive therapy. The current algorithm does not indicate the need for and timing of an HIV test, although in settings endemic for TB/HIV all children with symptoms suggestive of HIV infection and/or TB disease should be tested for HIV. Children of a parent known to be infected with HIV should also be tested. HIV testing should be done at the initial screening, because it influences the management of the child. If TB disease is excluded in an HIV-infected child, both TB and cotrimoxazole preventive therapy should be

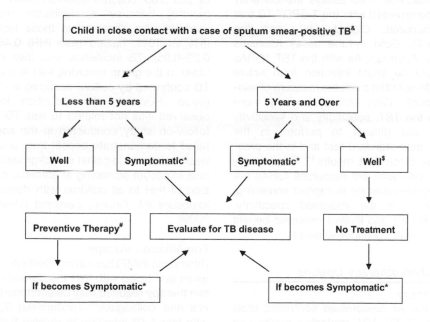

&Also consider if the mother or primary caregiver has sputum smear-negative pulmonary TB
*Symptomatic: If TB is suspected, refer to local guidelines on diagnosis of childhood TB
#Isoniazid 10/mg/kg daily for 6 months
$Unless the child is HIV-infected (in which case isoniazid 10/mg/kg daily for 6 months is indicated)

Fig. 1. Suggested approach to contact management when chest radiography and tuberculin skin testing are not readily available. (*Adapted from* World Health Organization. Guidance for national tuberculosis programmes on the management of tuberculosis in children. World Health Organization 2006; with permission. Available at: http://whqlibdoc.who.int/hq/2006/WHO_HTM_TB_2006.371_eng.pdf.)

provided and the child assessed for initiation of antiretroviral therapy. TB disease should be ruled out if the child develops symptoms suggestive of TB at any time.

A positive TST simply indicates TB infection and contributes no additional information other than a history of close contact with a case of infectious TB. The limitations of a negative TST test are well known especially in malnourished, HIV-infected, or sick children with possible disseminated disease. As a result of suboptimal sensitivity and because TST conversion can be delayed for 2 to 3 months, preventive therapy is indicated in all high-risk contacts irrespective of the initial TST result. Repeat TST may help to rule out the possibility of TB infection in an immune-competent child guiding early termination of preventive therapy, but this is rarely feasible in resource-limited settings. Interferon-gamma release assays (IGRAs) are an alternative to the TST. T cells are stimulated with *M tuberculosis*–specific antigens including early secreted antigenic target 6 (ESAT-6) and culture filtrate protein 10 (CFP-10), which are not found in *M bovis* BCG and most environmental mycobacteria. Two assays are currently available as commercial kits: the T-SPOT.*TB* test (Oxford Immunotec, Oxford, UK), and the QUANTIferon-TB Gold In-tube assay (Cellestis Ltd, Carnegie, Australia). As with the TST, IGRAs fail to differentiate latent infection from active disease and do not offer a reliable measure of reinfection. Although IGRAs are supposedly more specific than the TST, specificity and sensitivity assessments are difficult to perform in the absence of a gold standard test and in the presence of highly discordant results.[46–48] In nonendemic areas with sufficient resources IGRAs are currently recommended for immigrant screening, mainly because of the improved specificity. However, high cost and limited expected benefit precludes its use in TB-endemic areas.

Preventive Chemotherapy Options

INH monotherapy

A meta-analysis of randomized controlled trials that included 73,375 HIV-uninfected adults and children found that INH preventive therapy reduced the risk of disease by 60% (relative risk [RR] 0.40, 95% confidence interval [CI] 0.31–0.52) compared with placebo, and that there was no significant difference between 6- and 12-month courses.[49] A large prospective study over 30 years observed 1882 TB-infected children in the United States who received INH for 9 to 18 months and were followed up for a mean of 6.1 years.[50,51] Only 8 children developed overt disease,

a morbidity rate of 4.2/1000 persons; 7 of 8 were adolescents with pulmonary TB in whom re-infection could not be ruled out and one had documented INH resistance. None of the children infected before the age of 4 years developed disease, demonstrating high levels of protection compared with natural history data.[33] Available efficacy data support current recommendations for 6 to 9 months of INH. However, effective implementation requires strategies that will ensure optimal adherence. Most NTP manuals recommend screening of child contacts and provision of INH to at-risk children, but implementation is often nonexistent or very poor.[52] Even in nonendemic areas with adequate resources such as the United States, contact management does not always reach recommended targets of coverage.[53]

The efficacy of INH preventive therapy in adults with TB/HIV coinfection is discussed in detail in the next section. One study investigated the effect of universal INH given to all HIV-infected infants, irrespective of documented TB exposure.[54] The placebo arm was discontinued after recruitment of just 263 children (median follow-up of 5.7 months) because a significant reduction in mortality was observed in those receiving INH (8% vs 16%, hazard ratio (HR) 0.46, 95% CI 0.22–0.95). TB incidence was also significantly lower in the group receiving INH and all cases of TB confirmed by culture occurred in the placebo group. However, the reduction in mortality observed was not related to less TB disease. A follow-on study conducted in the same setting failed to demonstrate benefit from universal INH, when conducted against a background of meticulous exposure screening at enrollment and provision of INH to all children with documented TB exposure (M. Cotton, personal communication, 2009).

Combination therapy

Rifampicin (RMP) has strong sterilizing activity and when combined with INH the duration of preventive therapy required may be shortened.[55,56] Spyridis and colleagues[57] randomized 926 children with latent TB infection to receive 9 months INH versus 4 or 3 months INH/RMP dual therapy and followed them for at least 3 years. No child in any group developed TB disease or adverse reactions to therapy, but adherence was better with the shorter regimens. There are no similar data on HIV-infected children but data from adult studies including a large number of HIV-infected adults reported equivalence between 3 months INH/RMP and INH alone for 6 to 12 months.[58] Pyrazinamide (PZA) is another important sterilizing drug that is active against semi-dormant mycobacteria.[55,56] A combination of RMP/PZA for 2 to 3 months seems as efficacious as INH for 6 to 12 months in HIV-infected and uninfected adults,[59] but there are no similar data comparing efficacy in children.

Implementation of Contact Management

Despite the sound scientific basis underlying current recommendations and their enormous potential to reduce the burden of TB disease in children, contact screening and management rarely happen in resource-poor countries. Two recent studies from Malawi demonstrated that less than 10% of child TB contacts were screened or offered preventive therapy.[42,52] In those successfully screened, the prevalence of infection and suspected TB disease was high.[20] Opportunities for early TB diagnosis in symptomatic children and the provision of preventive therapy to asymptomatic contacts are frequently missed. Health care services are severely overburdened in resource-limited settings, especially those coping with concurrent TB and HIV epidemics, which emphasizes the need to identify pragmatic and feasible strategies for screening and the provision of preventive therapy. The screening process has often been a major hurdle because recommendations were often impossible to apply, making it locally irrelevant. As discussed, the screening process can be simplified to use clinical assessment alone. With this approach, screening can take place even in settings where access to TST and chest radiography is problematic; initial screening will require only 1 visit to the health service or a visit by a health care worker to the household, and the process can be decentralized to peripheral health centers where DOTS is applied.

To facilitate implementation and monitor the provision of preventive therapy to high-risk contacts, it may be sensible to add a box (**Fig. 2**) to the TB treatment card of all cases with positive sputum smears.[39] Achievable goals for practice could then be set and monitored by the NTP. In settings where health services are severely strained, the provision of preventive therapy could be restricted to the highest-risk groups. Data from the prechemotherapy era indicate that children infected before 2 years of age experience the greatest risk and that more than 95% of children who develop disease do so within 1 year of infection; therefore, it seems prudent to classify all children less than 3 years old as high-risk.[35] Those in contact with a index case with a positive sputum smear (or a primary caregiver with a negative sputum smear and pulmonary TB) would require preventive therapy. This restricted focus, compared with all children less than 5 years of age, should substantially reduce the workload and make the provision of preventive therapy to those at highest risk more feasible. Presently, all children with concomitant HIV infection are classified as high-risk and require a course of INH after each documented exposure to TB. Following initiation of antiretroviral therapy, those with undetectable viral loads and normal CD4 counts are less vulnerable, but immune recovery is never complete and heightened vigilance remains warranted.

The Millennium Development Goals aim to reduce mortality in children less than 5 years of age, and the prevalence of and deaths caused by TB by 2015. These targets deal with the overall burden of TB and its contribution to disease and death in young children. Treating child contacts should have an increasingly important place on the NTP agenda. At an international level, the political commitment to reduce the prevalence and severity of pediatric TB in endemic areas is growing, but at a national and regional level many obstacles remain. Although more resources

Name of contact	Age (years)	TB symptoms (Y/N)	Preventive therapy (Y/N)	TB treatment (Y/N)	TB registration number	Treatment outcome	HIV status (+ / - / NT)

Fig. 2. Proposed contact screening register to be added to the treatment card of all patients with a sputum smear-positive for TB. NT, not tested.

will be needed for implementation, many practical and logistical barriers can be overcome by using a simple decentralized screening process. Creative efforts are required to improve the visibility of pediatric TB as a public health concern and to raise awareness about the value of preventive therapy among caregivers, health care workers and policy makers.

ADULT PERSPECTIVE

As discussed earlier, complementary strategies must be considered to reduce the individual morbidity and mortality associated with TB in endemic areas and to limit the spread of the epidemic. Preventive therapy offers an attractive addition to the treatment of active disease. This section defines the groups most at risk, presents the evidence for treatment of latent infection and the more limited data on secondary prophylaxis, describes options for different drug regimens, and considers the 2 major challenges of adherence and exclusion of active TB. Managing contacts of patients with multidrug-resistant TB and the effect of antiretroviral therapy on TB prevention strategies are also discussed briefly.

Who Should Receive Preventive Therapy?

TB preventive therapy is recommended for high-risk groups including people living with HIV,[60] those on immune suppressive therapy,[61] renal dialysis and transplant patients,[62] and individuals in close contact with TB patients, including prisoners,[63] household contacts,[64] and health care staff.[65] In addition, individuals who migrate from endemic to nonendemic countries are usually screened and offered preventive therapy if latently infected with the aim of eradicating the pool of latent infection from which future disease may arise.[66]

HIV-infected individuals

Most of the recent work on screening and provision of preventive therapy has been conducted among people living with HIV. The incidence rate ratio (IRR) used by the WHO to reflect the relative risk of developing TB in HIV-infected individuals compared with HIV-uninfected people has recently been revised upwards.[1] In countries with a generalized HIV epidemic (ie, countries where the prevalence of HIV is more than 1% in the general population), the IRR is estimated to be 20.6 (95% CI 15.4–27.5) and this increases to 36.7 (95% CI 11.6–116) in countries where the prevalence of HIV in the general population is less than 0.1%.[1] People living with HIV are at risk of reactivating distant (latent) TB infection or

progressing to active TB after recent infection, at all levels of immunosuppression. In a retrospective cohort study in the South African gold mines, the relative risk of incident TB in HIV-infected individuals was 3 times that of HIV-uninfected individuals during the first 2 years after seroconversion, increasing to almost 10 after 10 years of HIV infection.[67] It was hoped that widespread use of antiretroviral therapy would reduce the risk of TB for those taking it, and although this is true the residual risk remains high with incident rate ratios 3 to 5 times that of the HIV-uninfected population.[68,69] Current CD4 cell count is the main predictor of TB risk and highly active antiretroviral therapy (HAART) strategies that minimize the time patients spend with CD4 cell counts less than a threshold of 500 cells/μL would seem to offer the best preventive strategy.[70]

HIV-uninfected individuals

The increased risk of TB in HIV-uninfected individuals with immunosuppression is highly variable. A review of the incidence of TB among patients with long-term steroid use found an increased risk of between 5 and 60 times that of the general population, although some studies had few cases.[71] Individuals exposed to multiple cases of TB, such as health care workers and people in institutional settings, have a higher risk of infection. A review of studies that evaluated the risk of TB infection and disease in health care workers in endemic countries reported IRRs ranging between 0.7 and 13.6 with annual nosocomial transmission risks of up to 11.3%.[72] Similar findings with lower overall risks have been reported in nonendemic countries.[73] During periods of high intensity exposure, such individuals might benefit from primary prophylaxis or treatment of latent infection if TST conversion occurs, although no randomized studies have been conducted. Among nurse trainees, those with an initial negative TST (previously uninfected) are at higher risk of disease development following TB exposure than those with pre-existing latent infection (TST positive), which may indicate that primary infection poses a greater risk than reinfection in young adults.[74]

Options for Preventive Therapy

Several drug regimens have been used as preventive therapy in adults including INH or RMP monotherapy and combination therapy with INH, RMP or PZA. Different durations have also been used ranging from 2 months for regimens containing RMP to more than 12 months with INH monotherapy.

HIV-infected individuals

A meta-analysis of 11 studies in HIV-infected individuals, including studies from TB-endemic and nonendemic countries, reported a 36% reduction in active TB (relative risk (RR) 0.64, 95% CI 0.51–0.81) for any drug combination, including all individuals regardless of TST result.[75] This meta-analysis found an overall reduction in the incidence of TB, but not in all-cause mortality. Benefit was greatest in those who were TST positive (RR 0.38, 95% CI 0.25–0.57); in those who were TST negative there was no statistically significant effect (RR 0.83, 95% CI 0.58–1.18). The studies varied in the drugs (INH, INH plus RMP, RMP plus PZA, or INH plus RMP plus PZA), the dosage (INH 300 mg/600 mg daily, INH 600/900 mg twice weekly, RMP 450/600 mg), the dosing interval (daily, twice weekly) and the duration (2–3 months for combination and 6–12 months for INH alone) of treatment provided. **Table 1** presents a summary of randomized trials that evaluated the value of TB preventive therapy in HIV-infected adults.[76–85] Studies of TST-negative and anergic individuals failed to show any benefit; head-to-head comparisons of different regimens showed no statistically significant differences in outcome.[59]

Observational studies from Haiti suggested a limited postpreventive therapy effect, dependent on the duration of INH monotherapy provided.[86] In studies from Zambia and Uganda, the duration of effect was approximately 3 years. In the Zambian study there was no difference between the INH or RMP/PZA regimens,[87] whereas in Uganda the RMP/INH/PZA regimen was found to have a longer duration of effect.[88] Both studies were added to the original trials and suffered excessive loss to follow-up. However, the limited duration of effect is not surprising because transmission in endemic areas is ongoing and preventive therapy offers no protection against new infections following cessation of therapy. The only way to protect vulnerable individuals against reinfection would be to consider prolonged or repeated courses of preventive therapy. A study in South Africa included continuous INH as 1 arm in a 4-arm randomized controlled trial, but failed to show that it was significantly more efficacious than a 6-month course of INH.[89] A larger study looking at the efficacy, safety, and tolerability of prolonged preventive regimens is still underway.

HIV-uninfected individuals

A Cochrane meta-analysis of 11 studies on preventive therapy in HIV-uninfected individuals included diverse risk groups.[49] Most of these studies used INH 300 mg daily for adults and the combined efficacy was a reduction in active TB of 60% (RR 0.4, 95% CI 0.31–0.52) compared with the placebo group. A review of 4 nonrandomized trials examining the efficacy of INH in patients treated with glucocorticosteroids reported mixed results.[71] Studies from India[90] and Mexico[91] reported benefit with INH preventive therapy, whereas studies from Hong Kong[92] and Japan[93] showed no benefit. Interpretation of these results is difficult because of the nonrandomized nature of the studies, different TB prevalence rates, and the low number of participants. In 1 randomized study of INH taken by renal transplant recipients for 12 months in Pakistan, a significantly decreased risk of TB was found in the first 2 years post-transplantation with no discontinuations because of drug toxicity.[94]

An International Union against TB trial conducted in Eastern Europe compared 3, 6 and 12 months of INH preventive therapy in individuals with fibrotic changes on chest radiography.[95] Only the 6- and 12-month regimens reduced the number of TB cases compared with placebo, with no difference between the 2 regimens. Subgroup analysis of adherent individuals showed increased benefit with the longer regimen, but adverse effects were more frequent. Evidence from large community level[7,96] and household contact studies[97] conducted in North America also suggested benefit from longer duration INH therapy, but there was no added benefit beyond 12 months. The large community trial conducted among the Inuit population in Alaska suggests that the protective effect of INH may persists for more than 10 years.[7,96] However, with this mass population–based intervention study, preventive therapy was implemented along with active case-finding and treatment of all diseased individuals, which eliminated the pool of latent infection and ongoing transmission at the same time.

Screening

TB screening is indicated to assess the risk of developing TB in the future and to exclude current active TB. Confidently excluding active TB before administration of preventive therapy is problematic, especially in individuals infected with HIV who are more likely to develop TB with negative sputum smear. Current recommendations are that a symptom screen and chest radiograph, if possible, should be used to exclude active TB in high-risk adults. The symptoms generally used include prolonged cough (prolonged or for 2–3 weeks), night sweats, fever, unintentional weight loss and chest pain or shortness of breath.

Table 1
Summary of randomized trials evaluating the benefit of different TB preventive therapy regimens in HIV-infected individuals

Study Location, Year Done[ref]	Number of Participants	% TST Positive	Treatment Provided	Duration in Months	TB rate/100 Person-Years	RR (95% CI)
Haiti, 1993[59]	58	66	INH/B6[a]	12	2.2	0.29 (0.09–0.91)
	60	42	B6 (12)	12	7.5	1
Kenya, 1997[86]	342	22	INH	6	4.29	0.92 (0.49–1.71)
	342	23.5	Placebo	6	3.86	1
Uganda, 1997[87,d]	536	100	INH	6	1.1	0.33 (0.14–0.77)
	556	100	INH/RMP	3	1.3	0.40 (0.18–0.86)
	463	100	INH/RMP/PZA	3	1.7	0.51 (0.24–1.08)
	464	100	Placebo	6	3.4	1
	395	Anergic[e]	INH	6	2.53	0.83 (0.34–2.04)
	323	Anergic[e]	Placebo	6	3.06	1
USA, 1997[88]	260	Anergic[e]	INH/B6	6	0.4	0.48 (0.12–1.91)
	257	Anergic[e]	Placebo/B6	6	0.9	1
Zambia, 1998[89]	350	23	INH	6[b]	2.74	0.56 (0.3–1.05)
	351	22	RIF/PZA	3[b]	3.16	0.65 (0.35–1.19)
	352	27	Placebo	6[b]	4.94	1
Haiti, 1998[90]	370	100	INH	6	1.7	N/A[c]
	370	100	RMP/PZA	2	1.8	N/A[c]
Haiti, Brazil, Mexico, USA 2000[91]	792	100	INH	12	1.1	1
	791	100	RMP/PZA	2	0.8	0.72 (0.40–1.31)
Haiti, 2001[92]	111	0	Placebo/B6	6	1.5	1.26 (0.36–4.37)
	126	0	INH/B6	6	1.9	1
Spain, 2003[93]	77	Anergic[e]	None		3.1	1
	83	Anergic[e]	INH	6	3.4	1.07 (0.24–4.80)
	82	Anergic[e]	RMP/INH	3	3.1	0.98 (0.22–4.40)
	77	Anergic[e]	RMP/PZA	2	1.2	0.39 (0.04–3.48)
South Africa, 2007[94]	50	Anergic[e]	Placebo	12[b]	11.6 (4.2–25.2)	1
	48	Anergic[e]	INH	12[b]	18 (8.2–34.1)	1.59 (0.57–4.49)

[a] Pyridoxine (vitamin B6).
[b] Twice weekly regimens.
[c] Not calculated in paper.
[d] Counted as 2 studies in meta-analysis: 1 for TST positives and 1 for anergic.
[e] Anergic was defined as being TST negative and also anergic to other common antigens on skin testing, eg, mumps, candida, tetanus and so forth.

However, the predictive values of this screening approach are variable and would be highly dependent on the symptom definitions used, the rigor with which it is performed, and the presence of severe immune compromise. Symptom-based screening will miss some cases of TB,[98] but chest radiographs are often unavailable in endemic areas and insistence on their use may limit access to preventive therapy. Routine chest radiographs increased the sensitivity in an extremely high-risk group of gold miners,[99,100] but its value has not been confirmed in a more generalized population with a lower prevalence of TB.[101] An important measure from a safety perspective is the negative predictive value of the screening test, which varies depending on the prevalence of TB in the population.[102] Reliably ruling out active TB remains a contentious area that requires ongoing surveillance and research to identify more accurate markers of disease. In HIV-infected individuals the benefit of preventive therapy has only been shown in those with a positive TST. IGRAs have replaced the TST in some high-income countries as a result of increased specificity,[103] but neither test is widely available in TB-endemic countries; in situations where they have been implemented, their use presented a significant barrier to therapy.[104]

OVERLAPPING ISSUES
Adherence

Adherence to preventive therapy is a major challenge in all populations studied. Preventive therapy does not provide immediate benefit to the patient, but may be associated with adverse effects that are unpleasant and immediately apparent. Highly variable adherence rates (20%–80%) have been reported, being higher in closely controlled trial settings than in real world situations.[104–107] Risk factors for nonadherence in adults include homelessness, male gender, age, and health beliefs.[108–110] Groups at highest risk of developing TB also have the greatest adherence challenges as a result of poverty, concomitant illness, or the need for additional chronic medication. In general, shorter duration regimens are strongly associated with increased adherence in adults,[81,111] although completion rates of shorter course combination therapy were not improved compared with 6 months of INH monotherapy in a retrospective study among migrants and refugees in Australia.[112] Measuring adherence is difficult. Most programs use pill collection and/or patient self-reporting. Urine testing for INH metabolites can be done using the Arkansas method or strip tests,[113] but added value may be limited if

only performed during scheduled visits. Cash and nutritional incentives have been shown to improve adherence.[107,114] Careful consideration should be given to optimal implementation strategies.

With children it is difficult to convince families of the need for 6 months or more of medication plus regular follow-up visits when the child is and remains well. Health workers are also not always convinced of the need for preventive therapy. In a recent survey of medical staff in 2 hospitals in New York, those trained in TB-endemic countries were less likely to treat latent TB infection than US-trained graduates despite both groups having similar knowledge of the recommendations.[115] A prospective study of South African children reported that of household TB contacts screened and advised to receive INH for 6 months, only 20% completed more than 4 months of unsupervised therapy.[116] In a separate retrospective study, adherence to INH/RMP for 3 months was significantly better than adherence to INH for 6 months (69.6% vs 27.6%, OR 4.97, 95% CI 2.40–10.36).[117] Experience from the United States and Greece also showed superior treatment completion rates among patients taking shorter courses of therapy compared with those taking INH for 9 months.[57,118] Because effectiveness is determined by efficacy and adherence, short-course combination regimens that are equivalent in efficacy to 6 to 9 months of INH under trial conditions may improve real life effectiveness. Alternative strategies to improve adherence, such as intermittent supervised therapy, also require further evaluation.

Adverse Events

It is important that preventive therapy is well tolerated. Adverse events reported with the use of preventive therapy are generally mild with few episodes of hepatotoxicity. A meta-analysis that compared INH with RMP/PZA in HIV-infected individuals found no difference in the number of adverse events or death.[59] However, there seems to be a major difference between the HIV-infected and uninfected groups in the incidence of adverse events with the RMP/PZA regimen. Combining trials performed among HIV-uninfected individuals showed that 8.2% of participants receiving RMP/PZA discontinued drugs because of severe hepatotoxicity compared with 1.7% of those receiving INH alone.[59] No mortality as a result of hepatotoxicity was reported, although cohort data collected in the United States did find an increased risk of hepatotoxicity and death following RMP/PZA preventive therapy and its use is no longer recommended.[119,120]

The major adverse events associated with first-line TB drugs in children were recently reviewed; in general, children tolerate TB drugs better than adults.[121] This may reflect differences in prevalence of other risk factors such as alcohol use or underlying hepatic disease, and/or differences in pharmacokinetics as serum levels are lower in children than in adults using the same mg/kg dosages.[122–124] Most reports of adverse events are with the use of INH alone, reflecting its long-standing and widespread use as preventive therapy. The major concern is hepatotoxicity and there are occasional case reports of severe INH-induced hepatitis and even hepatic failure.[118,125] However, prospective studies including large numbers of children using INH at daily dosages of 5 to 15 mg/kg for 6 to 12 months show that clinical hepatotoxicity is very rare. Jaundice was reported in 1 of more than 3500 children from studies using INH prophylaxis at 10 to 20 mg/kg.[51,57,126–131] Subclinical transient transaminase elevation is observed in 5% to 10% of children receiving INH,[130,131] the highest rates being reported in adolescents,[132] but routine monitoring is not recommended. An 11-year prospective trial conducted in Greece detected no serious drug-related adverse events with 9 months of INH or 3 to 4 months of RMP/INH.[57] RMP/INH dual therapy was also well tolerated in large observational studies from the United Kingdom.[133,134] Hepatotoxicity caused by RMP/PZA seems related to HIV infection status and age. Data in children are limited but standard first-line therapy that includes RMP and PZA is well tolerated and no hepatotoxicity was reported in 86 HIV-uninfected children who received 2 months of RMP/PZA preventive therapy.[135,136]

Creating Drug Resistance

The reason why accurate exclusion of TB disease is crucially important is that inadvertent treatment of active disease with 1 or 2 drugs could select for drug resistance. A systematic review of INH resistance amongst individuals who had received INH preventive therapy showed a relative risk of 1.45 (95% CI 0.85–2.47).[137] Although this is not a statistically significant finding, it represents a trend towards increased INH resistance, possibly as a result of secondary selection of INH resistant strains or a shift towards disease caused by primary resistant strains not responding to INH preventive therapy. Fear of inducing drug-resistant TB is the most frequently cited reason why countries are reluctant to implement INH

preventive therapy strategies.[100] This fear is not unfounded, because the exclusion of active disease can be extremely challenging in HIV-infected patients and effects that are nonsignificant in small scale trials may be amplified on a public health scale. INH is the most potent TB drug available and is crucial to rapidly reduce the organism load, which terminates transmission and protects companion drugs against resistance. Current evidence suggests that the standard 4-drug regimen used in adults should still be sufficient to effect cure in most patients with INH monoresistant disease,[138] although the theoretic risk of acquiring multidrug-resistant (MDR)-TB is increased. Good data collection from countries that have implemented universal INH preventive therapy in HIV-infected adults, such as Botswana, is vital to guide international policy.

The situation in young children is completely different. Children tend to develop pauci-bacillary disease, which implies a greatly reduced risk of acquiring drug resistance because the microbial load is low and drug penetration is good. In addition, young children rarely infect those around them and therefore the risk of transmitting drug-resistant disease within the community, should it develop, is minimal. Therefore concerns regarding the creation of drug resistance should not prevent the provision of preventive therapy to children.

Contact with Drug-resistant TB

Preventive therapy for close contacts of individuals with drug-resistant TB is more complex. A recent systematic review found no randomized trials and only 2 observational studies on close contacts of cases of drug-resistant TB.[139] One small retrospective study from Brazil used INH 400 mg daily for 6 months and found that fewer TST positive contacts developed TB in the treated group compared with the untreated group (OR 0.46, 95% CI 0.07–2.32).[140] The cases of TB that developed in the treated group had the same drug-resistance patterns as their presumed source cases, which is also true for children with drug-resistant TB, and demonstrates the need to take cognizance of drug resistance among likely source cases.[141] Drug-resistance patterns among children with TB provide an accurate measure of transmitted drug-resistant disease within communities.[142] Prospective surveillance data from Cape Town, South Africa, suggests an upward trend of drug-resistant TB among children,[143] with an over-representation of certain genotypes such as Beijing and Haarlem,[144] indicating successful transmission of these drug-resistant strains. The clinical presentation and basic principles guiding the management of drug-resistant disease are similar to those of drug-susceptible TB.

Monoresistance

Resistance to INH is usually the first step in the development of MDR; therefore, it is important from a public health perspective to monitor the prevalence of INH monoresistance. For the provision of preventive therapy to high-risk contacts of an infectious INH monoresistant index case, RMP alone for 4 months should suffice. Monoresistance to RMP is uncommon, although it seems more common among patients infected with HIV. INH preventive therapy should be sufficient for high-risk contacts of true RMP monoresistant cases. However, RMP resistance is frequently regarded as a marker for MDR and cases are usually managed as MDR-TB.

MDR

The term MDR-TB implies resistance to the most potent drugs in the first-line regimen, INH and RMP, with or without resistance to other TB drugs. The evidence base for the provision of preventive therapy to close contacts of MDR-TB cases is limited. Because second-line drugs are generally more toxic, a rational guide for preventive therapy would be to restrict this to high-risk contacts (children <3 years of age and those with severe immune compromise) and to use at least 2 drugs to which the organism is susceptible (or the presumed source case naive) for a duration of at least 6 months.[145] A single, prospective, cohort study in children reported a significant reduction in active disease among those receiving preventive therapy compared with those who did not (OR 0.2, 95% CI 0.04–0.94) using the strategy outlined earlier.[146] Extensive drug-resistant (XDR)-TB implies resistance to INH, RMP, the fluoroquinolones, and a second-line injectable agent such as kanamycin, amikacin, or capreomycin. Treatment options for these patients are extremely limited. Currently preventive therapy for XDR contacts is not advised, but in the light of possible low- or intermediate-level INH resistance, high-dose INH (15 mg/kg) may provide some protection to high-risk contacts.

Cost Effectiveness

Studies of TB preventive therapy in high- and low-income settings have found it to be cost effective and feasible, but clear program aims, adherence to guidelines, and high rates of preventive therapy are essential to achieve cost-effectiveness.[147–149] However, fears about drug resistance, feasibility concerns, and competing priorities have prevented most endemic countries from implementing wide-scale TB preventive therapy programs.

Screening for active TB in high-risk groups, especially HIV-infected populations, is not only an entry point for TB preventive therapy but also identifies TB cases who can be treated promptly thereby improving treatment outcomes and reducing transmission. In children, the identification of feasible strategies for the provision of preventive therapy to high-risk contacts provides an opportunity to reduce the massive pediatric disease burden in TB-endemic areas, although cost-effectiveness has not been formally assessed.

Options for HIV-infected Patients

Apart from treatment of latent infection, there is growing evidence that secondary preventive therapy, that is, prevention after a first episode of TB, can reduce the risk of recurrent TB among individuals infected with HIV in endemic areas.[100,150,151] Recurrent TB may occur as a result of relapse or reinfection and is common among children and adults infected with HIV in TB-endemic areas.[152,153] In a study from the South African mines, the incidence of recurrent TB was reduced by 55% among those who received INH (incidence rates 8.6 vs 19.1/100 person-years, IRR 0.45, 95% CI 0.26–0.78).[151] The efficacy of preventive therapy was unchanged after controlling for CD4 cell count, although the greatest benefit was derived among the more severely immune compromised. The number of person-years of INH preventive therapy required to prevent 1 case of recurrent TB among individuals with a CD4 cell count less than 200 cells/µL was 5; 19 for those with counts greater than 200 cells/µL. No similar study has been conducted in children infected with HIV.

Antiretroviral therapy reduces the incidence of TB in individuals infected with HIV especially those with the lowest CD4 counts.[154,155] However, the risk of developing TB while taking antiretroviral therapy remains higher than the risk for HIV-uninfected individuals. Randomized trials to establish the additional benefit of INH preventive therapy confirm that the combination has additive protective effect and that it is safe,[156,157] although data on TST-negative individuals and pregnant women are lacking. In children, early initiation of antiretroviral therapy provides clear survival benefit and reduces the likelihood of developing TB.[158,159] However, assessment of potential TB exposure should be routine at every follow-up visit, and with documented TB exposure, even if this occurs multiple times, INH preventive therapy is indicated in young or immune-suppressed children.

SUMMARY

Contact screening has an important role in identifying close contacts with TB who require treatment and those at risk for future disease who require preventive therapy. With limited resources and high rates of TB transmission, endemic countries need to focus on specific at-risk groups, whereas nonendemic countries may elect to provide preventive therapy to all individuals with documented TB infection and/or exposure. The major at-risk groups are young children and individuals infected with HIV. There is good evidence of efficacy and tolerance of preventive therapy in these populations, but adherence is a common problem and effective implementation is a major challenge.

Reliably excluding TB disease in individuals infected with HIV and the additional burden placed on already strained health care services require careful consideration. Where feasible strategies are implemented, the short- and long-term effects should be closely monitored. However, there are few complicating factors to consider in child TB contacts and the provision of preventive therapy to all high-risk children should be regarded as the standard of care, irrespective of the resources available.

REFERENCES

1. WHO Report. Global tuberculosis control. Epidemiology, strategy, financing. Geneva, Switzerland: World Health Organization; 2009.

2. Nunn P, Reid A, De Cock KM. Tuberculosis and HIV infection: the global setting. J Infect Dis 2007;196: S5–14.

3. Centres for disease Control and Prevention. Reported tuberculosis in the United States, 2006. Atlanta (GA). Available at: http://www.cdc.gov/tb/surv/surv2006/pdf/FullReport.pdf. Accessed June, 2009.

4. Van Rie A, Warren R, Richardson M, et al. Exogenous reinfection as a cause of recurrent tuberculosis after curative treatment. N Engl J Med 1999; 341:1174–9.

5. Charalambous S, Grant AD, Moloi V, et al. Contribution of reinfection to recurrent tuberculosis in South African gold miners. Int J Tuberc Lung Dis 2008;12: 942–8.

6. Verver S, Warren RM, Beyers N, et al. Rate of reinfection tuberculosis after successful treatment is higher than rate of new tuberculosis. Am J Respir Crit Care Med 2005;171:1430–5.

7. Comstock GW, Ferebee SH, Hammes LM. A controlled trial of community-wide isoniazid prophylaxis in Alaska. Am Rev Respir Dis 1967; 95:935–43.

8. Mack U, Migliori GB, Sester M, et al. LTBI: latent tuberculosis infection or lasting immune responses to M. tuberculosis? A TBNET consensus statement. Eur Respir J 2009;33:956–73.

9. Ehlers S. Lazy, dynamic or minimally recrudescent? On the elusive nature and location of the mycobacterium responsible for latent tuberculosis. Infection 2009;37:87–95.

10. Newton SM, Brent AJ, Anderson S, et al. Paediatric tuberculosis. Lancet Infect Dis 2008;8:499–510.

11. Marais BJ, Hesseling AC, Gie RP, et al. The burden of childhood tuberculosis and the accuracy of routine surveillance data in a high-burden setting. Int J Tuberc Lung Dis 2006;10:259–63.

12. Chintu C, Mudenda V, Lucas S, et al. Lung diseases at necropsy in African children dying from respiratory illnesses: a descriptive necropsy study. Lancet 2002;360:985–90.

13. Lawn SD, Bekker LG, Middelkoop K, et al. Impact of HIV infection on the epidemiology of tuberculosis in a peri-urban community in South Africa: the need for age-specific interventions. Clin Infect Dis 2006; 42:1040–7.

14. Marais BJ, Cotton M, Graham S, et al. Diagnosis and management challenges of childhood TB in the era of HIV. J Infect Dis 2007;196:S76–85.

15. Cotton MF, Schaaf HS, Lottering G, et al. Tuberculosis exposure in HIV-exposed infants in a high-prevalence setting. Int J Tuberc Lung Dis 2008; 12:225–7.

16. Grzybowski S, Barnett GD, Styblo K. Contacts of cases of active pulmonary tuberculosis. Bull Int Union Tuberc 1975;50:90–106.

17. Marks SM, Taylor Z, Qualls NL, et al. Outcomes of contact investigations of infectious tuberculosis patients. Am J Respir Crit Care Med 2000;162: 2033–8.

18. Kenyon TA, Creek T, Laserson K, et al. Risk factors for transmission of Mycobacterium tuberculosis from HIV-infected tuberculosis patients, Botswana. Int J Tuberc Lung Dis 2002;6:843–50.

19. Lienhardt C, Sillah J, Fielding K, et al. Risk factors for tuberculosis infection in children in contact with infectious tuberculosis cases in The Gambia, West Africa. Pediatrics 2003;111: e608–14.

20. Sinfield RL, Nyirenda M, Haves S, et al. Risk factors for TB infection and disease in young childhood contacts in Malawi. Ann Trop Paediatr 2006;26: 205–13.

21. Marais BJ, Obihara CC, Warren RW, et al. The burden of childhood tuberculosis: a public health perspective. Int J Tuberc Lung Dis 2005;9:1305–13.

22. Gopi PG, Subramani R, Narayanan PR. Trend in the prevalence of TB infection and ARTI after implementation of a DOTS programme in south India. Int J Tuberc Lung Dis 2006;10:346–8.

23. Salaniponi FM, Kwanjana J, Veen J, et al. Risk of infection with *Mycobacterium tuberculosis* in Malawi: national tuberculin survey 1994. Int J Tuberc Lung Dis 2004;8:718–23.

24. Bachtiar A, Miko TY, Machmud R, et al. Annual risk of tuberculosis infection in West Sumatra Province, Indonesia. Int J Tuberc Lung Dis 2008;12:255–61.

25. Middelkoop K, Myer L, Mark D, et al. Rates of tuberculosis transmission to children and adolescents in a community with a high prevalence of HIV infection among adults. Clin Infect Dis 2008; 47:349–55.

26. Kritzinger FE, den Boon S, Verver S, et al. No decrease in annual risk of tuberculosis infection in endemic area in Cape Town, South Africa. Trop Med Int Health 2009;14:136–42.

27. Marais BJ, Hesseling AC, Schaaf HS, et al. *Mycobacterium tuberculosis* transmission is not related to household genotype in a setting of high endemicity. J Clin Microbiol 2009;47:338–43.

28. Schaaf HS, Michaelis IA, Richardson M, et al. Adult-to-child transmission of tuberculosis: household or community contact? Int J Tuberc Lung Dis 2003;7:426–31.

29. Verver S, Warren RM, Munch Z, et al. Proportion of tuberculosis transmission that takes place in households in a high-incidence area. Lancet 2004;363:212–4.

30. Hauck FR, Neese BH, Panchal AS, et al. Identification and management of latent tuberculosis infection. Am Fam Physician 2009;79:879–86.

31. Pillay T, Khan M, Moodley J, et al. Perinatal tuberculosis and HIV-1: considerations for resource-limited settings. Lancet Infect Dis 2004;4:155–65.

32. Heyns L, Gie RP, Goussard P, et al. Nosocomial transmission of *Mycobacterium tuberculosis* in kangaroo mother care units: a risk in tuberculosis-endemic areas. Acta Paediatr 2006;95:535–9.

33. Marais BJ, Gie RP, Schaaf HS, et al. The natural history of childhood intra-thoracic tuberculosis: a critical review of literature from the pre-chemotherapy era. Int J Tuberc Lung Dis 2004;8:392–402.

34. Trunz BB, Fine P, Dye C. Effect of BCG vaccination on childhood tuberculous meningitis and miliary tuberculosis worldwide: a meta-analysis and assessment of cost-effectiveness. Lancet 2006;367:1173–80.

35. Marais BJ, Gie RP, Schaaf HS, et al. Childhood pulmonary tuberculosis – old wisdom and new challenges. Am J Respir Crit Care Med 2006;173: 1078–90.

36. Hesseling AC, Cotton MF, Jennings T, et al. High incidence of tuberculosis among HIV-infected infants: evidence from a South African population-based study highlights the need for improved tuberculosis control strategies. Clin Infect Dis 2009;48:108–14.

37. Madhi SA, Petersen K, Madhi A, et al. Increased disease burden and antibiotic resistance of bacteria causing severe community-acquired lower respiratory tract infections in human immunodeficiency virus type 1-infected children. Clin Infect Dis 2000;31:170–6.

38. Harries AD, Hargreaves NJ, Graham SM, et al. Childhood tuberculosis in Malawi: nationwide case-finding and treatment outcomes. Int J Tuberc Lung Dis 2002;6:424–31.

39. World Health Organization. Guidance for national tuberculosis programmes on the management of tuberculosis in children. Stop TB Partnership Childhood TB Subgroup. Geneva: World Health Organization; 2006. WHO/HTM/TB/2006.371.

40. Rieder HL. Interventions for tuberculosis control and elimination. Paris: International Union Against Tuberculosis and Lung Disease; 2002.

41. Centers for Disease Control and Prevention. Guidelines for the investigation of contacts of persons with infectious tuberculosis. MMWR Recomm Rep 2005;54(RR-15):16–8.

42. Nyirenda M, Sinfield R, Haves S, et al. Poor attendance at a child TB contact clinic in Malawi. Int J Tuberc Lung Dis 2006;10:585–7.

43. Marais BJ, Gie RP, Starke JR, et al. A proposed radiological classification of childhood intra-thoracic tuberculosis. Pediatr Radiol 2004;33:886–94.

44. The United States Public Health Service Tuberculosis Prophylaxis Trial collaborators. Prophylactic effects of isoniazid on primary tuberculosis in children. Am Rev Tuberc 1957;76:942–63.

45. Kruk A, Gie RP, Schaaf HS, et al. Symptom-based screening of child tuberculosis contacts: improved feasibility in resource-limited settings. Pediatrics 2008;121:e1646–52.

46. Davies MA, Connell T, Johannisen C, et al. Detection of tuberculosis in HIV-infected children using an enzyme-linked immunospot assay. AIDS 2009; 23:961–9.

47. Hesseling AC, Mandalakas AM, Kirchner LH, et al. Highly discordant T-cell responses in individuals with recent household tuberculosis exposure. Thorax 2008 [Epub ahead of print].

48. Marais BJ, Pai M. New approaches and emerging technologies in the diagnosis of childhood tuberculosis. Paediatr Respir Rev 2007;8:124–33.

49. Smieja MJ, Marchetti CA, Cook DJ, et al. Isoniazid for preventing tuberculosis in non-HIV infected persons. Cochrane Database Syst Rev 2000;(2): CD001363.

50. Hsu KH. Isoniazid in the prevention and treatment of tuberculosis. A 20-year study of the effectiveness in children. JAMA 1974;229:528–33.

51. Hsu KHK. Thirty years after isoniazid: its impact on tuberculosis in children and adolescents. JAMA 1984;251:1283–5.

52. Claessens NJ, Gausi FF, Meijnen S, et al. Screening childhood contacts of patients with smear-positive pulmonary tuberculosis in Malawi. Int J Tuberc Lung Dis 2002;6:362–4.

53. Reichler MR, Reves R, Bur S, et al. Evaluation of investigations conducted to detect and prevent transmission of tuberculosis. JAMA 2002;287:991–5.

54. Zar HJ, Cotton MF, Strauss S, et al. Effect of isoniazid prophylaxis on mortality and incidence of tuberculosis in children with HIV: randomised controlled trial. Br Med J 2007;334:136.

55. Mitchison DA. Role of individual drugs in the chemotherapy of tuberculosis. Int J Tuberc Lung Dis 2000;4:796–806.

56. Donald PR, Schaaf HS. Old and new drugs for the treatment of tuberculosis in children. Paediatr Respir Rev 2007;8:134–41.

57. Spyridis NP, Spyridis PG, Gelesme A, et al. The effectiveness of a 9-month regimen of isoniazid alone versus 3- and 4-month regimens of isoniazid plus rifampin for treatment of latent tuberculosis infection in children: results of an 11-year randomized study. Clin Infect Dis 2007;45:715–22.

58. Ena J, Valls V. Short course therapy with rifampicin plus isoniazid, compared with standard therapy with isoniazid, for latent tuberculosis: a meta-analysis. Clin Infect Dis 2005;40:670–6.

59. Gao XF, Wang L, Liu GJ, et al. Rifampicin plus pyrazinamide versus isoniazid for treating latent tuberculosis infection: a meta-analysis. Int J Tuberc Lung Dis 2006;10:1080–90.

60. Tuberculosis preventive therapy in HIV-infected individuals. A joint statement of the International Union Against Tuberculosis and Lung Disease (IUATLD) and the Global Programme on AIDS and the Tuberculosis Programme of the World Health Organization (WHO). Tuber Lung Dis 1994;75:96–8.

61. Chan YC, Yosipovitch G. Suggested guidelines for screening and management of tuberculosis in patients taking oral glucocorticoids – an important but often neglected issue. J Am Acad Dermatol 2003;49:91–5.

62. European Best Practice Guidelines for Renal Transplantation. European best practice guidelines for renal transplantation. Section IV: long-term management of the transplant recipient. IV.7.2. Late infections. Tuberculosis. Nephrol Dial Transplant 2002;17(Suppl 4):S39–43.

63. Centers for Disease Control and Prevention (CDC), National Center for HIV/AIDS, Viral Hepatitis, STD, and TB Prevention. Prevention and control of tuberculosis in correctional and detention facilities: recommendations from CDC. Endorsed by the Advisory Council for the Elimination of Tuberculosis, the National Commission on Correctional Health Care, and the American Correctional Association. MMWR Recomm Rep 2006;55(RR-9):1–44.

64. National Tuberculosis Controllers Association, Centers for Disease Control and Prevention (CDC). Guidelines for the investigation of contacts of persons with infectious tuberculosis. Recommendations from the National Tuberculosis Controllers Association and CDC. MMWR Recomm Rep 2005;54(RR-15):1–47.

65. Jensen PA, Lambert LA, Iademarco MF, et al. Guidelines for preventing the transmission of Mycobacterium tuberculosis in health-care settings. 2005. MMWR Recomm Rep 2005;(54):1–141.

66. Recommendations for prevention and control of tuberculosis among foreign-born persons. Report of the Working Group on Tuberculosis among Foreign-Born Persons. Centers for Disease Control and Prevention. MMWR Recomm Rep 1998;47(RR-16):1–29.

67. Glynn JR, Murray J, Bester A, et al. Effects of duration of HIV infection and secondary tuberculosis transmission on tuberculosis incidence in the South African gold mines. AIDS 2008;22:1859–67.

68. Brinkhof MW, Egger M, Boulle A, et al. Tuberculosis after initiation of antiretroviral therapy in low-income and high-income countries. Clin Infect Dis 2007;45:1518–21.

69. Lawn SD, Myer L, Bekker LG, et al. Burden of tuberculosis in an antiretroviral treatment programme in sub-Saharan Africa: impact on treatment outcomes and implications for tuberculosis control. AIDS 2006;20:1605–12.

70. Lawn SD, Myer L, Edwards D, et al. Short-term and long-term risk of tuberculosis associated with CD4 cell recovery during antiretroviral therapy in SA. AIDS 2009 [Epub ahead of print].

71. Falagas ME, Voidonikola PT, Angelousi AG. Tuberculosis in patients with systemic rheumatic or pulmonary diseases treated with glucocorticosteroids and the preventive role of isoniazid: a review of the available evidence. Int J Antimicrob Agents 2007;30:477–86.

72. Joshi R, Reingold AL, Menzies D, et al. Tuberculosis among health-care workers in low- and middle-income countries: a systematic review. PLoS Med 2006;3:e494.

73. Menzies D, Joshi R, Pai M. Risk of tuberculosis infection and disease associated with work in health care settings. Int J Tuberc Lung Dis 2007;11:593–605.

74. Bjartveit K. Olaf Scheel, Johannes Heimbeck: their contribution to understanding the pathogenesis and prevention of tuberculosis. Int J Tuberc Lung Dis 2003;7:306–11.

75. Woldehanna S, Volmink J. Treatment of latent tuberculosis infection in HIV infected persons. Cochrane Database Syst Rev 2004;(1):CD000171.

76. Pape JW, Jean SS, Ho JL, et al. Effect of isoniazid prophylaxis on incidence of active tuberculosis and

progression of HIV infection. Lancet 1993;342: 268–72.

77. Hawken MP, Meme HK, Elliott LC, et al. Isoniazid preventive therapy for tuberculosis in HIV-1-infected adults: results of a randomized controlled trial. AIDS 1997;11:875–82.

78. Whalen CC, Johnson JL, Okwera A, et al. A trial of three regimens to prevent tuberculosis in Ugandan adults infected with the human immunodeficiency virus. Uganda-Case Western Reserve University Research Collaboration. N Engl J Med 1997;337: 801–8.

79. Gordin FM, Matts JP, Miller C, et al. A controlled trial of isoniazid in persons with anergy and human immunodeficiency virus infection who are at high risk for tuberculosis. Terry Beirn Community Programs for Clinical Research on AIDS. N Engl J Med 1997;337:315–20.

80. Mwinga A, Hosp M, Godfrey Faussett P, et al. Twice weekly tuberculosis preventive therapy in HIV infection in Zambia. AIDS 1998;12:2447–57.

81. Halsey NA, Coberly JS, Desormeaux J, et al. Randomised trial of isoniazid versus rifampicin and pyrazinamide for prevention of tuberculosis in HIV-1 infection. Lancet 1998;351:786–92.

82. Gordin F, Chaisson RE, Matts JP, et al. Rifampin and pyrazinamide vs isoniazid for prevention of tuberculosis in HIV-infected persons: an international randomized trial. Terry Beirn Community Programs for Clinical Research on AIDS, the Adult AIDS Clinical Trials Group, the Pan American Health Organization, and the Centers for Disease Control and Prevention Study Group. JAMA 2000; 283:1445–50.

83. Fitzgerald DW, Severe P, Joseph P, et al. No effect of isoniazid prophylaxis for purified protein derivative-negative HIV-infected adults living in a country with endemic tuberculosis: results of a randomized trial. J Acquir Immune Defic Syndr 2001;28:305–7.

84. Rivero A, Lopez-Cortes L, Castillo R, et al. [Randomized trial of three regimens to prevent tuberculosis in HIV-infected patients with anergy]. Enferm Infecc Microbiol Clin 2003;21:287–92.

85. Mohammed A, Myer L, Ehrlich R, et al. Randomised controlled trial of isoniazid preventive therapy in South African adults with advanced HIV disease. Int J Tuberc Lung Dis 2007;11: 1114–20.

86. Fitzgerald DW, Morse MM, Pape JW, et al. Active tuberculosis in individuals infected with human immunodeficiency virus after isoniazid prophylaxis. Clin Infect Dis 2000;31:1495–7.

87. Quigley MA, Mwinga A, Hosp M, et al. Long-term effect of preventive therapy for tuberculosis in a cohort of HIV-infected Zambian adults. AIDS 2001;15:215–22.

88. Johnson JL, Okwera A, Hom DL, et al. Duration of efficacy of treatment of latent tuberculosis infection in HIV-infected adults. AIDS 2001;15:2137–47.

89. Martinson N, Barnes G, Msandiwa R, et al. Novel regimens for treating latent TB in HIV-infected adults in South Africa: a randomized clinical trial. In: 16th Conference on Retroviruses and Opportunistic Infections. 2009: Montreal.

90. Gaitonde S, Pathan E, Sule A, et al. Efficacy of isoniazid prophylaxis in patients with systemic lupus erythematosus receiving long term steroid treatment. Ann Rheum Dis 2002;61:251–3.

91. Hernandez-Cruz B, Ponce-de-Leon-Rosales S, Sifuentes-Osornio J, et al. Tuberculosis prophylaxis in patients with steroid treatment and systemic rheumatic diseases. A case-control study. Clin Exp Rheumatol 1999;17:81–7.

92. Mok MY, Lo Y, Chan TM, et al. Tuberculosis in systemic lupus erythematosus in an endemic area and the role of isoniazid prophylaxis during corticosteroid therapy. J Rheumatol 2005;32(4):609–15.

93. Kobashi Y, Matsushima T. Clinical analysis of pulmonary tuberculosis in association with corticosteroid therapy. Intern Med 2002;41:1103–10.

94. Naqvi R, Akhtar S, Noor H, et al. Efficacy of isoniazid prophylaxis in renal allograft recipients. Transplant Proc 2006;38:2057–8.

95. Efficacy of various durations of isoniazid preventive therapy for tuberculosis: five years of follow-up in the IUAT trial. International Union Against Tuberculosis Committee on Prophylaxis. Bull World Health Organ 1982;60:555–64.

96. Comstock GW, Baum C, Snider DE Jr. Isoniazid prophylaxis among Alaskan Eskimos: a final report of the bethel isoniazid studies. Am Rev Respir Dis 1979;119:827–30.

97. Ferebee SH, Mount FW. Tuberculosis morbidity in a controlled trial of the prophylactic use of isoniazid among household contacts. Am Rev Respir Dis 1962;85:490–510.

98. Hawken M, Nganga L, Meme H, et al. Is cough alone adequate to screen HIV-positive persons for tuberculosis preventive therapy in developing countries? Int J Tuberc Lung Dis 1999;3:540–1.

99. Day JH, Charalambous S, Fielding KL, et al. Screening for tuberculosis prior to isoniazid preventive therapy among HIV-infected gold miners in South Africa. Int J Tuberc Lung Dis 2006;10:523–9.

100. Churchyard GJ, Scano F, Grant AD, et al. Tuberculosis preventive therapy in the era of HIV infection: overview and research priorities. J Infect Dis 2007; 196:S52–62.

101. Mosimaneotsile B, Talbot EA, Moeti TL, et al. Value of chest radiography in a tuberculosis prevention programme for HIV-infected people, Botswana. Lancet 2003;362:1551–2.

102. Ayles H, Schaap A, Nota A, et al. Prevalence of tuberculosis, HIV and respiratory symptoms in two Zambian communities – implications for tuberculosis control in the era of HIV. PLoS One 2009;4: e5602.

103. Pai M, Zwerling A, Menzies D. Systematic review: T-cell-based assays for the diagnosis of latent tuberculosis infection: an update. Ann Intern Med 2008;149:177–84.

104. Lugada ES, Watera C, Nakiyingi J, et al. Operational assessment of isoniazid prophylaxis in a community AIDS service organisation in Uganda. Int J Tuberc Lung Dis 2002;6:326–31.

105. Munseri PJ, Talbot EA, Mtei L, et al. Completion of isoniazid preventive therapy among HIV-infected patients in Tanzania. Int J Tuberc Lung Dis 2008; 12:1037–41.

106. Szakacs TA, Wilson D, Cameron DW, et al. Adherence with isoniazid for prevention of tuberculosis among HIV-infected adults in South Africa. BMC Infect Dis 2006;6:97.

107. Tulsky JP, Pilote L, Hahn JA, et al. Adherence to isoniazid prophylaxis in the homeless: a randomized controlled trial. Arch Intern Med 2000;160: 697–702.

108. Lavigne M, Rocher I, Steensma C, et al. The impact of smoking on adherence to treatment for latent tuberculosis infection. BMC Public Health 2006;6:66.

109. Ngamvithayapong J, Uthaivoravit W, Yanai H, et al. Adherence to tuberculosis preventive therapy among HIV-infected persons in Chiang Rai, Thailand. AIDS 1997;11:107–12.

110. Tulsky JP, Hahn JA, Long HL, et al. Can the poor adhere? Incentives for adherence to TB prevention in homeless adults. Int J Tuberc Lung Dis 2004;8: 83–91.

111. Lardizabal A, Passannante M, Kojakali F, et al. Enhancement of treatment completion for latent tuberculosis infection with 4 months of rifampin. Chest 2006;130:1712–7.

112. MacIntyre CR, Ansari MZ, Carnie J, et al. No evidence for multiple-drug prophylaxis for tuberculosis compared with isoniazid alone in Southeast Asian refugees and migrants: completion and compliance are major determinants of effectiveness. Prev Med 2000;30: 425–32.

113. Schraufnagel DE, Stoner R, Whiting E, et al. Testing for isoniazid. An evaluation of the Arkansas method. Chest 1990;98:314–6.

114. Mangura BT, Passannante MR, Reichman LB. An incentive in tuberculosis preventive therapy for an inner city population. Int J Tuberc Lung Dis 1997; 1:576–8.

115. Hirsch-Moverman Y, Tsiouris S, Salazar-Schicchi J, et al. Physician attitudes regarding latent tuberculosis infection: international vs. U.S. medical graduates. Int J Tuberc Lung Dis 2006;10:1178–80.

116. Marais BJ, van Zyl S, Schaaf HS, et al. Adherence to isoniazid preventive chemotherapy in children: a prospective community-based study. Arch Dis Child 2006;91:762–5.

117. van Zyl S, Marais BJ, Hesseling AC, et al. Adherence to anti-tuberculosis chemoprophylaxis and treatment in children. Int J Tuberc Lung Dis 2006; 10:13–8.

118. Cook PP, Maldonado RA, Yarnell CT, et al. Safety and completion rate of short-course therapy for treatment of latent tuberculosis infection. Clin Infect Dis 2006;43:271–5.

119. McElroy PD, Ijaz K, Lambert LA, et al. National survey to measure rates of liver injury, hospitalization, and death associated with rifampin and pyrazinamide for latent tuberculosis infection. Clin Infect Dis 2005;41:1125–33.

120. Centers for Disease Control and Prevention (CDC), American Thoracic Society. Update: adverse event data and revised American Thoracic Society/CDC recommendations against the use of rifampin and pyrazinamide for treatment of latent tuberculosis infection–United States, 2003. MMWR Morb Mortal Wkly Rep 2003;52(31):735–9.

121. Frydenberg A, Graham SM. A review of toxicity of first-line drugs for treatment of tuberculosis in children. Trop Med Int Health, in press.

122. McIlleron H, Willemse M, Werely CJ, et al. Isoniazid plasma concentrations in a cohort of South African children with tuberculosis: implications for international pediatric dosing guidelines. Clin Infect Dis 2009;48:1547–53.

123. Schaaf HS, Willemse M, Cilliers K, et al. Rifampin pharmacokinetics in children, with and without human immunodeficiency virus infection, hospitalized for the management of severe forms of tuberculosis. BMC Med 2009;7:19.

124. Graham SM, Bell DJ, Nyirongo S, et al. Low levels of pyrazinamide and ethambutol in children with tuberculosis and impact of age, nutritional status, and human immunodeficiency virus infection. Antimicrob Agents Chemother 2006;50:407–13.

125. Lobato MN, Jereb JA, Starke JR. Unintended consequences: mandatory tuberculin skin testing and severe isoniazid hepatotoxicity. Pediatrics 2008;121:e1732–3.

126. Wu SS, Chao CS, Vargas JH, et al. Isoniazid-related hepatic failure in children: a survey of liver transplantation centers. Transplantation 2007;84: 173–9.

127. Dash LA, Comstock GW, Flynn JP. Isoniazid preventive therapy: retrospect and prospect. Am Rev Respir Dis 1980;121:1039–44.

128. Nakajo MM, Rao M, Steiner P. Incidence of hepatotoxicity in children receiving isoniazid chemoprophylaxis. Pediatr Infect Dis J 1989;8: 649–50.

129. Palusci VJ, O'Hare D, Lawrence RM. Hepatotoxicity and transaminase measurement during isoniazid chemoprophylaxis in children. Pediatr Infect Dis J 1985;14:144–8.

130. Beaudry PH, Brickman HF, Wise MB, et al. Liver enzyme disturbances during isoniazid chemoprophylaxis in children. Am Rev Respir Dis 1974;110: 581–4.

131. Rapp RS, Campbell RW, Howell JC, et al. Isoniazid hepatotoxicity in children. Am Rev Respir Dis 1978; 118:794–6.

132. Litt IF, Cohen MI, McNamara H. Isoniazid hepatitis in adolescents. J Pediatr 1976;89:133–5.

133. Ormerod LP. Reduced incidence of tuberculosis by prophylactic chemotherapy in subjects showing strong reactions to tuberculin testing. Arch Dis Child 1987;82:1005–8.

134. Ormerod LP. Rifampicin and isoniazid prophylactic chemotherapy for tuberculosis. Arch Dis Child 1998;78:169–71.

135. Magdorf K, Arizzi-Rusche AF, Geiter LJ, et al. Compliance and tolerance of new antitubercular short-term chemopreventive regimens in childhood–a pilot project. Pneumologie 1994;48: 761–4.

136. Priest DH, Vossel LF Jr, Sherfy EA, et al. Use of intermittent rifampin and pyrazinamide therapy for latent tuberculosis infection in a targeted tuberculin testing program. Clin Infect Dis 2004;39: 1764–71.

137. Balcells ME, Thomas SL, Godfrey-Faussett P, et al. Isoniazid preventive therapy and risk for resistant tuberculosis. Emerg Infect Dis 2006;12: 744–51.

138. LoBue PA, Moser KS. Isoniazid and rifampin-resistant tuberculosis in San Diego County, California, United States, 1993–2002. Int J Tuberc Lung Dis 2005;9:501–6.

139. Fraser A, Paul M, Attamna A, et al. Treatment of latent tuberculosis in persons at risk for multidrug-resistant tuberculosis: systematic review. Int J Tuberc Lung Dis 2006;10:19–23.

140. Kritski AL, Marques MJ, Rabahi MF, et al. Transmission of tuberculosis to close contacts of patients with multidrug-resistant tuberculosis. Am J Respir Crit Care Med 1996;153:331–5.

141. Schaaf HS, Gie RP, Beyers N. Primary drug-resistant tuberculosis in children. Int J Tuberc Lung Dis 2000;12:1149–55.

142. Schaaf HS, Marais BJ, Hesseling AC, et al. Childhood drug-resistant tuberculosis in the Western Cape Province of South Africa. Acta Paediatr 2006;95:523–8.

143. Schaaf HS, Marais BJ, Hesseling AC, et al. Surveillance of antituberculosis drug resistance among children from the Western Cape Province of South Africa–an upward trend. Am J Public Health 2009;99:1486–90.

144. Marais BJ, Victor TC, Hesseling AC, et al. Beijing and Haarlem genotypes are overrepresented among children with drug-resistant tuberculosis in the Western Cape Province of South Africa. J Clin Microbiol 2006;44:3539–43.

145. Schaaf HS. Drug-resistant tuberculosis in children. S Afr Med J 2007;97(Pt 2):995–7.

146. Schaaf HS, Gie RP, Kennedy M, et al. Evaluation of young children in contact with adult multidrug-resistant pulmonary tuberculosis: a 30-month follow-up. Pediatrics 2002;109: 765–71.

147. Diel R, Nienhaus A, Schaberg T. Cost-effectiveness of isoniazid chemoprevention in close contacts. Eur Respir J 2005;26:465–73.

148. Bell JC, Rose DN, Sacks HS. Tuberculosis preventive therapy for HIV-infected people in sub-Saharan Africa is cost-effective. AIDS 1999; 13:1549–56.

149. Macintyre CR, Plant AJ, Hendrie D. The cost-effectiveness of evidence-based guidelines and practice for screening and prevention of tuberculosis. Health Econ 2000;9:411–21.

150. Fitzgerald DW, Desvarieux M, Severe P, et al. Effect of post-treatment isoniazid on prevention of recurrent tuberculosis in HIV-1-infected individuals: a randomised trial. Lancet 2000;356:1470–4.

151. Churchyard GJ, Fielding K, Charalambous S, et al. Efficacy of secondary isoniazid preventive therapy among HIV-infected Southern Africans: time to change policy? AIDS 2003;17:2063–70.

152. Sonnenberg P, Murray J, Glynn JR, et al. HIV-1 and recurrence, relapse, and reinfection of tuberculosis after cure: a cohort study in South African mineworkers. Lancet 2001;358:1687–93.

153. Schaaf HS, Krook S, Hollemans DW, et al. Recurrent culture-confirmed tuberculosis in human immunodeficiency virus-infected children. Pediatr Infect Dis J 2005;24:685–91.

154. Badri M, Wilson D, Wood R. Effect of highly active antiretroviral therapy on incidence of tuberculosis in South Africa: a cohort study. Lancet 2002;359:2059–64.

155. Santoro-Lopes G, de Pinho AM, Harrison LH, et al. Reduced risk of tuberculosis among Brazilian patients with advanced human immunodeficiency virus infection treated with highly active antiretroviral therapy. Clin Infect Dis 2002;34:543–6.

156. Golub JE, Saraceni V, Cavalcante SC, et al. The impact of antiretroviral therapy and isoniazid preventive therapy on tuberculosis incidence in HIV-infected patients in Rio de Janeiro, Brazil. AIDS 2007;21:1441–8.

157. Golub JE, Pronyk P, Mohapi L, et al. Isoniazid preventive therapy, HAART and tuberculosis risk in HIV-infected adults in South Africa: a prospective cohort. AIDS 2009;23:631–6.

158. Walters E, Cotton MF, Rabie H, et al. Clinical presentation and outcome of tuberculosis in human immunodeficiency virus infected children on anti-retroviral therapy. BMC Pediatr 2008;8:1.

159. Violari A, Cotton MF, Gibb DM, et al. CHER Study Team. Early antiretroviral therapy and mortality among HIV-infected infants. N Engl J Med 2008; 359:2233–44.

Index

Clin Chest Med 30 (2009) 847–852
doi:10.1016/S0272-5231(09)00110-5
0272-5231/09/$ – see front matter © 2009 Elsevier Inc. All rights reserved.

Moving?

Make sure your subscription moves with you!

To notify us of your new address, find your **Clinics Account Number** (located on your mailing label above your name), and contact customer service at:

Email: journalscustomerservice-usa@elsevier.com

800-654-2452 (subscribers in the U.S. & Canada)
314-447-8871 (subscribers outside of the U.S. & Canada)

Fax number: 314-447-8029

Elsevier Health Sciences Division
Subscription Customer Service
3251 Riverport Lane
Maryland Heights, MO 63043

*To ensure uninterrupted delivery of your subscription, please notify us at least 4 weeks in advance of move.

United States Postal Service
Statement of Ownership, Management, and Circulation
(All Periodicals Publications Except Requester Publications)

1. Publication Title	2. Publication Number								3. Filing Date
Clinics in Chest Medicine	0	0	0	-	7	0	6		9/15/09

4. Issue Frequency	5. Number of Issues Published Annually	6. Annual Subscription Price
Mar, Jun, Sep, Dec	4	$251.00

7. Complete Mailing Address of Known Office of Publication *(Not printer)* *(Street, city, county, state, and ZIP+4®)*	Contact Person
Elsevier Inc. 360 Park Avenue South New York, NY 10010-1710	Stephen Bushing
	Telephone *(Include area code)*
	215-239-3688

8. Complete Mailing Address of Headquarters or General Business Office of Publisher *(Not printer)*

Elsevier Inc., 360 Park Avenue South, New York, NY 10010-1710

9. Full Names and Complete Mailing Addresses of Publisher, Editor, and Managing Editor *(Do not leave blank)*

Publisher *(Name and complete mailing address)*

John Schrefer, Elsevier, Inc., 1600 John F. Kennedy Blvd. Suite 1800, Philadelphia, PA 19103-2899

Editor *(Name and complete mailing address)*

Sarah Barth, Elsevier, Inc., 1600 John F. Kennedy Blvd. Suite 1800, Philadelphia, PA 19103-2899

Managing Editor *(Name and complete mailing address)*

Catherine Bewick, Elsevier, Inc., 1600 John F. Kennedy Blvd. Suite 1800, Philadelphia, PA 19103-2899

10. Owner *(Do not leave blank. If the publication is owned by a corporation, give the name and address of the corporation immediately followed by the names and addresses of all stockholders owning or holding 1 percent or more of the total amount of stock. If not owned by a corporation, give the names and addresses of the individual owners. If owned by a partnership or other unincorporated firm, give its name and address as well as those of each individual owner. If the publication is published by a nonprofit organization, give its name and address.)*

Full Name	Complete Mailing Address
Wholly owned subsidiary of	4520 East-West Highway
Reed/Elsevier, US holdings	Bethesda, MD 20814

11. Known Bondholders, Mortgagees, and Other Security Holders Owning or Holding 1 Percent or More of Total Amount of Bonds, Mortgages, or Other Securities. If none, check box → ☐ None

Full Name	Complete Mailing Address
N/A	

12. Tax Status *(For completion by nonprofit organizations authorized to mail at nonprofit rates) (Check one)*
The purpose, function, and nonprofit status of this organization and the exempt status for federal income tax purposes:
☐ Has Not Changed During Preceding 12 Months
☐ Has Changed During Preceding 12 Months *(Publisher must submit explanation of change with this statement)*

PS Form 3526, September 2007 (Page 1 of 3 (Instructions Page 3)) PSN 7530-01-000-9931 PRIVACY NOTICE: See our Privacy policy in www.usps.com

---

13. Publication Title	14. Issue Date for Circulation Data Below
Clinics in Chest Medicine	September 2009

15. Extent and Nature of Circulation		Average No. Copies Each Issue During Preceding 12 Months	No. Copies of Single Issue Published Nearest to Filing Date
a. Total Number of Copies *(Net press run)*		2851	2704
b. Paid Circulation (By Mail and Outside the Mail)	(1) Mailed Outside-County Paid Subscriptions Stated on PS Form 3541. *(Include paid distribution above nominal rate, advertiser's proof copies, and exchange copies)*	1425	1370
	(2) Mailed In-County Paid Subscriptions Stated on PS Form 3541 *(Include paid distribution above nominal rate, advertiser's proof copies, and exchange copies)*		
	(3) Paid Distribution Outside the Mails Including Sales Through Dealers and Carriers, Street Vendors, Counter Sales, and Other Paid Distribution Outside USPS®	699	673
	(4) Paid Distribution by Other Classes Mailed Through the USPS (e.g. First-Class Mail®)		
c. Total Paid Distribution *(Sum of 15b (1), (2), (3), and (4))*	→	2124	2043
d. Free or Nominal Rate Distribution (By Mail and Outside the Mail)	(1) Free or Nominal Rate Outside-County Copies Included on PS Form 3541	84	80
	(2) Free or Nominal Rate In-County Copies Included on PS Form 3541		
	(3) Free or Nominal Rate Copies Mailed at Other Classes Through the USPS (e.g. First-Class Mail)		
	(4) Free or Nominal Rate Distribution Outside the Mail (Carriers or other means)		
e. Total Free or Nominal Rate Distribution *(Sum of 15d (1), (2), (3) and (4))*	→	84	80
f. Total Distribution *(Sum of 15c and 15e)*	→	2208	2123
g. Copies not Distributed *(See instructions to publishers #4 (page #3))*	→	643	581
h. Total *(Sum of 15f and g)*	→	2851	2704
i. Percent Paid *(15c divided by 15f times 100)*		96.20%	96.23%

16. Publication of Statement of Ownership
☐ If the publication is a general publication, publication of this statement is required. Will be printed ☐ Publication not required
in the December 2009 issue of this publication.

17. Signature and Title of Editor, Publisher, Business Manager, or Owner	Date
Stephen R. Bushing	September 15, 2009
Stephen R. Bushing – Subscription Services Coordinator	

I certify that all information furnished on this form is true and complete. I understand that anyone who furnishes false or misleading information on this form or who omits material or information requested on the form may be subject to criminal sanctions (including fines and imprisonment) and/or civil sanctions (including civil penalties).

PS Form 3526, September 2007 (Page 2 of 3)